VOID

Library of
Davidson College

VISION AND THE BRAIN
The Organization of the Central Visual System

Research Publications:
Association for Research in Nervous and Mental Disease
Volume 67

ASSOCIATION FOR RESEARCH IN NERVOUS AND MENTAL DISEASE

OFFICERS—1987

Bernard Cohen, M.D.
President
Mt. Sinai School of Medicine
New York, NY

Ivan Bodis-Wollner, M.D.
Secretary-Treasurer
Mt. Sinai School of Medicine
New York, NY

Eric Heyer, M.D.
Assistant Secretary-Treasurer
Mt. Sinai School of Medicine
New York, NY

TRUSTEES

Melvin D. Yahr, M.D.
Chairman

Shervert Frazier, M.D.
Seymour S. Kety, M.D.
Paul McHugh, M.D.
Robert Michels, M.D.
Herbert Pardes, M.D.
Fred Plum, M.D.
Herman van Praag, M.D.
Dominick Purpura, M.D.
Lewis P. Rowland, M.D.
Albert J. Stunkard, M.D.
Stephen G. Waxman, M.D.

COMMISSION—1987

Ivan Bodis-Wollner, M.D.
New York, NY

Bernard Cohen, M.D.
New York, NY

Bela Julesz, Ph.D.
Murray Hill, NJ

Lloyd Kaufman
New York, NY

Anthony Movshon
New York, NY

Daniel Pollen
Worcester, MA

Pasko Rakic
New Haven, CT

Peter Schiller
Cambridge, MA

Torsten Wiesel
New York, NY

Vision and the Brain

The Organization of the Central Visual System

*Research Publications:
Association for Research
in Nervous and Mental Disease
Volume 67*

Editors

Bernard Cohen, M.D.
Ivan Bodis-Wollner, M.D.

*Department of Neurology
Mount Sinai School of Medicine
New York, New York*

Raven Press ● New York

Raven Press, 1185 Avenue of the Americas, New York, New York 10036

© 1990 by Raven Press, Ltd. All rights reserved. This book is protected by copyright. No part of it may be reproduced, stored in a retrieval system, or transmitted, in any form or by any means, electronic, mechanical, photocopy, or recording, or otherwise, without the prior written permission of the publisher.

Made in the United States of America

Library of Congress Cataloging-in-Publication Data

Vision and the brain : the organization of the central visual system / editors, Bernard Cohen, Ivan Bodis-Wollner.
    p. cm. — (Research publications / Association for Research in Nervous and Mental Disease ; v. 67)
    Includes bibliographical references and index.
    ISBN 0-88167-568-7
    1. Visual cortex. 2. Visual pathways. 3. Retina. I. Cohen, Bernard, 1929–   . II. Bodis-Wollner, Ivan, 1937–   III. Series: Research publications (Association for Research in Nervous and Mental Disease) : v. 67.
    [DNLM: 1. Brain—physiology. 2. Visual cortex—physiology. 3. Visual Perception—physiology. W1 RE233P v. 67 / WW 105 V8305]
    QP383.V57   1990
    612.8'4—dc20
    DNLM/DLC
    for Library of Congress   87-42968
                                                                                                                                        CIP

The material contained in this volume was submitted as previously unpublished material, except in the instances in which credit has been given to the source from which some of the illustrative material was derived.

Great care has been taken to maintain the accuracy of the information contained in the volume. However, neither Raven Press nor the editors can be held responsible for errors or for any consequences arising from the use of the information contained herein.

Materials appearing in this book prepared by individuals as part of their official duties as U.S. Government employees are not covered by the above-mentioned copyright.

9 8 7 6 5 4 3 2 1

RESEARCH PUBLICATIONS: ASSOCIATION FOR RESEARCH IN NERVOUS AND MENTAL DISEASE

I.	(1920)	*ACUTE EPIDEMIC ENCEPHALITIS (LETHARGIC ENCEPHALITIS)
II.	(1921)	*MULTIPLE SCLEROSIS (DISSEMINATED SCLEROSIS)
III.	(1923)	*HEREDITY IN NERVOUS AND MENTAL DISEASE
IV.	(1924)	THE HUMAN CEREBROSPINAL FLUID
V.	(1925)	*SCHIZOPHRENIA (DEMENTIA PRAECOX)
VI.	(1926)	*THE CEREBELLUM
VII.	(1922)	*EPILEPSY AND THE CONVULSIVE STATE (PART I)
	(1929)	*EPILEPSY AND THE CONVULSIVE STATE (PART II)
VIII.	(1927)	*THE INTRACRANIAL PRESSURE IN HEALTH AND DISEASE
IX.	(1928)	*THE VEGETATIVE NERVOUS SYSTEM
X.	(1929)	*SCHIZOPHRENIA (DEMENTIA PRAECOX) (COMMUNICATION OF VOL. V)
XI.	(1930)	*MANIC-DEPRESSIVE PSYCHOSIS
XII.	(1931)	*INFECTIONS OF THE CENTRAL NERVOUS SYSTEM
XIII.	(1932)	*LOCALIZATION OF FUNCTION IN THE CEREBRAL CORTEX
XIV.	(1933)	*THE BIOLOGY OF THE INDIVIDUAL
XV.	(1934)	*SENSATION: ITS MECHANISMS AND DISTURBANCES
XVI.	(1935)	*TUMORS OF THE NERVOUS SYSTEM
XVII.	(1936)	*THE PITUITARY GLAND
XVIII.	(1937)	*THE CIRCULATION OF THE BRAIN AND SPINAL CORD
XIX.	(1938)	*THE INTER-RELATIONSHIP OF MIND AND BODY
XX.	(1939)	*HYPOTHALAMUS AND CENTRAL LEVELS OF AUTONOMIC FUNCTION
XXI.	(1940)	*THE DISEASE OF THE BASAL GANGLIA
XXII.	(1941)	*THE ROLE OF NUTRITIONAL DEFICIENCY IN NERVOUS AND MENTAL DISEASE
XXIII.	(1942)	*PAIN
XXIV.	(1943)	*TRAUMA OF THE CENTRAL NERVOUS SYSTEM
XXV.	(1944)	*MILITARY NEUROPSYCHIATRY
XXVI.	(1946)	*EPILEPSY
XXVII.	(1947)	*THE FRONTAL LOBES
XXVIII.	(1948)	*MULTIPLE SCLEROSIS AND THE DEMYELINATING DISEASES
XXIX.	(1948)	*LIFE STRESS AND BODILY DISEASE
XXX.	(1950)	*PATTERNS OF ORGANIZATION IN THE CENTRAL NERVOUS SYSTEM
XXXI.	(1951)	*PSYCHIATRIC TREATMENT
XXXII.	(1952)	*METABOLIC AND TOXIC DISEASE OF THE NERVOUS SYSTEM
XXXIII.	(1953)	*GENETICS AND THE INHERITANCE OF INTEGRATED NEUROLOGICAL PSYCHIATRIC PATTERNS
XXXIV.	(1954)	*NEUROLOGY AND PSYCHIATRY IN CHILDHOOD
XXXV.	(1955)	*NEUROLOGIC AND PSYCHIATRIC ASPECTS OF DISORDERS OF AGING
XXXVI.	(1956)	*THE BRAIN AND HUMAN BEHAVIOR
XXXVII.	(1957)	*THE EFFECT OF PHARMACOLOGIC AGENTS ON THE NERVOUS SYSTEM
XXXVIII.	(1958)	*NEUROMUSCULAR DISORDERS
XXXIX.	(1959)	*MENTAL RETARDATION

XL.	(1960)	*ULTRASTRUCTURE AND METABOLISM OF THE NERVOUS SYSTEM
XLI.	(1961)	*CEREBROVASCULAR DISEASE
XLII.	(1962)	*DISORDERS OF COMMUNICATION
XLIII.	(1963)	*ENDOCRINES AND THE CENTRAL NERVOUS SYSTEM
XLIV.	(1964)	*INFECTIONS OF THE NERVOUS SYSTEM
XLV.	(1965)	*SLEEP AND ALTERED STATES OF CONSCIOUSNESS
XLVI.	(1968)	*ADDICTIVE STATES
XLVII.	(1969)	SOCIAL PSYCHIATRY
XLVIII.	(1970)	*PERCEPTION AND ITS DISORDERS
XLIX.	(1971)	*IMMUNOLOGICAL DISORDERS OF THE NERVOUS SYSTEM
50.	(1972)	NEUROTRANSMITTERS
51.	(1973)	BIOLOGICAL AND ENVIRONMENTAL DETERMINANTS OF EARLY DEVELOPMENT
52.	(1974)	AGGRESSION
53.	(1974)	BRAIN DYSFUNCTION IN METABOLIC DISORDERS
54.	(1975)	BIOLOGY OF THE MAJOR PSYCHOSES: A COMPARATIVE ANALYSIS
55.	(1976)	THE BASAL GANGLIA
56.	(1978)	THE HYPOTHALAMUS
57.	(1979)	CONGENITAL AND ACQUIRED COGNITIVE DISORDERS
58.	(1980)	PAIN
59.	(1981)	BRAIN, BEHAVIOR, AND BODILY DISEASE
60.	(1983)	GENETICS OF NEUROLOGICAL AND PSYCHIATRIC DISORDERS
61.	(1983)	EPILEPSY
62.	(1984)	EATING AND ITS DISORDERS
63.	(1985)	BRAIN IMAGING AND BRAIN FUNCTION
64.	(1986)	NEUROPEPTIDES IN NEUROLOGIC AND PSYCHIATRIC DISORDERS
65.	(1987)	MOLECULAR NEUROBIOLOGY IN NEUROLOGY AND PSYCHIATRY
66.	(1988)	LANGUAGE, COMMUNICATION, AND THE BRAIN
67.	(1990)	VISION AND THE BRAIN: THE ORGANIZATION OF THE CENTRAL VISUAL SYSTEM
68.	(1990)	IMMUNOLOGIC MECHANISMS IN NEUROLOGIC AND PSYCHIATRIC DISEASE

Titles marked with an (*) are out of print in the original edition. Some out-of-print volumes are available in reprint editions from Hafner Publishing Company, 866 Third Avenue, New York, N.Y. 10022.

Preface

The concept that vision is the integrated output of a series of subsystems, each of which is responsive to different attributes of the visual stimulus, has become a major theme driving research in visual sciences during the past 20 years. The goals of the conference, held in New York on December 4th and 5th, 1987 under the auspices of the Association for Research in Nervous and Mental Disease, and of this volume that arose from it, were to review recent work that illustrates the separate functioning of various parts of the visual system and to relate it wherever possible to clinical neuro-ophthalmology. In this preface we attempt to give a brief overview of the material presented in this volume, particularly as it relates to the central theme of the conference.

The idea that the visual system can be parceled into separate subsystems, each performing a discrete function, is not new. Thomas Young (1), by assigning individual colors to separate receptors, laid the foundation for the notion that there are separate channels that process various aspects of the visual signal. Descriptions of visual field deficits caused by injuries to the nervous system, particularly by gunshot wounds, provided important support for this notion. The work of Gordon Riddoch (2), among others, firmly established that there is "fragmentation" of visual function in patients with various forms of neurological disease. Such observations were important in revealing that there are discrete operations that are, in a sense, masked in the normal functioning of the visual system.

Studies on functional specificity and diversity in the visual system received strong impetus from the seminal work of Enroth-Cugell and Robson (3). Finding neurons with differing receptive fields, they proposed that there were three major classes of ganglion cells in the area centralis of the cat retina, X, Y, and W cells. They showed that the X and Y cells in the same retinal area respond differently to the same visual stimulus and that there is receptive field size diversity for each class of cells. Their findings suggested that the visual system has the requisite apparatus to perform a frequency analysis of the visual scene at the first level of input. Later it was shown that this retinal dichotomy extended into the geniculostriate system of the monkey as well (4), suggesting that sensing of color imposes additional channels of processing of visual information. Evidence has also been presented that indicates that the retinal disparity and signals of depth and movement in three dimensions, as well as signals related to form and motion, are separately represented in various parts of the cortex and subcortex of the visual system.

VISUAL INPUT: THE RETINA AND LATERAL GENICULATE NUCLEUS

Building on this foundation, the first part of the book is related to retinal organization and to the neurotransmitters utilized by retinal and geniculocortical neurons. The neuropharmacological diversity of the retina is reviewed by Karten and co-workers, who provided much of the original work on this subject. They show that retinal ganglion cells probably utilize a variety of neurotransmitters and suggest that this may reflect their functional diversity. Dowling, using electrophysiological and anatomical techniques, has shown that dopamine, one of the most studied of the retinal neurotransmitters, plays an important role in receptive field organization in lower vertebrates. It couples with a G protein through cyclic AMP to change the level of surround inhibition and mediate the sensitivity of the retina to light. Dowling postulates that this occurs by affecting glutamate channels in horizontal cells or by coupling or uncoupling gap junctions. Bodis-Wollner and co-workers have suggested somewhat different functional properties of the retinal dopaminergic subsystem in primates, employing other techniques, i.e., psychophysics, electroretinograms (ERGs), and visual evoked potentials. Although these interpretations are not exactly the same, both groups infer a modulatory role for dopamine in establishing receptive field properties of mammalian retinal ganglion cells. It is interesting that it is possible to bridge results from detailed cellular morphophysiology and behavior in offering new insights into function. Such crosstalk is one of the strengths of this book.

To understand the role of the microcircuitry in the lateral geniculate nucleus (LGN) as well as the function of specific subsystems, Schiller utilized the glutamate neurotransmitter analog, APB, to selectively block ionic channels related to on-center retinal ganglion cells and LGN cells. He demonstrated that the on- and off-center systems remain segregated up to the visual cortex. He concludes that the function of the on- and off-center channels is to provide rapid transfer of visual information related to contrast sensitivity via excitatory pathways. Pasik and colleagues review the literature on the putative neurotransmitters utilized by each of the known inputs to LGN and assess the possible role of these neurotransmitters in LGN function. They suggest that N-acetyl aspartyl glutamate (NAAG) may be an excitatory transmitter for the retinal ganglion cells acting on glutamate receptors.

CENTRAL PROCESSING: DEVELOPMENT AND AMBLYOPIA

Among the most important areas bridging visual neuroscience and clinical practice are developmental studies and amblyopia. Teller assesses current knowledge on development of visual function in human infants. She shows that although 1-month-old human infants can certainly see, they have limitations in stereovision, acuity, and color vision. This implies that there is a different time course for development of the various streams of information processing, particularly in the magno- and parvocellular systems.

The seminal studies of Wiesel and Hubel (5–7) in the late 1950s demonstrated that sensory deprivation had physiological and structural effects on development of the visual cortex. This line of study has been expanded by Cynader and colleagues who have applied detailed pharmacological techniques to the study of the visual cortex of the cat after visual deprivation. They show that various receptors undergo different changes in distribution during postnatal development, particularly with regard to the critical period for cortical plasticity. Their work suggests that pharmacological differences after visual deprivation are important and must be taken into account in understanding and formulating therapeutic approaches to amblyopia.

STUDIES ON ORGANIZATION OF THE CENTRAL VISUAL SYSTEM

Livingstone synthesized psychophysical and anatomical data to suggest the importance of segregating luminance and color opponent functions in the visual cortex. She proposes a separation of the color system into subsystems that recognize hue and color form, relating this to anatomic structures revealed by cytochrome oxidase staining called "blobs." She postulates that the geniculocortical visual system can be subdivided into three components: a pathway for movement and stereoscopic depth, a pathway for high resolution static form perception, and a pathway concerned with color (but not movement), shape discrimination, or stereopsis. She further suggests a distinction between color contrast and luminance contrast, particularly as revealed by psychophysics.

Hildreth introduces a theoretical structure to explain how the flow field is sensed. She demonstrates that techniques of artificial intelligence can provide insight into the way that groups of neurons process information for motion. Although there is not as yet a direct correlation with studies of cellular activity in motion-sensing regions of the visual system, such as in the medial temporal cortex, nevertheless it is possible to relate her analytic models to physiological data of the type developed by Movshon et al. (8) to derive general concepts for velocity field computation.

Related to separation of channels for processing information about motion and form, Grüsser and co-workers studied the ability of normal subjects, of patients with right- and left-hemisphere lesions, and of schizophrenics to distinguish a fundamental aspect of form: recognition of the human face. A localized deficit in facial recognition, prosopagnosia, is rare but occurs after lesions of the basal and mesial occipitotemporal regions. Grüsser et al. demonstrate that facial recognition is also impaired after other cerebral lesions.

Surprisingly, schizophrenic patients had more difficulty in recognizing faces than normals. Evoked potentials were utilized to provide quantitative information about the nature of facial recognition in normals and patients.

THE VISUAL-OCULOMOTOR INTERFACE: SACCADES, PURSUIT, AND OPTOKINETIC NYSTAGMUS

Although the eyes move to subserve vision, until recently there was little information or interest in the interface between the visual and oculomotor systems. Major steps have now been taken to define this interface in the monkey. Not surprisingly, the diversity of the subsystems represented in the visual system is also reflected in the oculomotor system. Pathways that carry activity for slow and rapid eye movements are largely separate at many locations in the CNS, and it is possible to study them in isolation. Goldberg and Segraves show that portions of the visual system that are used to localize targets in extrapersonal space, i.e., the prefrontal cortex and frontal eye fields, have a close topographic link to the superior colliculus. Electrical stimulation demonstrated connections from the frontal cortex to the superior colliculus. They also showed that animals had deficits in making saccades to remembered targets after frontal lobe lesions. Together the frontal eye fields and the superior colliculus are essential parts of the saccadic system. As Schiller and co-workers (9) demonstrated previously, when lesions involve both the frontal eye fields and the colliculi, monkeys hold their eyes centered and immobile, and it is not possible for them to orient to eccentric targets by making saccadic eye movements.

Wurtz and co-workers review evidence that the middle temporal (MT) and medial superior temporal (MST) areas are related to visual motion processing. They show that cells in these regions are active during pursuit eye movements and that lesions of these regions cause deficits in ocular pursuit. Thus, processing for saccades and pursuit movements is separate at several important locations in the cerebral cortex. In addition, the separation in visual processing for motion and form appears to be reflected in oculomotor function, particularly at locations where ocular pursuit movements are generated.

Although it is known that the subcortical visual system is important for visual processing in lateral-eyed animals, the role of the subcortical visual system in primate vision has been unclear. Cohen et al. demonstrated that the optokinetic response to movement of the visual surround could be selectively elicited by electrical stimulation of the nucleus of the optic tract (NOT). Lesions of this nucleus caused a loss of these components, including optokinetic afternystagmus (OKAN). It was inferred that NOT is the input pathway to the vestibular nuclei for retinal slip related to head movement, which supports the vestibulo-ocular reflex during head turning and locomotion. Wurtz and co-workers demonstrated that optokinetic nystagmus (OKN) was affected by MT/MST lesions. Presumably, information about visual motion processed in the MT/MST regions is sent to subcortical regions to support gaze stabilization during head movements. Cohen suggested that clinical conditions exist in which NOT lesions affect the generation of OKN and OKAN.

NEW TECHNIQUES FOR STUDY OF THE VISUAL SYSTEM

Several authors have provided insight into the function of the overall system utilizing imaging techniques in association with psychophysical studies and new evoked potential techniques. Raichle shows that measurement of blood flow with PET scanning can demonstrate areas of the cerebral cortex that are strongly activated during normal vision. He combined it with image averaging and statistical techniques to measure the differences. The technique will be useful for studying activation of the cerebrum during complex tasks involving vision and visual memory. Kaufman and Williamson report a new evoked potential technique, magneto-encephalography (MEG), which should be useful in studying details of visual processing in the cortex. They found evidence for parallel processing in channels for high and low spatial frequencies and have also identified several new areas where visual information appears to be processed. Maffei and Fiorentini summarize their studies on the pattern electroretinogram (PERG). They show that the PERG is related to activity of retinal ganglion cells, although it may not directly originate in this layer. The PERG is sensitive to increased intraocular pressure, retinal ischemia, and lesions of the optic nerve. As a result of their work, PERG has become a useful measurement in clinical diagnosis of visual disorders.

PATHOLOGY OF THE CENTRAL VISUAL SYSTEM

The specificity of some visual subsystems becomes particularly apparent in various types of visual system pathology. Bodis-Wollner reviews work to demonstrate that spatial contrast sensitivity is reduced in Parkinson patients and that this deficit can be reversed with administration of dopaminergic drugs. Studies utilizing 1-methyl-4-phenyl 1,2,3,6-tetrahydropyridine (MPTP) in monkeys were consistent with these conclusions. (MPTP is an agent that creates a pharmacological and behavioral model of parkinsonism in primates.) Regan addresses the question of whether visual deficits in patients with multiple sclerosis provide evidence for parallel processing. Individual channels that respond to the size of retinal images were first inferred in psychophysical studies by Campbell and colleagues (10,11) in 1968. Clinical studies established the validity of this spatial frequency channel concept by demonstrating the vulnerability of one or another spatial frequency channels without affecting visual acuity (12). Studies by Regan and colleagues on patients with multiple sclerosis (13), reviewed in this chapter, provide further indication that this idea is viable and indicate that deficits in such patients can often be analyzed using such concepts.

It is perhaps not surprising that Alzheimer's disease, which has widespread effects on various classes of neurons in the brain, also causes changes in the retina. Sadun and Bassi, utilizing the stain, paraphenylene diamine (PPD), demonstrate degeneration of retinal ganglion cells and suggest that the process is selective to the channel carrying the input of the magnocellular elements. They suggest that the type of visual deficits that occur in Alzheimer patients supports their hypothesis.

SUMMARY

It is now clearly established that segregation exists in the primary visual pathways for information conveying individual colors, sizes, and other modalities of visual stimuli such as shape and form. Much of the material in this book is related to questions concerning the different anatomy, physiology, pharmacology, and pathophysiology of these specific visual functions, because they are the currency of modern visual science. Further diversity is to be expected as we understand more about neuropharmacology, neurophysiology, and neuroanatomy, and new correlations of function with neurochemical and neuroanatomical subdivisions will undoubtedly come from such work. It seemed important to hold this conference at a time when there was so much new information about segregation of function in various subsystems of the central visual system. By splitting the system apart, many additional insights have been gained. However, the ultimate and most sophisticated aim still remains to be realized, that is, how the subsystems interact and are utilized to enable to see.

Bernard Cohen
Ivan Bodis-Wollner

REFERENCES

1. Young T. On the theory of light and colours. *Philos Trans R Soc Lond* 1802;92:12–48.
2. Riddoch G. Dissociation of visual perceptions due to occipital injuries, with especial reference to appreciation of movement. *Brain* 1917;40:15–53.
3. Enroth-Cuggell C, Robson JG. The contrast sensitivity of retinal ganglion cells of the cat. *J Physiol (Lond)* 1966;187:517–552.
4. Kaplan E, Shapley RM. X- and Y-cells in the lateral geniculate nucleus of macaque monkeys. *J Physiol (Lond)* 1982;330:125–143.
5. Wiesel TN, Hubel DH. Effects of visual deprivation on morphology and physiology of cells in the cat's lateral geniculate body. *J Neurophysiol* 1963;26:978–993.
6. Wiesel TN, Hubel DH. Single-cell responses in striate cortex of kittens deprived of vision in one eye. *J Neurophysiol* 1963;26:1003–1017.
7. Wiesel TN, Hubel DH. Comparison of the effects of unilateral and bilateral eye closure on cortical unit responses in kittens. *J Neurophysiol* 1965;28:1029–1040.

8. Movshon JA, Adelson EH, Gizzi MS, Newsome WT. The analysis of moving visual patterns. In: Chagas C, Gattas R, Gross CG, eds. *Pattern recognition mechanisms.* Rome: Vatican Press, 1985;117–151.
9. Schiller PH, True SD, Conway JL. Deficits in eye movements following frontal eye-field and superior colliculus ablations. *J Neurophysiol* 1980;44:1175–1189.
10. Campbell SW, Green DC. Optical and retinal factors affecting visual resolution. *J Physiol (Lond)* 1965;181:576–593.
11. Campbell SW, Robson JG. Application of Fourier analysis to the visibility of gratings. *J Physiol (Lond)* 1968;197:551–566.
12. Bodis-Wollner I. Visual acuity and contrast sensitivity in patients with cerebral lesions. *Science* 1972;178:769–771.
13. Regan D. Visual information channeling in normal and disordered vision. *Psychol Rev* 1984;89:407–444.

Acknowledgments

We thank the members of the Advisory Committee, Drs. Harvey Karten, Anthony Movshon, Pasko Rakic, Peter Schiller, Torsten Wiesel, and Robert Wurtz for their expert counsel. We also thank Olie Westheimer for efficiently planning and executing the conference.

Contents

1 Functional and Pharmacological Organization of the Retina: Dopamine, Interplexiform Cells, and Neuromodulation
John E. Dowling

19 Biochemical and Morphological Heterogeneity of Retinal Ganglion Cells
Harvey J. Karten, Kent T. Keyser, and Nicholas C. Brecha

35 The On and Off Channels of the Visual System
Peter H. Schiller

43 Chemically Specified Systems in the Dorsal Lateral Geniculate Nucleus of Mammals
Pedro Pasik, Ricardo Molinar-Rode, and Tauba Pasik

85 Neural Mechanisms Underlying Modifiability of Response Properties in Developing Cat Visual Cortex
M. Cynader, C. Shaw, G. Prusky, and F. Van Huizen

109 The Development of Visual Function in Infants
Davida Y. Teller

119 Segregation of Form, Color, Movement, and Depth Processing in the Visual System: Anatomy, Physiology, Art, and Illusion
Margaret Livingstone

139 The Neural Computation of the Velocity Field
Ellen C. Hildreth

165 Brain Mechanisms for Recognition of Faces, Facial Expression, and Gestures: Neuropsychological and Electroencephalographic Studies in Normals, Brain-Lesioned Patients, and Schizophrenics
Otto-Joachim Grüsser, Nina Kirchhoff, and Alexander Naumann

195 The Role of the Frontal Eye Field and Its Corticotectal Projection in the Generation of Eye Movements
Michael E. Goldberg and Mark A. Segraves

211 Cortical Visual Motion Processing for Oculomotor Control
Robert H. Wurtz, Hidehiko Komatsu, Dwayne S. G. Yamasaki, and Max R. Dürsteler

233 Contribution of the Nucleus of the Optic Tract to Optokinetic Nystagmus and Optokinetic Afternystagmus in the Monkey: Clinical Implications
Bernard Cohen, Daniel Schiff, and Jean Buettner

257 Developing a Functional Anatomy of the Human Visual System with Positron Emission Tomography
Marcus E. Raichle

271 Neuromagnetic Localization of Neuronal Activity in Visual and Extravisual Cortex
Lloyd Kaufman and Samuel J. Williamson

289 The Pattern Electroretinogram in Animals and Humans: Physiological and Clinical Applications
L. Maffei and A. Fiorentini

297 The Visual System in Parkinson's Disease
Ivan Bodis-Wollner

317 To What Extent Can Visual Deficits Caused by Multiple Sclerosis Be Understood in Terms of Parallel Processing?
D. Regan

331 The Visual System in Alzheimer's Disease
Alfredo A. Sadun and Carl J. Bassi

349 Subject Index

Contributors

Carl J. Bassi
Departments of Ophthalmology and
  Neurosurgery
University of Southern California
  School of Medicine
Doheny Eye Institute
1355 San Pablo Street
Los Angeles, California 90033

Ivan Bodis-Wollner
Department of Neurology, Box 1052
Mount Sinai School of Medicine
One Gustave Levy Place
New York, New York 10029

Nicholas C. Brecha
Departments of Anatomy and Cell
  Biology and Medicine
University of California at
  Los Angeles
Los Angeles, California 90024

Jean Buettner
Department of Physiology
University of Munich
Munich, West Germany

Bernard Cohen
Department of Neurology, Box 1135
Mount Sinai School of Medicine
1 East 100th Street
New York, New York 10029

M. Cynader
Department of Ophthalmology
VGH/UBC Eye Care Centre
University of British Columbia
2550 Willow Street
Vancouver, British Columbia
Canada V5Z 3N9

John E. Dowling
Department of Cellular
  and Developmental Biology
The Biological Laboratories
Harvard University
16 Divinity Avenue
Cambridge, Massachusetts 02138

Max R. Dürsteler
Laboratory of Sensorimotor Research
National Eye Institute
National Institutes of Health
Building 10, Room 10C101
Bethesda, Maryland 20892

A. Fiorentini
Istituto di Neurofisiologia del CNR
Via S. Zeno, 51
56100 Pisa, Italy

Michael E. Goldberg
Laboratory of Sensorimotor Research
National Eye Institute
National Institutes of Health
Building 10, Room 10C101
Bethesda, Maryland 20892

Otto-Joachim Grüsser
Department of Physiology
Freie Universität Berlin
Arnimallee 22
1 Berlin 33, West Germany

Ellen C. Hildreth
Massachusetts Institute of Technology
Artificial Intelligence Laboratory
545 Technology Square
Cambridge, Massachusetts 02139

Harvey J. Karten
Department of Neurosciences, M-008
University of California at San Diego
La Jolla, California 92093

Contributors

Lloyd Kaufman
Neuromagnetism Laboratory
Departments of Psychology and
  Physics
New York University
2 Washington Place
New York, New York 10003

Kent T. Keyser
Department of Neurosciences, M-008
University of California at San Diego
La Jolla, California 92093

Nina Kirchhoff
Department of Physiology
Freie Universität Berlin
Arnimallee 22
1 Berlin 33, West Germany

Hidehiko Komatsu
Laboratory of Sensorimotor Research
National Eye Institute
National Institutes of Health
Building 10, Room 10C101
Bethesda, Maryland 20982

Margaret Livingstone
Department of Neurobiology
Harvard Medical School
25 Shattuck Street
Boston, Massachusetts 02115

L. Maffei
Istituto di Neurofisiologia del CNR
Via S. Zeno, 51
56100 Pisa, Italy

Ricardo Molinar-Rode
Neurobiology Graduate Program
Mount Sinai School of Medicine
One Gustave Levy Place
New York, New York 10029

Alexander Naumann
Department of Physiology
Freie Universität Berlin
Arnimallee 22
1 Berlin 33, West Germany

Pedro Pasik
Departments of Neurology and
  Anatomy
Mount Sinai School of Medicine
One Gustave Levy Place
New York, New York 10029

Tauba Pasik
Department of Neurology
Mount Sinai School of Medicine
One Gustave Levy Place
New York, New York 10029

G. Prusky
Department of Ophthalmology
VGH/UBC Eye Care Centre
University of British Columbia
2550 Willow Street
Vancouver, British Columbia
Canada V5Z 3N9

Marcus E. Raichle
Mallinckrodt Institute of Radiology
Department of Neurology and
  Neurological Surgery
McDonnell Center for Studies of
  Higher Brain Function
The Washington University
  Medical Center
St. Louis, Missouri 63110

D. Regan
Department of Psychology
York University
4700 Keele Street
North York, Ontario
Canada M3J 1P3

Alfredo A. Sadun
Departments of Ophthalmology and
  Neurosurgery
University of Southern California
  School of Medicine
Doheny Eye Institute
1355 San Pablo Street
Los Angeles, California 90033

Daniel Schiff
Department of Neurology, Box 1135
Mount Sinai School of Medicine
One Gustave Levy Place
New York, New York 10029

CONTRIBUTORS

Peter H. Schiller
Department of Brain and Cognitive
  Sciences, E25-634
Massachusetts Institute of Technology
77 Massachusetts Avenue
Cambridge, Massachusetts 02139

Mark A. Segraves
Laboratory of Sensorimotor Research
National Eye Institute
National Institutes of Health
Building 10, Room 10C101
Bethesda, Maryland 20892

C. Shaw
Department of Ophthalmology
VGH/UBC Eye Care Centre
University of British Columbia
2550 Willow Street
Vancouver, British Columbia
Canada V5Z 3N9

Davida Y. Teller
Departments of Psychology and
  Physiology/Biophysics, NI-25
University of Washington
Seattle, Washington 98195

F. Van Huizen
Department of Ophthalmology
VGH/UBC Eye Care Centre
University of British Columbia
2550 Willow Street
Vancouver, British Columbia
Canada V5Z 3N9

Samuel J. Williamson
Neuromagnetism Laboratory
Departments of Psychology and
  Physics
New York University
2 Washington Place
New York, New York 10003

Robert H. Wurtz
Laboratory of Sensorimotor Research
National Eye Institute
National Institutes of Health
Building 10, Room 10C101
Bethesda, Maryland 20892

Dwayne S. G. Yamasaki
Laboratory of Sensorimotor Research
National Eye Institute
National Institutes of Health
Building 10, Room 10C101
Bethesda, Maryland 20892

Association for Research in Nervous and Mental Disease

Members

A

Abrams, Bernard M.
Abrams, Gary M.
Adams, Raymond
Adelman, Lester S.
Adler, Lenard A.
Agranoff, B. W.
Ahuwalia, Brij M.S.
Aiken, Robert D.
Airing, Charles D.
Aita, John F.
Allen, Marshall B., Jr.
Allen, Richard
Almaleh, Hassan
Alter, Milton
Alvord, Ellsworth C., Jr.
Anderson, Milton H.
Anderson, Paul J.
Anderson, William W.
Andriola, Mary
Andy, Orlando J.
Angrist, Burton
Ansari, Khurshed A.
Asbury, Arthur
Auerbach, Sanford
Auth, Thomas L.
Ayala, Giovanni

B

Baker, Robert N.
Baldessarini, Ross J.
Ball, Stanley M.
Ballweg, Gail P.
Bank, Arnold
Barchi, Robert L.
Barclay, Laurie
Barlow, Charles F.
Barlow, John S.
Barnes, Karen L.
Barnett, H. J. M.
Barrett, Robert E.
Bartle, Harvey, Jr.
Baska, Richard E.
Batkin, Stanley
Battista, Arthur A.
Becker, Donald P.
Bell, Robert L.
Bender, Adam N.
Benjamin, Vallo
Berg, Seymour
Bergmann, Kenneth
Berl, Soll
Bertrand, Claude
Bick, Katherine L.
Biele, Flora H.
Blankfein, Robert J.
Black, Samuel P. W.
Blass, John Paul
Block, Jerome M.
Boath, Carl
Bodis-Wollner, Ivan
Bohn, Martha
Boldrey, Edwin B.
Borrus, Joseph C.
Bosley, Thomas McCarthy
Brannon, William, Jr.
Bray, Patrick F.
Breitner, John C. S.
Brendler, Samuel J.
Bridger, Wagner
Bridgers, Samuel L. II
Brill, A. Bertrand
Brill, Charles B.
Britton, Carolyn Barley
Brodie, Jonathan D.
Brooks, Chandler
Brosin, Henry
Broughton, Roger J.
Brown, Dennis
Brown, Lucy L.
Brundy, Joseph
Brust, John C. M.
Bruun, Bertel
Budabin, Murray
Bullard, Dexter M., Jr.
Burger, Andrew
Burke, Robert E.
Buschke, Herman
Butler, Ian J.

C

Cadet, Jean Lud
Cafferty, Maureen S.
Camp, Walter A.
Cancro, Robert
Carmichael, Miriam
Caronna, John J.
Carpenter, William T., Jr.
Carruthers, Richard R.
Carton, Charles A.
Catel, James
Cattanach, George S.
Caviness, Verne S., Jr.
Cedarbaum, Jesse M.
Charlton, Maurice H.

xxi

Charney, Jonathan Z.
Chase, Richard A.
Chase, Thomas N.
Chawluk, John B.
Chokroverty, Sudhansu
Cicero, Theodore J.
Clark, William K.
Coccaro, Emil F.
Coddon, David R.
Cohen, Bernard
Cohen, Jeffrey
Cohen, Norman
Cohen, Robert A.
Cohen, Sidney M.
Cohen, Stanley L.
Cohen, Wendy Ellen
Cohn, Robert
Cole, Andrew James
Cole, Malvin
Cole, Monroe
Collins, William F., Jr.
Conomy, John Paul
Cook, David G.
Cook, Patricia
Cook, Stuart D.
Correll, James W.
Cote, Lucien
Couch, James R.
Critides, Samuel D.
Cullis, Paul Anthony
Cummings, Jeffrey L.
Cuthill, John

D

Dale, Robert T.
Damasio, Antonio
Damasio, Hanna
Daroff, Robert B.
Davey, Lycurgus M.
David, Noble
Davis, Kenneth L.
DeFries, Zira
DeGirolami, Umberto
Delaney, John F.
DeNapoli, Robert A.
Denckla, Martha B.
Denker, Peter G.
Derby, Bennett M.
DeVivo, Darryl
Diamond, Mark S.
Diamond, Sidney
Dodge, Philip R.

Dodson, William E.
Donaldson, James O.
Drachman, David
Dreifuss, Fritz E.
Duane, Drake D.
Dubin, Louis L.
Dunstone, David C.
Duvoisin, Roger
Dyken, Mark L.
Dyken, Paul

E

Earls, Felton James
Easton, J. Donald
Ebers, George C.
Echlin, Francis A.
Ecker, Arthur D.
Edelson, Alan
Edwards, Diana Dow
Effron, Abraham S.
Eisenberg, Leon
Elizan, Teresita S.
Elliott, M. Marcus
Epstein, Fred
Erba, Giuseppe
Escer, Robert A.
Everts, William H.

F

Fahn, Stanley
Faillace, Louis A.
Falci, Thomas
Feinberg, Irwin
Feindel, William
Feldman, Daniel S.
Feldman, Martin
Feringa, Earl R.
Ferriss, Gregory S.
Fetell, Michael
Finkelhor, Howard B.
Finley, Knox H.
Fish, Irving
Fishman, Donald
Flamm, Eugene S.
Fleming, T. Corwin
Flicker, David J.
Fogelson, M. Harold
Foley, Kathleen M.
Folstein, Marshall
Folstein, Susan
Forrest, David V.
Forster, George
Frazier, Shervert H.

Friedhoff, Arnold J.
Friedman, Richard C.
Frosch, William A.
Funkenstein, H. Harris

G

Gandy, Samuel E.
Garofalo, Michael, Jr.
Garvin, John S.
Gascon, Generoso G.
Geller, Lester M.
Gendelman, Seymour
Gershon, Samuel
Ghetti, Bernardino
Ghilardi, Maria Felice
Ghobrial, Mona
Gibbs, James
Giblin, Dennis R.
Gillen, H. W.
Gilman, Sid
Gilroy, John
Glusman, Murray
Gold, Arnold P.
Goldberg, Allan
Goldberg, Harold H.
Goldin, Gurston D.
Goldstein, Murray
Gottschalk, Louis A.
Grabow, Jack D.
Grebb, Jack A.
Green, David
Green, Martin A.
Greenberg, Alvin D.
Greenberg, Jack O.
Greenwood, Robert S.
Greer, Melvin
Gretter, Thomas
Gross, David
Gross, Paul T.
Grossman, Robert
Gumnit, Robert J.
Gutmann, Ludwig
Guynn, Robert William
Guze, Samuel

H

Haase, Gunter R.
Hackett, Earl R.
Haddad, Raef
Hale, Mahlon A.
Hamburg, David A.
Hamill, Robert W.
Hammill, James F.

MEMBERS

Hanna, George R.
Harbison, John W.
Harriman, Christian, Jr.
Hasenbush, Lester
Hass, William Karl
Hauser, W. Allen
Hayward, James Neil
Healton, Edward B.
Helfer, Lewis M.
Hershey, Linda A.
Heyer, Eric
Hinterbuchner, L. P.
Hirano, Asao
Hoehn, Margaret
Hoenig, Eugene M.
Hoff, Julian T.
Hoffman, Julius
Hoffman, Stephen F.
Hogan, Edward L.
Hogan, Patrick A.
Holmes, Gregory L.
Horenstein, Simon
Horowitz, Steven
Housepian, Edgar M.
Hudson, Charles J.
Hunter, Ralph W.

I
Iadecola, Costantino

J
Jacobs, Erwin M.
Jacobs, Lawrence D.
Jacobson, Sherwood A.
Jacquet, Yasuko R.
Jaffe, Joseph
Jammes, J. L.
Jeub, Robert P.
Joh, Tong H.
Johnson, Anne B.
Johnson, Richard T.
Jonas, Saran
Jones, H. Royden, Jr.
Joynt, Robert J.
Jubelt, Burk

K
Kaelber, William W.
Kandel, Eric R.
Kaplan, Lawrence I.
Kaplan, Harry A.
Karliner, William
Kase, Carlos S.

Kattah, Jorge C.
Katzman, Robert
Kaye, Edward M.
Keller, N. J.
Kellner, Charles H.
Kennedy, Charles
Kenny, John Thomas
Kessler, Robert M.
Khurana, Ramesh
Kienast, N. M.
King, Arthur
Kinkel, William R.
Kirschberg, Gordon
Klass, Donald W.
Klee, Claude Elise B.
Klein, Donald
Koenig, Harold
Koenigsberger, M. R.
Koeppen, Arnulf H.
Kofman, Oscar
Kolar, Oldrich Jan
Kolodny, Edwin H.
Korein, Julius
Kornfeld, Mario
Krieger, Howard P.
Kreinsky, Michael M.
Kupersmith, Mark J.
Kurtzke, John F.

L
Landau, William M.
Lapovsky, Arthur
Lautin, Andrew
Lavenstein, Bennett
Layzer, Robert
Lederman, J. Richard
Lehrer, Gerard M.
Leiberman, James S.
Leibowitz, Sarah
Lepore, Frederick E.
Lesse, Stanley
Leven, Harvey Steven
Levens, Arthur J.
Leventhal, Carl M.
Levine, Irving M.
Levy, David E.
Levy, Lewis L.
Levy, Susan R.
Levy, Walter J.
Lewis, Linda D.
Liberson, Vladimir
Lightfoote, William

Lipkin, Lewis E.
Lisak, Robert Philip
Liss, Leopold
Livingston, E. Arthur
Loman, Julius
Lombroso, Cesare T.
Lubic, Lowell G.
Lublin, Fred, D.

M
Madonick, Moses
Madow, Michael
Maertens, Paul
Maker, Howard
Malitz, Sidney
Mancall, Elliott L.
Mandel, Martin M.
Maniscalco, Anthony G.
Manyam, Bala
Markham, Charles H.
Martin, Herbert L.
Martin, Joseph
Martinez, Leonardo
Mashman, Jan
Massey, Edward Wayne
Massey, Janice
Mastri, Angeline R.
Matthysse, Steven
Mattson, Richard
Mayer, Richard F.
Mayeux, Richard
McDowell, Fletcher H.
McGee, Thomas P.
McGillicuddy, John
McHenry, John T.
McHugh, Paul R.
McIlroy, William J.
McKee, Mary Ann
McKinney, Alexander S.
McKinney, William M.
McMasters, Robert E.
Mearin, Robert J.
Meisel, Arthur M.
Mendelson, Jack H.
Mendoza, Marina R.
Merlis, Jerome K.
Meyer, John Sterling
Meyerson, Arthur T.
Michels, Robert
Michaelson, W. Jost
Mickel, Hubert S.
Miller, Claude H.

MEMBERS

Miller, James R.
Millichap, J. G.
Milner, Brenda
Mitsumoto, Hiroshi
Mohr, J. P.
Mohs, Richard C.
Mondell, Brian E.
Moossy, Jon
Mora, Sol N.
Morantz, Robert A.
Moros, Daniel A.
Morris, Charles T.
Moshe, Solomon L.
Moskowitz, Michael A.
Mumford, Robert S.
Munsat, Theodore L.
Myers, Gary J.
Myler, H. Richard

N

Nastuck, William L.
Natelson, Benjamin
Nathanson, Morton
Neumann, Meta
Nilaver, Gajanan
Norsa, Luigia

O

O'Brien, Joseph L.
Okazaki, Haruo
Onofrj, Marco C.
Osborn, Morris

P

Pacella, Bernard
Paddison, Richard M.
Pappas, Carol L.
Pardes, Herbert
Pasamanick, Benjamin
Pasik, Pedro
Paul, Norman
Pavlakis, Steven
Payne, Richard
Pearl, Richard
Pearlson, Godfrey D.
Pedley, Timothy
Penn, Audrey S.
Penry, J. Kiffin
Perlo, Vincent P.
Petajan, Jack
Peterson, Arthur L.
Peterson, Patti L.
Piepmeier, Joseph

Pietrucha, Dorothy M.
Pincus, Jonathan
Pinney, Edward L., Jr.
Pittman, Hal W.
Pitts, Ferris N., Jr.
Plaitakis, Andreas
Pleasure, David
Plum, Fred
Pollock, George H.
Porrino, Linda J.
Posner, Jerome B.
Posner, Michael
Prensky, Arthur L.
Price, Richard
Prince, David A.
Prioleau, George R., Jr.
Prockof, Leon D.
Prohovnik, Isak
Purpura, Dominick P.

R

Rabiner, A. M.
Raichle, Marcus E.
Raine, Cedric S.
Rainer, John D.
Rakic, Pasko
Ramachandran, Tarakad
Ransohoff, Joseph
Rao, Ajyaraman
Rapin, Isabelle
Raskin, Neil H.
Rasmussen, Theodore
Reichlan, Seymour
Reife, Ross A.
Reis, Donald J.
Reivich, Martin
Richards, Nelson G.
Richardson, Edward P.
Richter, Ralph W.
Rinsley, Donald B.
Roberts, M. P., Jr.
Robinson, Robert G.
Roizin, Leon
Rose, Arthur, L.
Rose, Augustus S.
Rosenbaum, David
Rosenberg, Edwin M.
Rosenberg, Roger N.
Rosenblum, Jay A.
Rosenthal, Jesse
Rosenthal, Norman E.
Rosomoff, Hubert L.

Ross, Emanuel
Rothballer, Alan
Rowan, James A.
Rowland, Lewis P.
Rubenstein, Alan
Ruff, Robert L.
Rumberg, Joan

S

Sabshin, James K.
Sackeim, Harold A.
Sackler, Mortimer D.
Sage, Jacob I.
Salmoiraghi, G. C.
Saloman, Michael
Samuels, Stanley
Saper, Joel R.
Sattin, Albert
Sax, Daniel S.
Schanzer, Bernard
Schapiro, Daniel
Schatz, Norman J.
Schaumburg, Herbert
Schear, Myrna J.
Schildkraut, Joseph J.
Schlezinger, Nathan
Schoenberg, Bruce
Schuelein, Marianne
Schulman, Elliott A.
Sciarra, Daniel
Seelye, Edward E.
Selby, Roy C.
Selverstone, Bertram
Selzer, Michael E.
Sencer, Walter
Shamoian, Charles A.
Shanzer, Stefan
Shapiro, Mortimer F.
Shapiro, Sidney K.
Shapiro, William R.
Sheremata, William A.
Sherman, David G.
Sherwin, Ira
Shouldson, Ira
Shriver, Joyce
Shuter, Eli R.
Sibley, William A.
Sidell, Alvin
Siekert, Robert G.
Siever, Larry Joseph
Silberberg, Donald H.
Silberfarb, Peter

Silberstein, Marsha M.
Silberstein, Stephen
Siller, Everard J.
Silverstein, Allen
Singer, Robert P.
Singh, Avtar
Singh, Baldev Kaur
Siris, Joseph H.
Sivak, Mark
Slosberg, Paul S.
Slotwiner, Paul
Small, Iver F.
Smith, G. Bushnell
Smith, Carolyn B.
Smith, Gerard P.
Smith, Michael
Snider, Ray S.
Snyder, Lawrence H.
Sobin, Allan
Sobol, Norman J.
Sokoloff, Louis
Solomon, Gail
Solomon, Seymour
Spencer, Dennis D.
Spencer, Susan S.
Sprague, James
Sprofkin, Bertram H.
Sroka, Hava
Stadlan, Emmanuel M.
Staley, Robert
Starbuck, Helen L.
Stein, Martin H.
Stein, Marvin
Stern, Yakov
Stewart, Bruce
Stewart, James G.
Stunkard, Albert J.
Sugerman, A. Arthur
Sullivan, Daniel Carl
Sumner, Austin J.
Sung, Joo Ho
Suter, Cary G.
Swanson, David W.
Sweeney, M.D.
Sweet, Richard
Syed, Athar H.

T

Taren, James A.
Tarsy, Daniel
Tcheupdijian, Leon
Tejera, Gertrude
Tellez, Isabel
Terry, Robert D.
Thal, Leon J.
Thomas, Madison H.
Thompson, Hartwell
Thompson, Raymond K.
Thorner, Melvin
Thurston, Jean H.
Timberlake, William H.
Tolge, Bruno P.
Tolosa, Eduardo
Tourian, Ara
Triedman, M. Howard
Tsai, Luke Y.
Tuchman, Alan J.
Tucker, Jolyon S.
Twitchell, Thomas E.

V

Valsamis, Marius
Van Der Velde, Christian
Van Praag, Herman M.
Vigman, Melvin
Vincent, Frederick

W

Wagman, Irving H.
Wall, James H.
Wallner, Julius M.
Walton, Norman
Waltz, Arthur G.
Wanger, Stephen L.
Ward, Arthur
Warner, Carolyn
Watson, Robert
Waxman, Stephen G.
Wechsler, Adam F.

Weinberg, Harold
Weinberger, Jesse
Weiner, Herbert
Weinreb, Herman J.
Weiss, Arthur H.
Weissman, William
West, Louis Jolyon
Westbrook, Edward
Wharton, Ralph N.
Whetsell, William
Wiener, Jill
Wilk, Ronald
Williams, Robert L.
Williams, Shirley Y.
Wilson, Barbara
Wilson, William
Winkler, Howard A.
Winokur, George
Winsberg, Bertrand G.
Wishnow, Donald E.
Wisniewski, Henry
Wolfson, Leslie I.
Wolkin, Adam
Woodall, J. Martin
Woolsey, Joyce E.
Woolsey, Robert M.
Wright, Jesse H.
Wright, R. Lewis
Wurtman, Richard L.

Y

Yaskin, H. Edward
Yatsu, Frank
Young, Robert C.

Z

Zervas, Nicholas
Ziegler, Dewey
Zier, Adolfo
Zimmerman, Earl A.
Ziskind, Eugene
Zitrin, Arthur

MEMBERS

Senior Members

A
Ackerman, Sigurd H.
Adler, Alexandra
Aird, Robert B.
Amols, William

B
Badal, Daniel W.
Baker, A. B.
Beach, Frank A.
Bell, H. Craig
Berry, Richard G.
Binger, Carl
Blau, Abram
Bodian, David
Borkowski, Winslow J.
Boshes, Louis D.
Botelho, Stella Y.
Brody, Matthew
Brown, Joe R.
Buckley, Paul J.
Busse, Ewald W.

C
Cahs, Paul
Carter, Sidney
Chambers, William W.
Chusidm, Joseph
Cobb, Cully A.
Cowen, David
Culleton, James F.

D
Davis, Hollowell
DeJong, Russell N.
Denbo, Elic A.
Donnelly, John
Dunstone, H. Carter

E
Eberhart, John
Englisch, Robert
Epstein, Samuel H.
Evans, Harrison S.

F
Farmer, Thomas W.
Felix, Robert H.
Fields, William

Flexner, Louis B.
Foley, Joseph M.
Frank, Karl
Friedman, Arnold P.

G
Galbraith, James
Gates, Edward M.
Glaser, Gilbert
Goldman, Douglas
Greenhill, Maurice
Grinker, Roy R., Sr.

H
Hamilton, Francis
Hare, Clarence C.
Heath, Robert G.
Hinsey, Joseph C.
Holmes, Thomas
Hovde, Christian A.
Hudson, Robert J.

J
Jarcho, Leonard

K
Kabat, Elvin A.
Kalinowsky, Lothar B.
Kaplan, Harold
Kety, Seymour
Kies, Marion W.
Kolb, Lawrence
Kral, Vartech

L
Lakke, Hohannes P.W.F.
Larrabee, Martin G.
Lebensohn, Zigmond M.
Levin, Jules
Levy, Daniel
Lipin, Theodore
Livingston, Robert E.
Lowry, Oliver H.

M
MacPherson, Donald J.
Madow, Leo
Malmo, Robert B.
Masland, Richard L.

McKnight, William K.
McNerney, John C.
Menninger, Karl A.
Michael, Stanley
Millikan, Clark
Moore, Matthew T.

N
Nardini, John E.
Negrin, Juan, Jr.
Nurnberger, John

O
Oldberg, Eric
Osborne, Raymond L.
Osler, Geoffrey F.

P
Palmer, Edwin J.
Parker, Joseph
Pasik, Tauba
Perret, George
Peterson, Arthur
Pietri, Raoul
Pisetsky, Joseph
Pope, Alfred

R
Rabb, Preston
Randt, Clark T.
Rasmussen, Theodore
Richter, Curt P.
Robinson, Franklin
Roich, D.
Roseman, E.
Ross, Alexander T.
Rottersman, William
Ruesch, Jurgen

S
Sabin, Albert B.
Schlesinger, Edward
Schumacher, George
Senerchia, Fred, Jr.
Shenkin, Henry A.
Simon, John
Singer, Marcus
Smith, Wilbur K.
Soriano, Victor

Spotnitz, Hyman
Stafford-Clark, David
Stellar, Stanley
Sweet, William H.

T

Thompson, George N.
Tissenbaum, Morris
Tornay, Anthony
Trufant, Samuel
Tucker, Weir M.

W

Waggoner, Raymond W.
Wang, S. C.
Warner, Francis
Weickhardt, George D.
Whelan, Joseph L.
Williams, Ernest
Wittson, Cecil L.
Woodbury, Dixon M.
Woolsey, Clinton H.

Y

Yahr, Melvin D.
Yorshis, Morris

Z

Zfass, Isadore S.
Zubin, Joseph

Constitution and Bylaws

ASSOCIATION FOR RESEARCH IN NERVOUS AND MENTAL DISEASE, INC.

As revised in 1954 and amended in 1964, 1976, and 1978 by the members of the annual executive sessions

CONSTITUTION

ARTICLE I

Name

The Association shall be known as the "Association for Research in Nervous and Mental Disease, Incorporated."

ARTICLE II

Objects

The objects of the Association are to encourage, promote, foster, and assist investigations and research in nervous and mental disease and to prepare, print, issue, and distribute publications based upon such investigations and research.

ARTICLE III

Members

The membership of the Association for Research in Nervous and Mental Disease, Inc., shall consist of active, sustaining, and senior members.

ARTICLE IV

Officers

The officers of the Association shall be a President, First Vice-President, Second Vice-President, Secretary-Treasurer, and Assistant Secretary-Treasurer. The officers shall be elected by the members of the Association at the annual meeting to serve for one year.

ARTICLE V

Board of Trustees

There shall be a Board of Trustees consisting of twelve elected members with the President and Secretary-Treasurer of the Association acting as ex-officio members of the Board of Trustees. The Board of Trustees shall elect one of its elected members as its Chairman.

ARTICLE VI

Commission

The members of the Commission shall consist of individuals appointed by the President and approved by the Board of Trustees, to serve for the current year. The members of the Commission need not belong to the Association.

The Commission shall sit with the President at the annual meeting to hear the papers presented before the Association, may participate in the discussion of the contributions, and question the authors of the papers presented before the Association.

ARTICLE VII

Meetings

The time and place of the annual meeting shall be determined by the Board of Trustees.

ARTICLE VIII

Amendments

Amendments to this Constitution shall be made in the following manner: The proposed amendment shall be presented in writing, signed by at least three members of the Association, and submitted to the Board of Trustees at least thirty days before the current annual meeting. At the current annual meeting the Board of Trustees shall report to the Association upon said proposed amendment with their recommendation. The amendment shall then be voted upon and two-thirds of all votes cast at the meeting shall be necessary for the adoption of the amendment.

BYLAWS

ARTICLE I

Election of Trustees: Duties of Trustees

At each annual meeting a member of the Association shall be elected to the Board of Trustees of the Association for a term of seven years to replace members whose terms have expired. Members of the Board of Trustees shall be eligible for re-election.

The Board of Trustees shall have general charge of the affairs, funds, and property of the Association. It shall have full power and it shall be its duty to carry out the purposes of the Association according to the Charter, Constitution and Bylaws. A majority of its members shall constitute a quorum.

The Chairman of the Board of Trustees shall be the Chief Executive Officer of the Association.

ARTICLE II

Election of Officers: Duties of Officers

The officers of the Association shall be elected by a majority of the members present at the Executive Session of the annual meeting and shall serve for one year. Officers shall be eligible for re-election. Vacancies occurring in any office shall be filled by the Board of Trustees for the unexpired term until the next annual election.

The President: The President shall be responsible for the preparation of the scientific program, shall preside at the annual meeting, recommend to the Board of Trustees the appointment of the members of the Commission, call meetings of the Commission, and shall perform all duties customary to his office.

The First Vice-President: In the absence of the President, the First Vice-President shall discharge all the duties of the President.

The Second Vice-President: In the absence of the President and the First Vice-President, the Second Vice-President shall discharge all the duties of the President.

The Secretary-Treasurer: The Secretary-Treasurer shall issue notices of and keep records of the proceedings of all Executive and Scientific meetings of the Association and of the meetings of the Board of Trustees; shall notify officers, members of the Commission and members of Committees of their election; certify official records, keep a list of members; issue notices of all meetings; and perform all duties which may be required of him by the Board of Trustees, the President and Vice-Presidents. He shall be responsible for and keep account of all funds of the Association and make disbursements as directed by the Board of Trustees.

The Assistant Secretary-Treasurer: The Assistant Secretary-Treasurer shall act as an assistant to the Secretary-Treasurer and shall have power to act as the Secretary-Treasurer in the absence or during any disability of the Secretary-Treasurer.

ARTICLE III

Nomination and Election of Members: Qualification for Election

All members in good standing of neurologic or psychiatric societies or of societies devoted to basic research related to neurology or psychiatry in the United States and

Canada are eligible for membership in the various classes of membership of the Association upon being proposed by one and seconded by another member in good standing in the Association.

Proposals for election to membership must be reviewed by the Committee on Admissions and declared approved or disapproved. Such favorable or unfavorable action shall be reviewed by the Board of Trustees and the Board of Trustees shall then elect by majority vote those individuals whom they approve. Candidates acted upon unfavorably by the Committee on Admissions may be elected to membership by the unanimous vote of the Board of Trustees. Candidates shall become members following election by the Board of Trustees and upon payment of dues.

Sustaining and Active members shall be individuals who are engaged in the practice of neurology, neurologic surgery, psychiatry or who are engaged in research in these areas. Classification as a Sustaining or Active member depends upon the choice of the individual.

Individuals not fully qualified under the provisions of the preceding paragraphs may, under special circumstances, be elected to membership in the organization.

Senior membership shall consist of those who have been members in good standing for twenty-five years and who have reached the age of sixty-five years. Transfer to Senior membership of qualified Sustaining or Active members of the Association shall be optional. Members in good standing not possessing the preceding qualifications may, under exceptional circumstances, be eligible for transfer to Senior membership at the discretion of the Board of Trustees.

ARTICLE IV

Committees

A Nominating Committee of three members shall be appointed by the Chairman of the Board of Trustees prior to the annual meeting of the Association and the names of these members of the committee shall appear on the printed program. It shall be the duty of the Nominating Committee to nominate a President, First Vice-President, Second Vice-President, Secretary-Treasurer, Assistant Secretary-Treasurer, a member of the Board of Trustees, a member of the Admissions Committee, a member of the Committee on Public Relations, and such other offices as the Association may from time to time desire.

A committee on Admissions shall consist of three members, each member to serve for a period of three years. Each year a new member shall be elected at the Executive Session to replace the senior member of the Committee. All proposals for membership shall be submitted to the Committee for recommendation and those that are approved by the Committee shall then be forwarded to the Board of Trustees for final action.

An Auditing Committee of three members shall be appointed by the Chairman of the Board of Trustees prior to each annual meeting. It shall be the duty of the Auditing Committee to examine the accounts of the Treasurer and to report to the Association at its annual meeting.

A Committee on Public Relations shall consist of three members, each member to serve for a period of three years. Each year a new member of the Committee shall be elected at the Executive Session to replace the senior member of the Committee. The Committee on Public Relations shall be responsible for all matters of public relations particularly in connection with the lay and medical press and the relations of the Association with governmental and lay organizations.

ARTICLE V

Meetings

The Executive Session of each annual meeting shall be arranged by the Board of Trustees and the scientific program shall be organized by the President of the Association. Twenty-five members shall constitute a quorum at the Executive Session at the annual meeting. Robert's Rules of Order, Revised, shall govern all meetings of the Association, except where otherwise specifically provided by the Constitution and/or Bylaws of the Association.

Meetings of the Board of Trustees shall be held whenever called by its Chairman or at the request of three of its members. A majority of the Board of Trustees shall constitute a quorum.

ARTICLE VI

Dues

The dues for Sustaining and Active members shall be determined annually by the Board of Trustees. Senior and Associate members will not be subject to the payment of annual dues or assessments. Dues may be remitted, under special circumstances, by action of the Board of Trustees on request of an Active member.

Any member who shall fail for one year to pay his dues, may, after due notification by registered letter from the Treasurer, have his name stricken from the list of members at the discretion of the Board of Trustees, unless said dues be paid within thirty days of the date of mailing the notice. The Trustees shall be empowered to excuse any member from the payment of dues for reasons deemed by them to be good and sufficient.

ARTICLE VII

Amendments

These Bylaws may be amended in the same manner and with the same procedure as outlined for an amendment to the Constitution. Amendments of the Bylaws may also, if urgently needed, be made by unanimous action of the Board of Trustees. Such amendments, however, to continue effective must be approved at the Executive Session of the next annual meeting of the Association.

VISION AND THE BRAIN
The Organization of the Central Visual System

Research Publications:
Association for Research in Nervous and Mental Disease
Volume 67

Functional and Pharmacological Organization of the Retina: Dopamine, Interplexiform Cells, and Neuromodulation

John E. Dowling

Department of Cellular and Developmental Biology, The Biological Laboratories, Harvard University, Cambridge, Massachusetts 02138

Our understanding of the vertebrate retina has increased significantly during the past 30 years. The synaptic contacts made by the retinal neurons are known in some detail as well as the response properties of most of the classes of retinal cells. Thus, it is now possible to suggest how the receptive field organization of the various retinal ganglion cells is established by the synaptic interactions occurring between the retinal neurons (1).

Figure 1 is a summary diagram showing the circuitry underlying the formation of on-center, off-center, and on-off ganglion cells in the retina. This diagram pertains predominantly to cone pathways; rod pathways differ between species and are not as well-known as are the cone pathways (but see [2]). I begin with the on- and off-center cells, which, as has been known since the studies by Horace Barlow (3) and Stephen Kuffler (4) in the early 1950s, have a center-surround organization. Illumination of the receptive field center yields an on- or an off-response, whereas illumination of the periphery of the receptive field yields a response of opposite polarity; that is, upon surround illumination, an off-response is generated in an on-center cell and an on-response in an off-center cell.

We now know that these two ganglion cell types receive input from two types of bipolar cells (5): on-center cells receive input from bipolar cells that depolarize in response to illumination of the center of their receptive fields and the off-center cells receive input from bipolar cells that hyperpolarize in response to central receptive field illumination (6,7). These two bipolar cell types in turn receive their input from the photoreceptors, and thus the division of on- and off-channels in the visual system begins at the photoreceptor-bipolar synapse. Both bipolar cell types also show a center-surround receptive field organization (5) so that the basic receptive field organization of the on- and off-center ganglion cell is established already at the level of the bipolar cell.

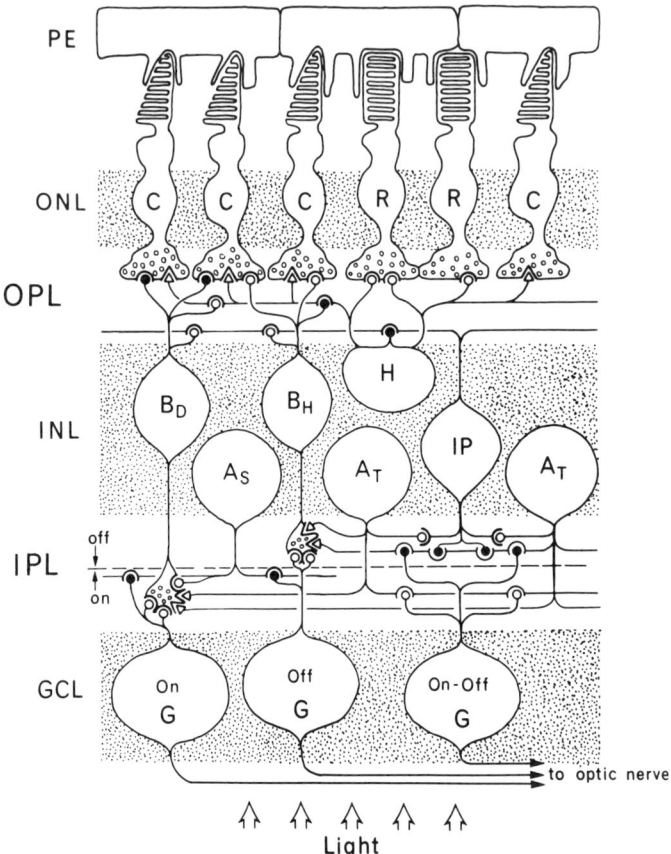

FIG. 1. Summary diagram illustrating the basic cellular and synaptic organization of the vertebrate retina. Two synaptic layers, the outer and inner plexiform layers (OPL and IPL) are interspersed between three cellular layers, the outer and inner nuclear layers and ganglion cell layers (ONL, INL, and GCL). The cell bodies (perikarya) of the cone and rod photoreceptors (C and R) make up the ONL; horizontal (H), bipolar (B), amacrine (A), and interplexiform (IP) cell perikarya make up the INL. Ganglion cell perikarya (G) make up the GCL. Excitatory synapses (○), inhibitory synapses (●), and reciprocal synapses (▲) are indicated in each plexiform layer. Two types of bipolar cells are indicated, those that depolarize in response to spot illumination (B_D), and those that hyperpolarize to spot illumination (B_H). Because depolarizing bipolars terminate in the lower half of the IPL, most on-responses are generated in that part of the IPL. Conversely, most off-responses are generated in the upper part of the IPL where the hyperpolarizing bipolars terminate. Two types of amacrine cells are also indicated, those that respond to light with sustained potentials (A_S) and those that respond with transient potentials (A_T). Through the synaptic interactions occurring in each synaptic layer, the receptive field properties of the on- and off-center ganglion cells and on-off ganglion cells are formed. (From ref. 1.)

The surround responses of the bipolar cells are provided by the horizontal cells, which are inhibitory interneurons that extend processes widely in the outer plexiform layer. Horizontal cells exert their inhibitory effects either by feeding back onto the receptors (8) or by antagonizing directly the bipolar cells (9), or both, and one horizontal cell can antagonize both types of bipolar cell (10). This has been shown by injecting hyperpolarizing current into horizontal cells, which induces depolarizing responses in center-hyperpolarizing bipolar cells and hyperpolarizing responses in center-depolarizing bipolar cells. Thus, the receptive field center of the bipolar cell reflects the direct input of receptors into the bipolar cells, whereas the antagonistic receptive field surround response reflects receptor to horizontal to bipolar cell input.

In the inner plexiform layer, amacrine cells interact with both bipolar terminals and ganglion cell dendrites (11). Two types of amacrine cell response are known: those that respond with sustained responses to light and others that respond transiently to retinal illumination (5,12,13). Amacrine cell input to ganglion cells may contribute to antagonistic surround mechanisms and may also impart more complex properties to the ganglion cell receptive fields, such as orientation selectivity (14). Ganglion cells that receive little input from amacrine cells show response and receptive field properties like bipolar cells. These cells give sustained responses to illumination and show a center-surround organization. Ganglion cells that receive more amacrine cell input show more transient responses and often more complex receptive field properties. The main difference between X- and Y-type ganglion cells in cat and P- and M-type ganglion cells in monkey may relate to the amount of amacrine cell input they receive (15).

There are some ganglion cells that receive most, if not all, of their input from amacrine cells (16,17). The example best known is the on-off, direction-sensitive ganglion cell studied extensively in rabbit. This cell responds well to spots of light passing across retina in one (the preferred) direction but not at all, or is actively inhibited, by spots of light moving in the opposite direction (null direction). The on-off ganglion cell receives excitatory input from amacrine cells that release acetylcholine (ACh) (19,20) and inhibitory input from amacrine cells that release γ-aminobutyric acid (GABA) (14). On-off ganglion cells that lack substantial inhibitory input from GABAergic amacrine cells are movement sensitive but not direction sensitive (14).

INTERPLEXIFORM CELLS AND NEUROMODULATION

The last cell type in the diagram, the interplexiform cell, is a more recently discovered cell (21). It is a centrifugal neuron, receiving all of its input in the inner plexiform layer, whereas most of its output is in the outer plexiform layer on horizontal cells and bipolar cells (22). This cell has interested us for some time for two main reasons. First, we have been curious as to the role of such a centrifugal neuron in the retina and second, in a number of species it contains and presumably releases dopamine (21). Dopamine in many parts of the brain acts as a neuromodulator; it exerts its action on postsynaptic cells through receptors that are linked to the enzyme adenylate cyclase. The resulting changes in intracellular cyclic AMP levels mediate the effects of dopamine by altering the properties of postsynaptic neurons.

All of the other synaptic interactions described above appear mediated by classic neurotransmitters; that is, the substances released at these synapses act directly on postsynaptic membranes to alter conductances to one or a few ions. For example, receptors and bipolar cells appear to release L-glutamate, horizontal cells and many amacrines release GABA, excitatory amacrine cells release ACh, etc. (1). However, it is now well established that there are many neuroactive substances released from retinal neurons, and the guess is that many if not most of these substances, including the monoamines and the peptides, serve as neuromodulators in the retina. What kinds of functions do they play?

The system in which we have studied this question is the fish retina. The reason for this is twofold. Most interplexiform cells in teleost fish are dopaminergic (21), and horizontal cells in fish, the primary target of the interplexiform cells, are especially large allowing for many kinds of experimental manipulations. Figure 2 shows a summary of the circuitry of interplexiform cells in fish. They receive their input in the inner plexiform layer from amacrine cells and centrifugal fibers, whereas in the outer plexiform layer they make numerous junctions on horizontal cells and a few synapses on bipolar cells (22,23). We have focused our attention on the effects of dopamine on horizontal cells.

As noted above, horizontal cells are inhibitory interneurons that form the antagonistic surround responses of bipolar cells. Another feature of horizontal cells is that they are extensively coupled electrically (24,25). The extensive electrical coupling between horizontal cells serves to increase the receptive field size of cells, and this means that stimulation of the retina over a wide area influences horizontal cells.

EFFECTS OF DOPAMINE ON HORIZONTAL CELLS

What does dopamine do to horizontal cells? Two principal effects have been demonstrated: (a) a reduction in the light responsiveness of the cell (26,27) and (b) an uncoupling of electrical junctions between the cells (28–30). This is shown in Fig. 3. Records from one experiment are shown in Fig. 3a and a summary of several experiments is shown in Fig. 3b (31). In the experiment shown Fig. 3a, a carp retina was presented alternately with spot (0.8 mm diameter) and full-field stimuli, while an intracellular recording was made from a horizontal cell. Spot stimuli probe the coupling between cells, and full-

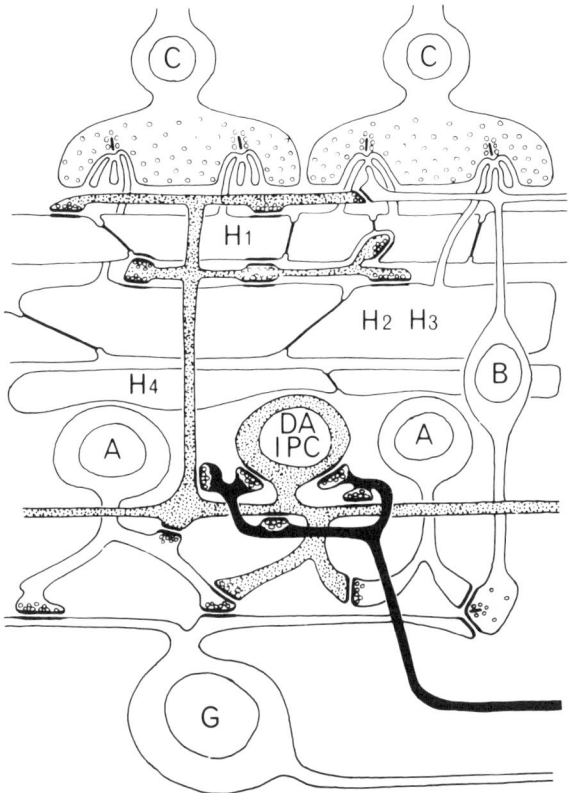

FIG. 2. Schematic diagram of the synaptic connections of the interplexiform cells (IP) in the white perch retina. The input to these neurons is in the inner plexiform layer from amacrine cells (A) and centrifugal fibers (filled processes). The interplexiform cell processes make synapses onto amacrine cell processes in the inner plexiform layer, but they never contact the ganglion cells (G) or their dendrites. In the outer plexiform layer, the processes of the interplexiform cells make synapses mainly onto the cone horizontal cells (H1, H2, and H3) and occasionally onto bipolar cell dendrites. The interplexiform cell processes have never been observed to make synapses on or receive input from the photoreceptors, nor have synapses been seen between interplexiform cell processes and rod horizontal cells (H4). C, cone photoreceptor. (From ref. 23.)

field stimuli evaluate the light sensitivity of the cell. Initially the spot and full-field stimuli were adjusted in intensity to give equal amplitude responses. Since horizontal cells are much more responsive to large fields (because of the electrical coupling between the cells), the intensity of the spot was considerably brighter than was the full-field stimulus. Following superfusion of the retina with dopamine for approximately 30 sec at a concentration of 200 μM, the horizontal cell depolarized slightly (~3 mV), the response to the spot increased by more than threefold and the response to full-field illumination

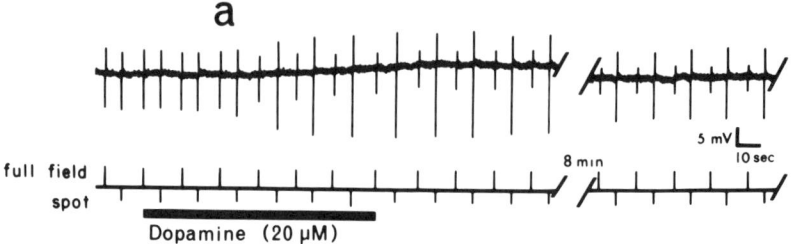

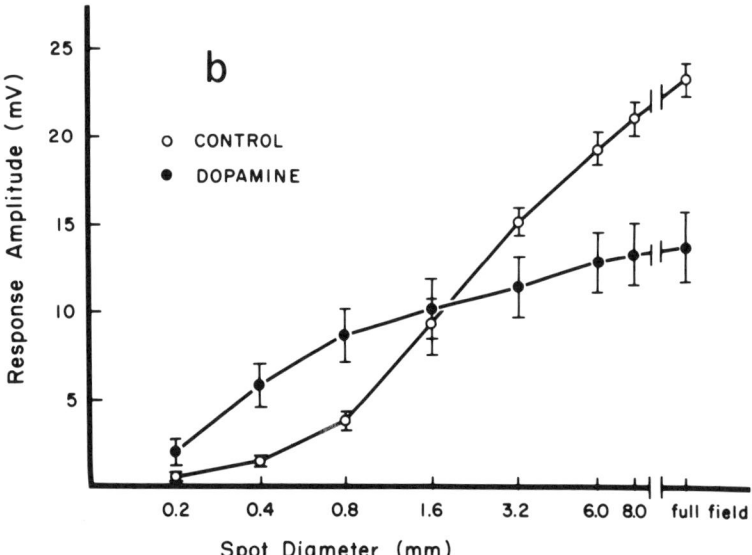

FIG. 3. a: Intracellular records of carp horizontal cell responses to spot and full-field white-light stimuli before, during, and after the addition of dopamine (20 μM) to the superfusion medium. The spot (0.8 mm in diameter) and full-field stimuli were presented as an alternating pair and adjusted before dopamine application to generate responses of approximately equal amplitudes. Dopamine caused the responses to spot stimuli to increase in amplitude, and the responses to full-field stimuli to decrease in amplitude. Recovery from these drug effects requires an average of approximately 15 min. Note that dopamine also caused the horizontal cell to depolarize slightly. **b:** Average horizontal cell response amplitudes as a function of stimulus spot diameter. The stimuli were centered in the middle of the cell's receptive field and were at an intensity that generated a half-maximal response when a full-field stimulus was used. Dopamine application caused average response amplitudes to small spot stimuli to be significantly larger and average response amplitudes to large spot and full-field stimuli to be significantly smaller. (From ref. 27.)

decreased by approximately one-third. These effects were long lasting; 8 to 9 min after dopamine infusion ceased, changes in response amplitudes to both spot and full-field stimuli were still pronounced.

Figure 3b shows in graph form the effects of dopamine on the receptive field profile and responsiveness of carp horizontal cells. These data show that with small spots (0.2–0.8 mm diameter) dopamine significantly increases response amplitudes, whereas with large spots (3.2–8 mm) and full-field illumination, dopamine significantly decreases response amplitudes. The increase in response amplitude to small spot stimuli can be readily explained by decreased electrical coupling between horizontal cells. That is, less current can flow from horizontal cells in the illuminated area to cells in the dark surrounding regions, and thus a larger voltage is recorded in cells in the illuminated area. However, the decreased responsiveness to large and full-field stimuli cannot be explained on this basis. With full-field stimuli, little current flow should occur between adjacent horizontal cells because all horizontal cells are receiving equal input from the photoreceptors and they should all be at the same potential. Thus, altering the strength of coupling between cells should not have effects on responses elicited with full-field stimuli. Therefore, Fig. 3b shows that dopamine induces at least two independent effects on horizontal cells; decreased responsiveness of the cell to light stimuli and decreased electrical coupling between adjacent horizontal cells.

DOPAMINE ACTS VIA CYCLIC AMP

How is dopamine exerting these effects? It is difficult to analyze the mechanisms underlying such effects in the intact retina because of the numerous interactions, both electrical and chemical, between the cells. Thus, we turned to isolated horizontal cells that are maintained in culture. It is relatively easy to isolate cells from the vertebrate retina by incubation of the retina in tissue culture medium (L-15) containing a protease (papain), followed by trituration of the retina with small bore pipettes. Figure 4 shows freshly isolated horizontal cells from the white perch retina obtained in this way and placed into tissue culture dishes containing fresh medium (32). Four types of horizontal cells can be distinguished; three of these are cone horizontal cells (H1–H3) and one is a rod horizontal cell (H4). The dopaminergic interplexiform cells make synapses only onto cone horizontal cells, and present evidence indicates that dopamine causes similar effects on all three types of cone horizontal cells.

In early experiments with isolated horizontal cells from the carp retina, it was found that at physiological concentrations (<300 μM), dopamine altered neither membrane potential nor membrane resistance (33). This immediately suggested that the effects of dopamine on horizontal cells were not mediated directly, but by a second messenger such as cyclic AMP.

Evidence that the dopamine receptors on horizontal cells are linked to

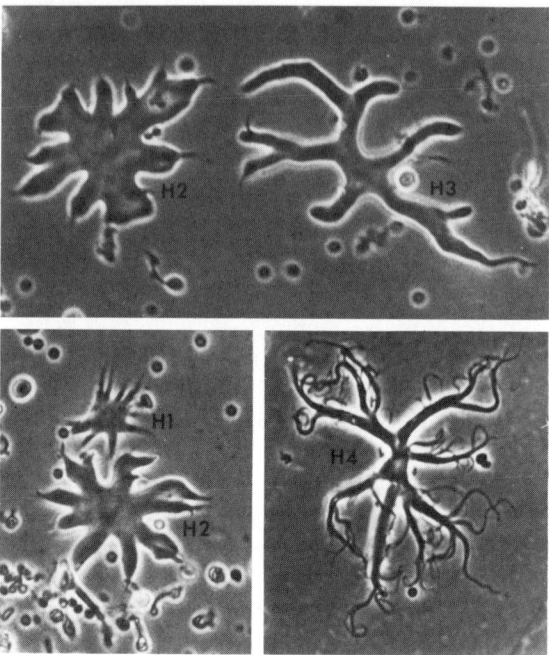

FIG. 4. Four morphologically distinct types of horizontal cells (H1–H4) are observed in cultures of the white perch retina. The four types appear to correspond to the four layers of horizontal cells typically seen in radial sections of this retina. The H1 cells are most distally positioned in the retina, whereas the H2 cells are found in the second layer. The H3 and H4 cells are more proximally located. The H1, H2, and H3 cells are cone-driven horizontal cells, whereas the H4 is a rod-driven horizontal cell. (From ref. 32.)

adenylate cyclase was provided by preparing purified fractions of isolated carp horizontal cells and determining cyclic AMP content after exposure to dopamine (Fig. 5) (34). Fractions containing rod photoreceptors demonstrated substantial basal levels of cyclic AMP, but their cyclic nucleotide content was unaffected by dopamine in the incubating medium. On the other hand, fractions enriched in horizontal cells showed very low basal levels of cyclic AMP; however, there was a graded increase in cyclic AMP levels with increasing concentrations of dopamine in the incubating medium. Approximately 10 μM of dopamine was required to half-saturate the system, which is the same concentration of dopamine required to half-saturate cyclic AMP accumulation in the intact retina. These experiments showed not only that there are dopamine receptors linked to adenylate cyclase on isolated horizontal cells, but that these receptors are not altered significantly by the isolation of the horizontal cells from the retina. Thus, the failure of dopamine to alter the membrane potential or resistance of isolated horizontal cells could not be attributed to a loss of dopamine receptors from the cells.

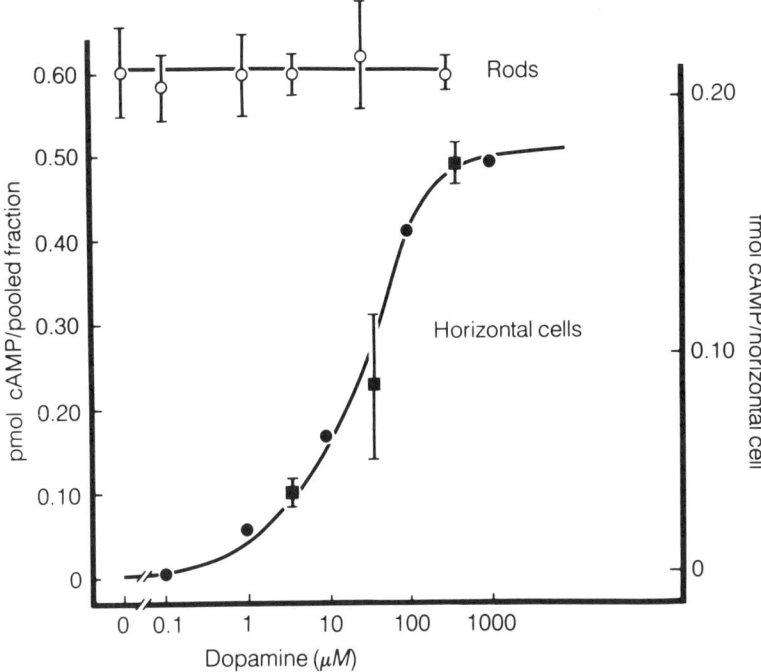

FIG. 5. Effects of various concentrations of dopamine on cyclic AMP content of purified fractions of isolated horizontal cells and rod cells from the carp retina. All fractions were preincubated in Ringer's solution containing 2 mM isobutylmethylxanthine (a phosphodiesterase inhibitor) for 3 min and then incubated in Ringer's solution containing dopamine for 5 min. Results expressed as femtomoles of cyclic AMP per horizontal cell are based on the assumption of 3,000 horizontal cells per fraction. Standard errors of the mean are provided for those points based on three or more experiments. Dopamine caused a graded increase in cyclic AMP content in the horizontal cell fractions, but not in the rod cell fractions. (From ref. 34.)

How dopamine via cyclic AMP may alter the light sensitivity of horizontal cells was suggested by experiments carried out on single white perch horizontal cells (35). The rationale for these experiments was as follows: Since horizontal cells receive input directly from the photoreceptors, could it be that dopamine and cyclic AMP alter the sensitivity of the horizontal cells to the photoreceptor neurotransmitter, namely L-glutamate? It was found that both dopamine and cyclic AMP significantly enhance ionic conductance changes elicited in isolated horizontal cells by L-glutamate or kainate, a glutamate analogue (Fig. 6). For these experiments, the horizontal cells were voltage clamped with patch electrodes and currents measured across the cell membrane in response to the application of dopamine, kainate, cyclic AMP or a combination of these agents. The application of dopamine itself (200 μM) to isolated horizontal cells induced no significant change in membrane conductance (top traces). The lower traces show the conductance changes induced in

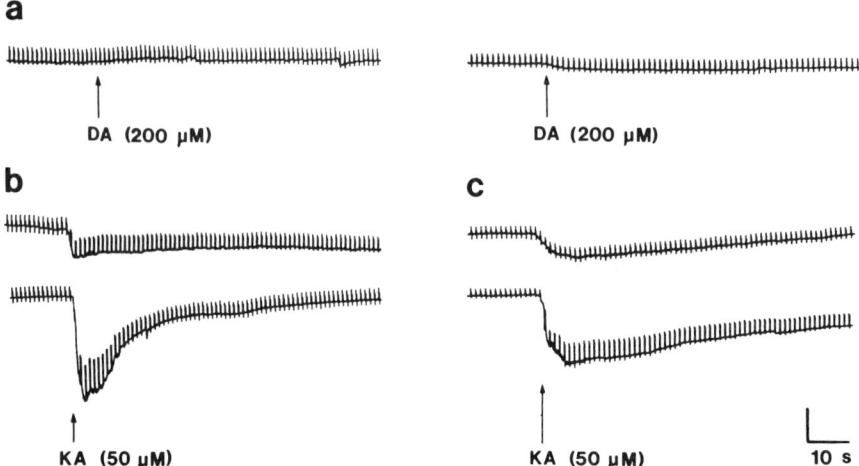

FIG. 6. Effects of dopamine (DA) and cyclic AMP on ionic conductances mediated by kainate (KA) (a glutamate agonist) in perch horizontal cells maintained in culture. **a:** The application of short (~0.5 sec) pulses of dopamine (200 μM) to horizontal cells caused no significant changes in membrane conductance. **b,c:** Kainate- (50 μM) induced conductances before (upper traces) and a few minutes after (lower traces) the application of a pulse of dopamine (b) or cyclic AMP (c) to horizontal cells. Both dopamine (200 μM) and cyclic AMP (500 μM) enhanced the kainate-mediated conductances by two- to threefold. (From ref. 35.)

these cells by kainate (50 μM) before and 2 to 3 min after the application of a pulse of Ringer's containing 200 μM dopamine or 500 μM cyclic AMP to the cells. In both cases the currents induced by kainate were enhanced by more than twofold.

Figure 7 summarizes the data obtained in these experiments, expressed as enhancement of kainate current as a function of various treatments. A control response to kainate (50 μM) was first determined and then 2 to 3 min after application of a pulse of Ringer's or Ringer's containing a test agent, the current induced by the control dose of kainate was remeasured. Both dopamine and cyclic AMP induced approximately a doubling of the kainate current in cone horizontal cells. However, neither dopamine nor cyclic AMP affected the kainate current in rod horizontal cells, an expected result because rod horizontal cells do not receive dopaminergic input. The effects of dopamine on cone horizontal cells were blocked by haloperidol, a dopamine antagonist, and serotonin, an indoleamine, caused no enhancement of kainate current in horizontal cells.

An explanation for the *decrease* in light responsiveness of horizontal cells following dopamine application to the intact retina is as follows: The light response of the horizontal cell results from a reduction in the release of transmitter from the photoreceptor. Dopamine, by enhancing the potency of the photoreceptor transmitter, renders the light-induced reduction of transmitter release from the receptors less effective and thus decreases the amplitude

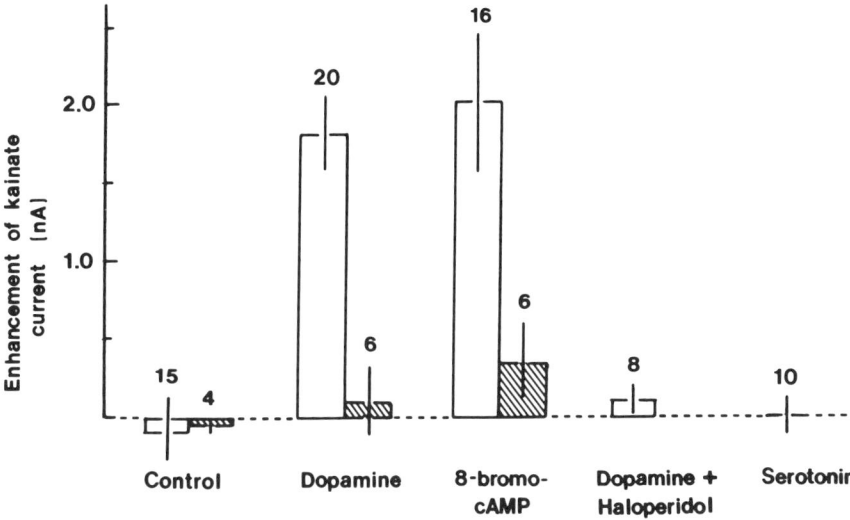

FIG. 7. The effects of dopamine, 8-bromo-cyclic AMP, and dopamine plus haloperidol and serotonin on kainate-induced currents in cultured cone and rod horizontal cells from the white perch retina. For each cell tested, the amount of kainate ejected was first adjusted to give a nonsaturating response (0.3–2.5 nA). This dose was used in all subsequent applications of kainate to that cell. A pulse of Ringer's containing dopamine (200 μM), 8-bromo-cyclic AMP (500 μM), dopamine plus haloperidol or serotonin (500 μM) was then applied, followed by repeated applications of kainate. Values plotted represent the difference between the initial response and the largest kainate-induced current observed after exposure to the test agent. *Open bars* represent cone horizontal cells, *shaded bars* represent rod horizontal cells. Number of cells tested in each condition is indicated above the bars. Rod horizontal cells were not tested in the haloperidol and serotonin experiments. Error bars denote s.e.m. See text.

of the cell's response to light. These observations may also provide an explanation for the paradoxical observation that dopamine usually depolarizes horizontal cells in the intact retina (Fig. 3), but has no consistent effect on membrane potential or conductance of isolated horizontal cells (Fig. 6). Since the ongoing release of photoreceptor transmitter continually depolarizes horizontal cells, dopamine, by facilitating the action of the transmitter, would depolarize horizontal cells in the intact retina, but have no effects on isolated cells in culture when transmitter is absent.

The effects of dopamine and cyclic AMP on the electrical coupling between horizontal cells can also be studied with isolated cells, but for such experiments pairs of overlapping cells of the same subtype are required (36). In most culture dishes, such pairs can be found and quantitative measures of the electrical coupling between the cells determined. Figure 8 illustrates an experiment on a pair of cultured white perch horizontal cells. Both cells were voltage clamped with patch electrodes and the potential of one of the cells, the driver cell (lower record), was shifted by 20 mV with current pulses. In response to dopamine, the cells uncoupled, as shown by the decrease in

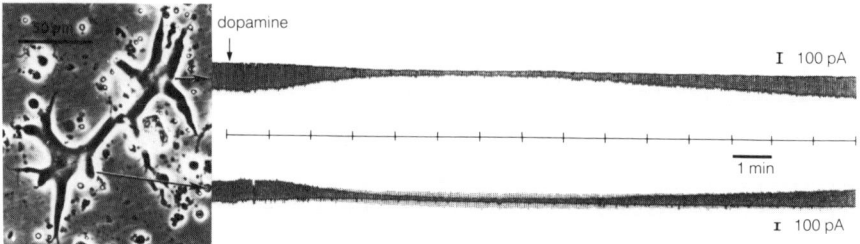

FIG. 8. Effects of dopamine on an electrically coupled pair of white perch horizontal cells maintained in culture **(left).** Both cells were voltage clamped at −60 mV with patch electrodes and current pulses were applied to the driver cell (lower trace) to shift the membrane potential +20 mV. A pulse of Ringer's solution containing dopamine was applied to the cell pair. The cells gradually uncoupled, as shown by the decrease in the magnitude of the clamp current pulses passed into the follower cell (upper trace), which reflects the decreased conductance of the junctional membrane, and the decrease in magnitude of the current pulses required to depolarize the driver cell by 20 mV, which reflects the increased resistance of the driver cell. (From ref. 36.)

magnitude of the pulses recorded in both cells. The pulses in the follower cell (upper trace) became smaller because of the decreased conductance of the gap junctional membrane; the magnitude of the pulses in the driver cell (lower trace) decreased because of the increased input resistance of the cell. Before the application of the dopamine pulse, a junctional resistance of approximately 80 MΩ was measured. After drug application, there was a latency of approximately 30 sec before uncoupling began. Cells were maximally uncoupled after approximately 4 min, at which point the junctional resistance had risen to approximately 660 MΩ. Coupling between the cells remained low for approximately 1 min and then slowly increased. After approximately 14 min, the junctional resistance had recovered to approximately 100 MΩ. For other cell pairs tested in this way, or following the injection of cyclic AMP into one of the cells, junctional resistance increased from control levels of 20 to 60 MΩ to as much as 300 to 700 MΩ.

How cyclic AMP modifies gap junctional conductance between horizontal cells is not known. In other cyclic AMP-mediated systems, protein phosphorylation is involved (37). Cyclic AMP activates specific kinases that in turn phosphorylate particular proteins. Phosphorylation is known to alter the properties of proteins, and it may be that phosphorylation of gap junctional membrane proteins alters the conductance of the junction. Recent experiments have shown that the injection of the catalytic subunit of cyclic AMP-dependent kinase into horizontal cells uncouples pairs of horizontal cells maintained in culture, a finding supporting this hypothesis (38).

A summary scheme of how dopamine influences both light responsiveness of, and electrical coupling between, horizontal cells is shown in Fig. 9. Dopamine interacts with receptors that are linked to the enzyme adenylate cyclase through a G protein. Activation of adenylate cyclase results in the conversion of ATP to cyclic AMP. Cyclic AMP, in turn, interacts with kinases

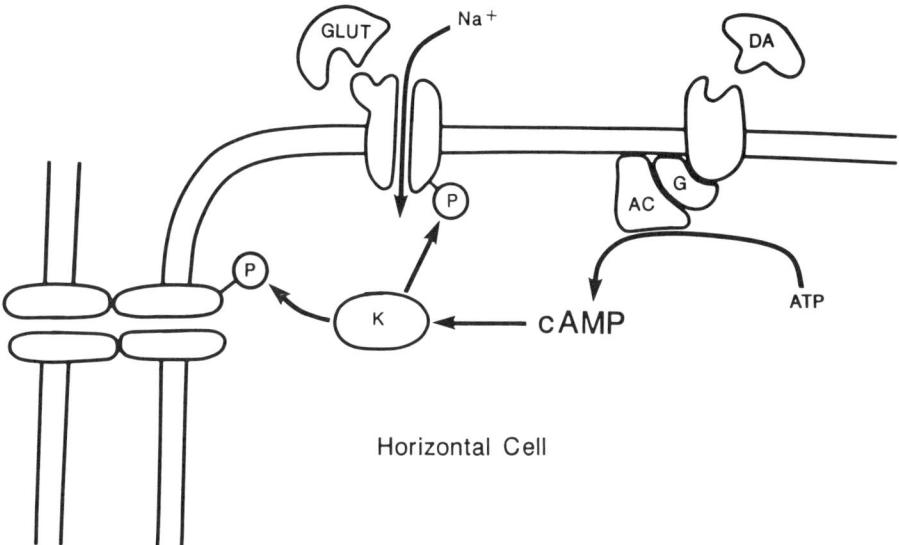

FIG. 9. Summary scheme showing how dopamine, acting via cyclic AMP, may influence the responsiveness of horizontal cells to L-glutamate (the photoreceptor transmitter) and the electrical coupling between horizontal cells. Dopamine (DA) interacts with receptors that are linked to the enzyme adenylate cyclase (AC) via a G protein. Activation of adenylate cyclase results in the conversion of ATP to cyclic AMP. The cyclic AMP interacts with kinases (K) that phosphorylate (P) the glutamate (Glut) channels or the gap junction channels. See text.

that phosphorylate the glutamate channels or the gap junction channels. We propose that phosphorylation of the glutamate channel enhances the conductance induced by the interaction of L-glutamate or a glutamate analogue with the channel (Fig. 6), whereas phosphorylation of the gap junction channels reduces their conductance. As yet we have no direct evidence for phosphorylation of the L-glutamate channels in horizontal cells upon dopamine treatment, but Douglas McMahon in our laboratory has shown phosphorylation of presumed gap junctional proteins following dopamine application to the white perch retina.

THE ROLE OF DOPAMINE IN RETINAL FUNCTION

What is the significance of the dopamine-mediated modulation of horizontal cells? What role might it play in visual function? Overall, the action of dopamine on horizontal cells is to diminish the effectiveness of the cell in mediating lateral inhibitory effects in the outer plexiform layer of the retina. Decreasing the light responsiveness of the cell and shrinking its receptive field size are effective ways of lessening the inhibitory influences of horizontal cells. Since horizontal cells form the antagonistic surround responses of the bipolar and receptor cells, a decrease in bipolar and receptor cell surround responses is to be expected following dopamine application, and such changes have been observed (26). Furthermore, it has long been known that following prolonged periods of darkness, the antagonistic surrounds of many ganglion cells are reduced in strength or even eliminated. This was first shown by Barlow, Fitzhugh, and Kuffler (39) in the cat and a similar phenomenon also occurs in the frog and the rabbit (40,41). This change in field organization does not relate to a switch from cone to rod vision, and the mechanisms that underlie the alteration in center-surround organization of ganglion cells are unknown. An obvious speculation is that interplexiform cells and/or dopamine play such a role and regulate the strength of lateral inhibition and center-surround antagonism in the retina as a function of adaptive state.

Evidence in favor of such an idea has been provided by examining the receptive field profiles of horizontal cells in the carp retina following short (30–40 min) and long (100–120 min) periods of time in complete darkness (27,31). As shown in Fig. 10, the receptive field profile of horizontal cells in retinas maintained for long periods of time in the dark is distinctly different from those profiles measured from horizontal cells in retinas maintained in the dark for short periods of time. The profiles from retinas kept in prolonged

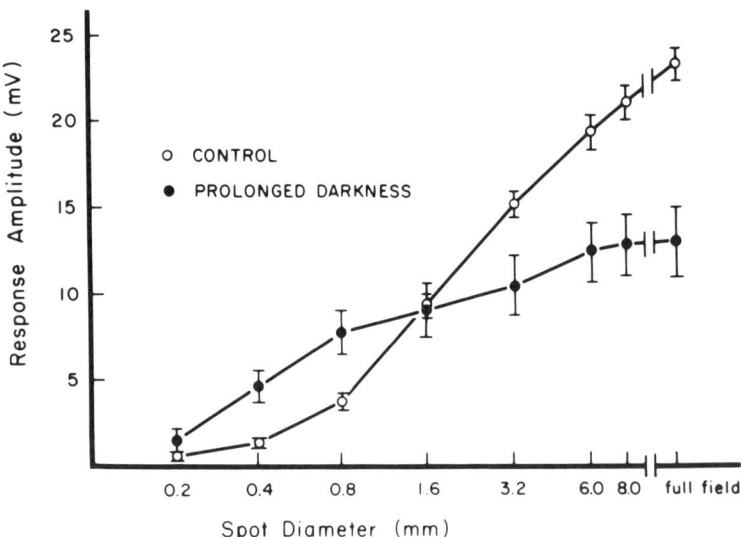

FIG. 10. Average carp horizontal cell response amplitudes as a function of stimulus spot diameter following 30–40 min in the dark (control) and following 100–120 min in the dark (prolonged darkness). Prolonged darkness, like dopamine, caused average response amplitudes to small spot stimuli to be significantly larger, and response amplitudes to large spot stimuli to be significantly smaller. (From ref. 27.)

darkness closely resemble those of horizontal cells from control retinas exposed to dopamine.

The effects of prolonged darkness on the electrical coupling between horizontal cells in the white perch retina is shown even more directly in Fig. 11 (42). In these experiments, the fluorescent dye, Lucifer yellow, was injected into one horizontal cell in intact retinas. In the short-term dark-adapted retina (top micrograph), the fluorescent dye spread to many surrounding cells, indicating extensive coupling between the horizontal cells. In prolonged dark-adapted retinas (bottom micrograph), dye was observed only in the injected cell and a few surrounding cells. Furthermore, the fluorescence seen in the

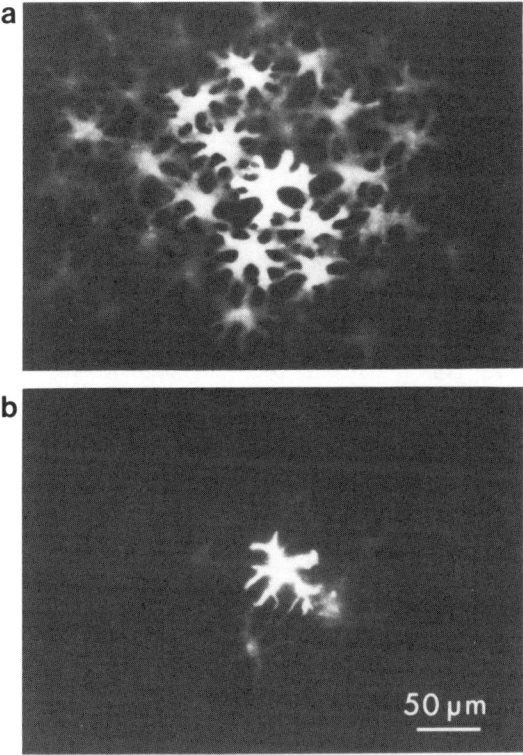

FIG. 11. a: Lucifer yellow injected cells in a short-term dark-adapted white perch retina. The dye was presumably injected into the H2 cell in the center of the micrograph that shows the brightest fluorescence. The dye diffused into a large number of surrounding cells; i.e., a considerable amount of dye coupling is seen. This cell was injected for 14 min with 20 nA hyperpolarizing current pulses. b: Lucifer yellow injected cells in a prolonged dark-adapted white perch retina. The injected cell (center) is of the H2 type with short, stout processes, slightly branched at the endings. Dye diffused into only a few surrounding cells, and these cells show only weak fluorescence. This cell was injected for 15 min with 20 nA hyperpolarizing current pulses. Fluorescence micrograph calibration bar is 50 μM. (From ref. 42.)

surrounding cells was comparatively weak, indicating significantly diminished coupling between the horizontal cells. These experiments, like those shown in Fig. 10, suggest that after a prolonged period of time in the dark, dopamine is released tonically from the interplexiform cells.

To summarize, the interplexiform cells and dopamine appear to modulate horizontal cell activity as a function of the light history of the retina. In the light and in short-term darkness, the interplexiform cells are turned off and horizontal cells function maximally. In prolonged darkness, the interplexiform cells become active, releasing dopamine, which depresses horizontal cell activity. Thus, lateral inhibition and surround antagonism are reduced under these conditions, making the retina a better photodetector, but, presumably, at the expense of visual acuity.

This system may be a model for neuromodulation both in the retina and elsewhere. The dopaminergic interplexiform cells in the fish retina, like other presumed neuromodulatory neurons, are relatively rare cells, making up no more than a few percent of the cells in the inner nuclear layer. However, they spread processes widely in both plexiform layers, and in the outer plexiform layer they make abundant synapses on the horizontal cells. Dopamine has no direct effects on membrane voltage or resistance of the horizontal cells, but it activates, through specific dopamine receptors, the enzyme adenylate cyclase that increases cyclic AMP levels within the cell. The cyclic AMP mediates multiple effects in the cell, including a decrease in its light responsiveness and a shrinkage of its receptive field. These effects diminish the lateral inhibition mediated by the horizontal cells in the outer plexiform layer and reduce center-surround antagonism in receptor, bipolar, and presumably other neurons. It is important to emphasize that dopamine and the interplexiform cells do not mediate the center-surround antagonism but modulate its strength. Thus, enhancing or blocking dopaminergic activity in the retina does not change the basic receptive field organization of retinal cells; instead it alters the balance of center and surround responses.

What might be the role of other neuromodulatory substances and neurons in the retina? Evidence that these neurons, like interplexiform cells, make specific synaptic connections has been provided in several instances (43,44). This suggests that there may be modulatory control of many, if not all, of the major excitatory and inhibitory neurons and pathways in the retina and brain. Tests of such ideas are needed and the retina appears to be an ideal part of the central nervous system in which to determine the role of neuromodulators in brain function.

ACKNOWLEDGMENTS

This work has been supported in part by NIH grants EY-00811 and EY-00824. I thank Stephanie Levinson for typing the manuscript and Patricia Sheppard for preparing the figures.

REFERENCES

1. Dowling JE. *The retina: an approachable part of the brain.* Cambridge, MA: Harvard University Press, 1987.
2. Kolb H, Nelson R. Rod pathways in the retina of the cat. *Vision Res* 1983;23:301–312.
3. Barlow HB. Summation and inhibition in the frog's retina. *J Physiol* 1953;119:69–88.
4. Kuffler SW. Discharge patterns and functional organization of mammalian retina. *J Neurophysiol* 1953;16:37–68.
5. Werblin FS, Dowling JE. Organization of the retina of the mudpuppy, *Necturus maculosus*. II. Intracellular recording. *J Neurophysiol* 1969;32:339–355.
6. Miller RF, Dacheux RF. Synaptic organization and ionic basis of on and off channels in mudpuppy retina. III. A model of ganglion cell receptive field organization based on chloride-free experiments. *J Gen Physiol* 1976;67:679–690.
7. Naka K-I. Functional organization of catfish retina. *J Neurophysiol* 1977;40:26–43.
8. Baylor DA, Fuortes MGF, O'Bryan PM. Receptive fields of single cones in the retina of the turtle. *J Physiol* 1971;214:256–294.
9. Dowling JE, Werblin FS. Organization of retina of the mudpuppy, *Necturus maculosus*. I. Synaptic structure. *J Neurophysiol* 1969;32:315–338.
10. Sakuranaga M, Naka K-I. Signal transmission in the catfish retina. I. Transmission in the outer retina. *J Neurophysiol* 1985;53:373–389.
11. Dowling JE, Boycott BB. Organization of the primate retina: electron microscopy. *Proc R Soc [Biol]* 1966;166:80–111.
12. Kaneko A. Physiological studies of single retinal cells and their morphological identification. *Vision Res (Suppl)* 1971;3:17–26.
13. Toyoda J, Hashimoto H, Ohtsu K. Bipolar-amacrine transmission in the carp retina. *Vision Res* 1973;13:295–307.
14. Caldwell JH, Daw HW, Wyatt HJ. Effects of picrotoxin and strychnine on rabbit retinal ganglion cells: lateral interactions for cells with more complex receptive fields. *J Physiol* 1978;276:277–298.
15. Victor JD, Shapley RM. The nonlinear pathway of Y ganglion cells in the cat retina. *J Gen Physiol* 1979;74:671–689.
16. Dowling JE. Synaptic organization of the frog retina: an electron microscopic analysis comparing the retinas of frogs and primates. *Proc R Soc [Biol]* 1968;170:205–228.
17. West RW, Dowling JE. Synapses onto different morphological types of retinal ganglion cells. *Science* 1972;178:510–512.
18. Barlow HB, Hill RM, Levick WR. Retinal ganglion cells responding selectively to direction and speed of image motion in the rabbit. *J Physiol* 1964;173:377–407.
19. Ariel M, Daw NW. Pharmacological analysis of directionally sensitive rabbit retinal ganglion cells. *J Physiol* 1982;324:161–185.
20. Masland RH, Mills JW, Cassidy C. The functions of acetylcholine in the rabbit retina. *Proc R Soc [Biol]* 1984;223:121–139.
21. Ehinger B, Falck B, Laties AM. Adrenergic neurons in teleost retina. *Z Zellforsch* 1969;97:285–297.
22. Dowling JE, Ehinger B. Synaptic organization of the amine-containing interplexiform cells of the goldfish and *Cebus* monkey retina. *Science* 1975;188:270–273.
23. Zucker CL, Dowling JE. Centrifugal fibers synapse on interplexiform cells in the teleost retina. *Nature* 1987;330:166–168.
24. Yamada E, Ishikawa T. The fine structure of the horizontal cells in some vertebrate retinae. *Cold Spring Harbor Symp Quant Biol* 165;30:383–392.
25. Kaneko A. Electrical connexions between horizontal cells in the dogfish retina. *J Physiol* 1971;213:95–105.
26. Hedden WL, Dowling JE. The interplexiform cell system. II. Effects of dopamine on goldfish retinal neurons. *Proc R Soc [Biol]* 1978;201:27–55.
27. Mangel SC, Dowling JE. Responsiveness and receptive field size of carp horizontal cells are reduced by prolonged darkness and dopamine. *Science* 1985;229:1107–1109.
28. Teranishi T, Negishi K, Kato S. Dopamine modulates S-potential amplitude and dye-coupling between external horizontal cells in carp retina. *Nature* 1983;301:243–246.

29. Teranishi T, Negishi K, Kato A. Regulatory effect of dopamine on spatial properties of horizontal cells in carp retina. *J Neurosci* 1984;4:1271–1280.
30. Piccolino M, Neyton J, Gerschenfeld HM. Decrease of gap junction permeability induced by dopamine and cyclic adenosine 3',5'-monophosphate in horizontal cells of turtle retina. *J Neurosci* 1984;4:2477–2488.
31. Mangel SC, Dowling JE. The interplexiform horizontal cell system of the fish retina: effects of dopamine, light stimulus and time in the dark. *Proc R Soc [Biol]* 1987;23:91–121.
32. Dowling JE, Pak MW, Lasater EM. White perch horizontal cells in culture: methods, morphology and process growth. *Brain Res* 1985;360:331–338.
33. Lasater EM, Dowling JE. Carp horizontal cells in culture respond selectively to L-glutamate and its agonists. *Proc Natl Acad Sci USA* 1982;79:936–940.
34. Van Buskirk R, Dowling JE. Isolated horizontal cells from carp retina demonstrate dopamine-dependent accumulation of cyclic AMP. *Proc Natl Acad Sci USA* 1981;78:7825–7829.
35. Knapp AG, Dowling JE. Dopamine enhances excitatory amino acid-gated conductances in retinal horizontal cells. *Nature* 1987;325:437–439.
36. Lasater EM, Dowling JE. Dopamine decreases conductance of the electrical junctions between cultured retinal horizontal cells. *Proc Natl Acad Sci USA* 1985;82:3025–3029.
37. Greengard P. *Cyclic nucleotides, phosphorylated proteins, and neuronal function*. New York: Raven Press, 1978.
38. Lasater EM. Retinal horizontal cell gap junctional conductance is modulated by dopamine through a cyclic AMP-dependent protein kinase. *Proc Natl Acad Sci USA* 1987;84:7319–7323.
39. Barlow HB, FitzHugh R, Kuffler SW. Change of organization of the receptive fields of the cat's retina during dark adaptation. *J Physiol* 1957;137:338–354.
40. Donner KO, Reuter T. Visual adaptation of the rhodopsin rods in the frog's retina. *J Physiol* 1968;199:59–87.
41. Masland RH, Ames A III. Responses to acetylcholine of ganglion cells in an isolated mammalian retina. *J Neurophysiol* 1976;39:1220–1235.
42. Tornqvist K, Yang X-L, Dowling JE. Modulation of cone horizontal cells activity in the teleost fish retina. III. Effects of prolonged darkness and dopamine on electrical coupling between horizontal cells. *J Neurosci* 1988;8:2279–2288.
43. Holmgren-Taylor I. Electron microscopical observations on the indoleamine-accumulating neurons and their synaptic connections in the retina of the cat. *J Comp Neurol* 1982;208:144–156.
44. Yazulla S, Studholme KM, Zucker CL. Synaptic organization of substance P-like immunoreactive amacrine cells in goldfish retina. *J Comp Neurol* 1985;231:232–238.

Vision and the Brain,
edited by B. Cohen and I. Bodis-Wollner.
Raven Press, Ltd., New York © 1990.

Biochemical and Morphological Heterogeneity of Retinal Ganglion Cells

*Harvey J. Karten, *Kent T. Keyser, and †Nicholas C. Brecha

Department of Neurosciences, University of California at San Diego, La Jolla, California 92093, and †Departments of Anatomy and Cell Biology and Medicine, University of California at Los Angeles, Los Angeles, California 90024

The vertebrate retina is a highly stratified structure containing five major categories of neurons: photoreceptor, horizontal, bipolar, amacrine, and ganglion cells. Studies within the past decade have revealed the existence of a variety of classical neurotransmitters as well as many neuropeptides within the retina. Immunohistochemical analysis of the retina has demonstrated that some of the five major cell types of the retina may consist of as many as 15 to 20 subtypes, with a precise correspondence between the morphology and biochemical content of many of the individual subtypes of neurons. These findings have led to major advances in understanding the operations of the inner retina, particularly the inner plexiform layer (IPL).

The IPL is a complex region of synaptic interaction of bipolar, amacrine, and ganglion cells, with a dramatic, although covert, pattern of lamination. The output of ganglion cells is determined by the complex biochemical and electrical information that they receive from amacrine and/or bipolar cells and by the specific neurotransmitter receptors produced by the ganglion cells themselves. Similarly, the information received by central visual structures is determined by the immediate and long-term effects of substances released by the retinal ganglion cells (RGCs). Recent research on this topic has indicated that RGCs may contain any of a wide variety of transmitters/modulators, including substance P (frog, chick, rabbit), enkephalin (frog), cholecystokinin (frog, pigeon), bombesin (frog), dopamine (cat, pigeon), serotonin (elasmobranch, chicken), and glutamate (pigeon, rat, cat). Each biochemically distinct class of RGCs may terminate in separate, defined domains within a single central target. Comparison of data derived from different methodologies and various species strongly indicates that we still do not know the full range of RGC transmitters and/or modulators. Identifying RGC transmitters is of vital importance to understanding the information content of retinal input to central visual areas.

The heterogeneity of RGCs has been further emphasized by the finding that their expression of specific receptors and second messengers, their responses to injury, and their selective ability to regenerate may vary as widely as do their input and content of neurotransmitters.

MORPHOLOGICAL CLASSIFICATION OF RGCs

Ramón y Cajal's (1) morphological studies of the vertebrate retina, using the Golgi method, were of landmark significance for two major reasons. Foremost was that they formed the basis of his proposal of the neuron doctrine. For students of the visual system, however, his studies are the foundation of all that followed during the next century. Indeed, the continuing importance of Cajal's study of the retina is reflected in the realization that many of the most novel morphological findings of the past decade often proved to be validations of Cajal's earlier suggestions. Cajal showed that cells of the retina were extremely diverse in their morphology, differing not only in the size of their somata, but even more strikingly in the organization of their dendritic trees. Cajal stressed the importance of the laminar organization of the IPL, emphasizing its pentalaminar nature in many species. He described an extraordinary heterogeneity of ganglion cell morphology and illustrated various types of ganglion cells that arborized in only a single lamina and others that branched in two or more laminae of the IPL. This astonishing variety of cell types remained largely unexplored for many decades. Even as basic an issue as the presence of lamination in the IPL was long ignored, until combined physiological and morphological studies revealed an important aspect of lamination of the IPL in relationship to bipolar, amacrine, and ganglion cells (2–4). These studies demonstrated that cells arborizing in the outer portion of the IPL were off cells, whereas those arborizing in the inner part of the IPL were on cells.

TARGET SPECIFICITY OF RGCs

Cajal (1), Lettvin et al. (5), and others emphasized that morphologically different types of RGCs selectively project to individual central targets. The development of effective retrogradely transportable markers in the 1970s provided a means of obtaining the first direct evidence in support of this notion. For example, Karten et al. (6) demonstrated that the displaced ganglion cells of Dogiel (7) were the sole source of input to the nucleus of the basal optic root of the accessory optic system in birds (Fig. 1).

More recently, a variety of morphological and histochemical methods have been used to identify other types of ganglion cells that project to specific central targets. Some of these will be discussed in a later section.

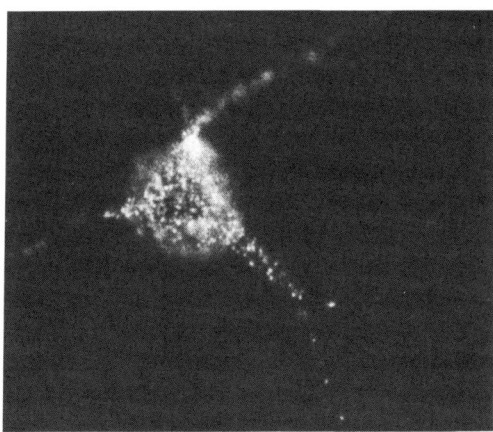

FIG. 1. A ganglion cell in the pigeon retina 5 days after rhodamine-labeled beads were injected into the accessory optic system.

ELECTROPHYSIOLOGY AND CELL TYPOLOGY: ENTERING THE MODERN ERA

Studies of the physiological characteristics of single ganglion cells were first carried out by Hartline (8). He found that some ganglion cells in the frog responded with increased activity (on cells) when a light was presented to a restricted area of the retina. He referred to this area as the receptive field of the ganglion cell. Other cells, the off cells, exhibited increased activity when light was turned off. Still other cells exhibited transient responses at both the onset and cessation of light stimuli. These were termed on-off cells.

Independent studies by Barlow (9) and Kuffler (10), both published in 1953, demonstrated that the receptive fields of RGCs were composed of both a central area and a surround area. Stimulation of the surround antagonized the center response. Furthermore, Barlow noted that on-off ganglion cells in frogs were exquisitely sensitive to moving stimuli. He suggested that these cells might be referred to as "fly detectors." Maturana et al. (11) later expanded on the idea that many cells were sensitive to well-defined stimuli and demonstrated that ganglion cells may respond maximally to any of a wide array of stimulus combinations. Small moving objects might elicit responses from one type of cell, whereas another type might respond to a dark curved edge moving across the receptive field. Other investigators extended such studies to the rabbit retina and found similar diversity in ganglion cell responses. Among rabbit ganglion cells were some that were sensitive to objects moving in a certain direction in the receptive field. Others exhibited orientation selectivity in that a bar of light moving across the receptive field might be effective if it was oriented horizontally but ineffective if it was oriented vertically.

The complexity of ganglion cell physiological characteristics was further demonstrated by Enroth-Cugell and Robson (12). They showed that cat on-center and off-center ganglion cells each exhibited two types of responses to sinusoidal stimuli. One type of cell, which they termed X cells, linearly summated the responses to illumination in different areas of the receptive field. The other type, Y cells, summated responses to such illumination nonlinearly (13). Other cells that appeared different from both X and Y cells were termed W cells (14). Further differentiation of cells was suggested on the bases of such criteria as sustained versus transient activity in response to particular stimuli (13) and brisk or sluggish responses to stimuli of increasing intensity (15). Cleland and Levick (15) also suggested that the brisk sustained cells were X cells and that the brisk transient cells corresponded to Y cells.

Other investigators attempted to correlate specific morphological classes of ganglion cells in the cat retina with cells classified previously by physiological criteria. Boycott and Wässle (16) described a class of cells with large somata and sparsely branched dendrites that they termed α cells. They demonstrated that these cells were Y cells. Other cells that they termed β cells were smaller in all respects than α cells at equivalent retinal locations and were suggested to be X cells. They also suggested that their γ cells corresponded to W cells. An important consequence of their work was the demonstration of a systematic gradation of the size of both α and β cells with increasing distance from the central area.

Thus, there are a number of possible ganglion cell classification schemes based on physiological or morphological properties. However, each of the schemes suffers from drawbacks in terms of both general applicability (e.g., many mammalian retinae do not have a cell comparable to Y cells of the cat) and acceptance. Therefore, there is a need for a more generally applicable scheme based on characteristics that can be studied in the ganglion cells of all animals. Dowling (17) suggested that a classification based on the ways in which receptive fields are formed may be the most appropriate.

GANGLION CELL TRANSMITTERS

Although RGCs are among the most intensively studied neurons of the nervous system, surprisingly little is known of the transmitter(s) employed by them at their central sites of termination. This is reflected in frequent references to their purportedly single common transmitter. However, the actual identity of the RGC transmitters are still the subject of speculation and study. There is immunohistochemical evidence of glutamate immunoreactivity in ganglion cells, but the widespread distribution of endogenous glutamate has prompted cautious interpretation of these results. Recently, Yu et al. (18) suggested that some ganglion cells in the rabbit may contain significant amounts of γ-aminobutyric acid (GABA) immunoreactivity. This latter suggestion also requires additional investigation before it is accepted. In principle, however, there is no *a priori* reason to insist that all ganglion cells release only amino acids.

There has been some progress in identifying a series of nonamino acid transmitter-related molecules in specific subsets of RGCs. Their actions at the terminals of RGC are still poorly understood, and although some of these substances are capable of altering the postsynaptic activity of target cells, they do not fulfill all the necessary criteria to be proven to act as neurotransmitters. The two major categories of substances found to be contained within specific subtypes of RGCs include (a) catecholamine-synthesizing enzymes, indicative of the presence of one of several possible catecholamines, and (b) several neuropeptides, including substance P, bombesin, cholecystokinin, enkephalin, neurotensin/LANT-6, and possibly neuropeptide Y.

Tyrosine hydroxylase (TH), the rate-limiting enzyme necessary for the synthesis of dopamine, norepinephrine, and epinephrine, has been localized in RGCs in the pigeon (19; Keyser et al., *in preparation*). TH-positive cells in the ganglion cell layer (Fig. 2) were identified as ganglion cells based on their content of retrogradely transported markers initially deposited in the accessory optic nucleus (nBOR of pigeon), optic tectum, and ventral nucleus of the lateral geniculate complex (Fig. 3). TH-positive RGCs appear to constitute less than 1% of all ganglion cells but are highly selective in their central distribution. Similar-appearing cells with clearly identifiable axons that could be followed to the optic nerve head have been observed in the ganglion cell layer of elasmobranchs (20) and several mammals, including ferrets (Keyser et al., *unpublished observations*). Other investigators have reported the presence of catecholamine-synthesizing enzymes in cells in the ganglion cell layer of rats, but the identity of these cells as ganglion cells has not been confirmed (21–23). The nature of the particular catecholamine produced by RGCs has not yet been identified. As in the case of the more extensively studied avian retina, the total number of TH-positive cells in the ganglion cell layer of rats appears to be small.

The neuropeptides constitute an extremely diverse group of biologically active molecules. Although their systemic effects on the physiology of animals has been extensively documented, their effects on neurons have proved difficult to characterize. Several substances, such as substance P, are often excitatory in nature. Others, such as enkephalin, have profound influence in alleviating pain, but their cellular mechanism of action is still unknown. In a series of studies on the frog retinotectal system, Kuljis and Karten (24,25) were able to demonstrate that RGCs of the frog contained a variety of neuropeptides, including substance P, cholecystokinin, enkephalin, and bombesin. Each of these substances was contained in different populations of RGCs. The axons of the different populations terminated in different layers of the contralateral optic tectum. Subsequently, Ehrlich et al. (26) demon-

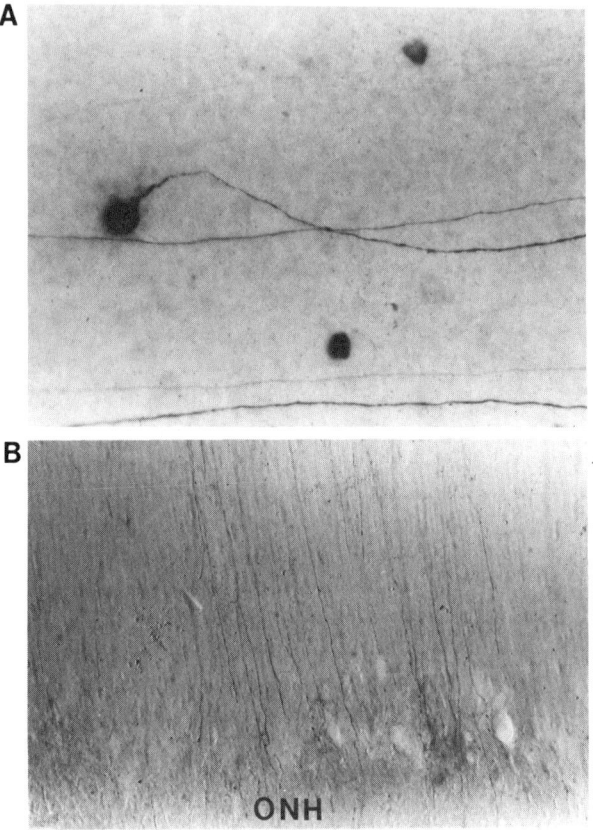

FIG. 2. A: A tyrosine hydroxylase immunoreactive cell in the ganglion cell layer of the pigeon retina. Both the cell body and its axon are visible. The axon could be traced toward the optic nerve head. **B:** A photomicrograph of the optic fiber layer near the optic nerve head in a pigeon retina. TH-positive axons can be seen to enter the optic nerve head.

strated the presence of a population of substance P immunoreactive ganglion cells in the chick retina (Fig. 4). Their dendrites were found to arborize in layer 5 of the IPL and terminate in a single layer of the optic tectum, layer 3 (Fig. 5). Brecha and co-workers (27) discovered a major population of substance P immunoreactive ganglion cells in the rabbit and demonstrated their pattern of termination in the lateral geniculate nucleus and the superior colliculus (Fig. 6). Eldred et al. (28) found significant amounts of LANT-6 immunoreactivity in ganglion cells of birds and reptiles. Karten and co-workers (*in preparation*) have evidence that selective subpopulations of CCK-containing ganglion cells in the chick project to a single subnucleus of the dorsal nucleus of the lateral geniculate complex.

One of the most striking features of these various studies using antibodies

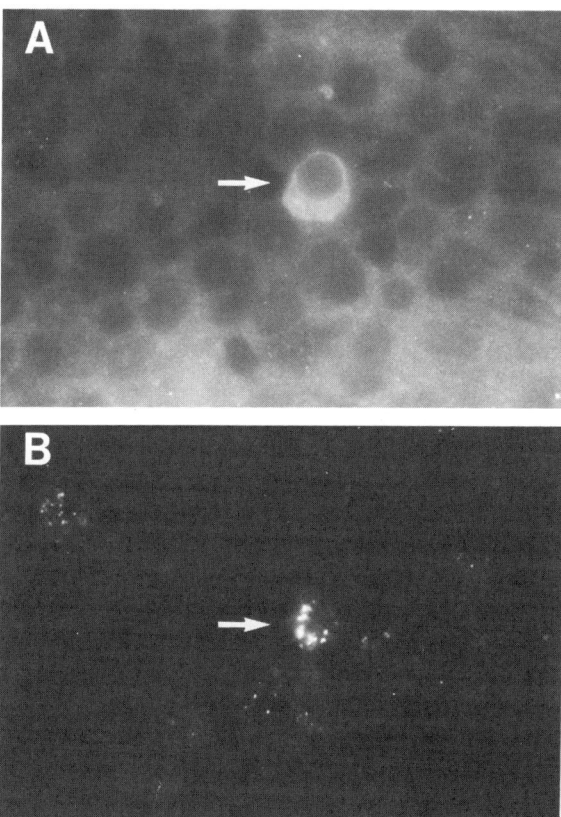

FIG. 3. Tyrosine hydroxylase immunoreactivity in a cell in the ganglion cell layer of the pigeon retina. The animal had received an injection of rhodamine-labeled beads in the contralateral tectum 5 days earlier. **A:** A TH-positive cell in the ganglion cell layer. **B:** The same cell exhibits rhodamine bead fluorescence.

directed against specific neuropeptides is the finding that specific populations of RGCs contain particular neuropeptides. Although we do not know the cellular effects of each of these neuropeptides, the fact that the terminals of biochemically distinct populations of ganglion cells are restricted to certain central retinal targets might indicate that each of these classes of ganglion cells has different effects on their targets. This attitude differs from our earlier notion that suggested that all RGCs released the same compounds at their terminals, and the information transferred at the synapse could be predicted on the basis of firing frequency of ganglion cells. In this earlier formulation, although ganglion cells might differ widely in their responses to various stimuli, they shared a common transmitter molecule. Our present findings impose a much more complex set of variables that must be understood in order to clarify the operations of the visual system.

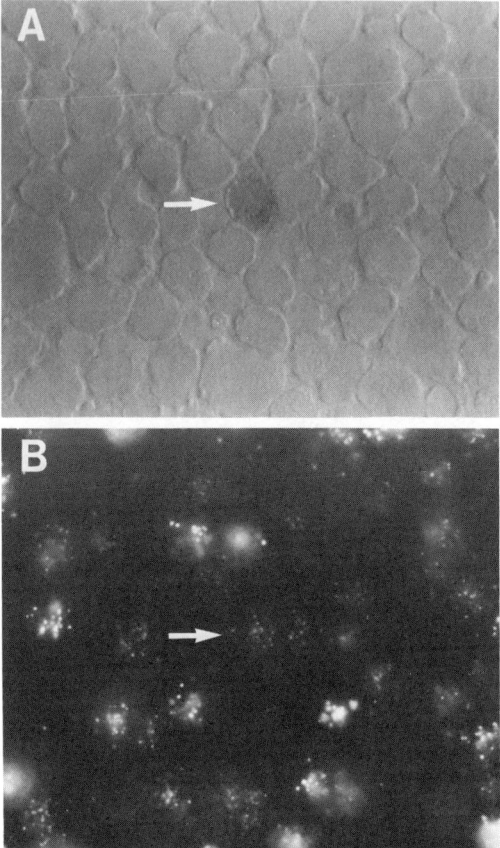

FIG. 4. Substance P immunoreactivity in the chick retina. The animal had received an injection of fluorescent label in the contralateral tectum 4 days earlier. **A:** A substance P-labeled ganglion cell in the ganglion cell layer. **B:** The same cell exhibits rhodamine bead fluorescence.

COMPONENTS OF THE IPL AND RECEPTOR SPECIFICITY IN GANGLION CELLS

Recent studies have finally begun to provide some indication of the diversity of potential transmitters/modulators synthesized and presumably released by RGCs at their central terminations. However, progress has been more modest on the far more difficult issue of the microcircuitry within the IPL, and the specific inputs to each of the different types of ganglion cells.

The major inputs to ganglion cells are provided by bipolar and amacrine cells. Although the bipolar cell transmitters have not been investigated thoroughly, they are thought to be predominantly glutamatergic (i.e., they release glutamate at their synaptic endings on ganglion and amacrine cells [29]). How-

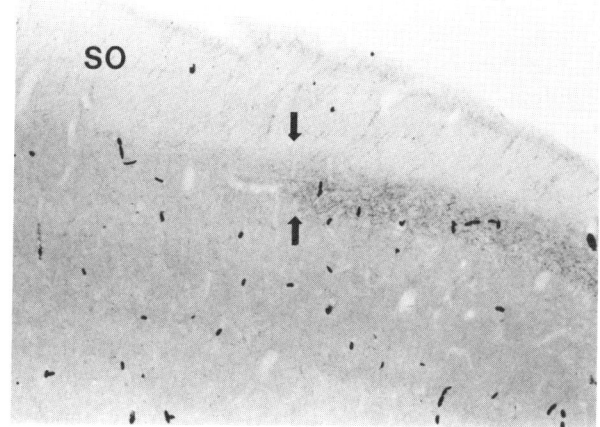

FIG. 5. Substance P immunoreactivity in the dorsal optic tectum of the chick 12 days after a lesion of the contralateral retina. The *arrows* mark the boundary between the affected and unaffected regions. SO, stratum opticum.

ever, the finding that a category of bipolar cells in birds exhibits serotonin-like immunoreactivity and accumulates indolealkyl amines suggests the possibility of additional bipolar cell transmitters, some of which may colocalize with glutamate immunoreactivity.

Relatively little is known about amacrine cells, but they have been found to be extremely diverse in morphology and transmitter/peptide content. Various types are cholinergic, GABAergic, dopaminergic, serotonergic, and adrenergic. Others contain any one of a dazzling diversity of peptides. These may

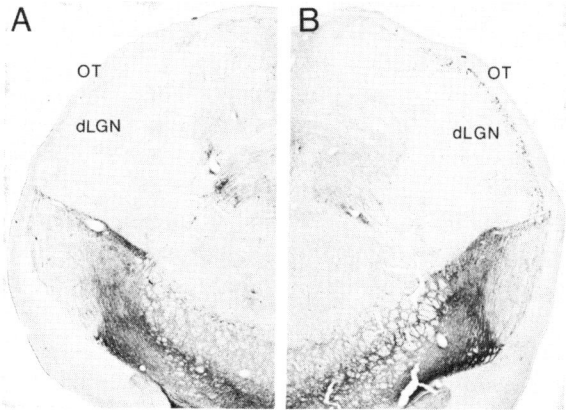

FIG. 6. Distribution of tachykinin-like immunoreactivity in the dorsal lateral geniculate nucleus (dLGN) of the rabbit. In normal animals, immunoreactivity is mainly confined to a thin plexus adjacent to the optic tract (OT) in the superficial portion of the dLGN as illustrated in **B**. This plexus is eliminated after optic nerve transection as illustrated in **A**. (From ref. 27.)

include substance P, enkephalin, neurotensin, somatostatin, vasoactive intestinal polypeptide, cholecystokinin, neuropeptide Y, glucagon, thyrotropin-releasing hormone, corticotrophin-releasing factor, and others. Several instances of individual cell types containing two or more of these peptides or combinations of a peptide and a nonpeptide transmitter have been described. Generally, however, each morphologically distinct subtype of amacrine cells with arborizations limited to sharply bounded laminae of the IPL exhibits a characteristic peptide content. The restricted distribution of these arbors necessarily limits their potential contacts to those ganglion cells that arborize in the same layers.

The present level of analysis of transmitter localization within the IPL mainly provides information regarding the laminar distribution of dendrites of cells that contain the various putative transmitters/modulators. The lack of information concerning the postsynaptic targets of biochemically distinct classes of amacrine and bipolar cells continues to pose one of the most intractable problems in the analysis of retinal organization. Although it is possible to serially reconstruct neurons contributing to the IPL, and thus identify their various afferent and efferent relationships, in practice this is an overwhelmingly burdensome task. It has been done in several instances by Sterling, and others, but remains a technologically demanding and time-consuming procedure.

However, a new approach to this problem has gradually emerged during the past decade as a result of studies of the distribution of specific receptor molecules for different transmitters. Previously, studies addressing this issue relied on the use of radiolabeled ligands that bound to receptor sites, or at least near such sites. For example, radio-iodinated α-bungarotoxin was used to attempt to identify the location of the presumed nicotinic acetylcholine receptors (30–32). Unfortunately, autoradiographic localization of radioligands in the retina often does not provide the spatial resolution necessary to permit detection of single cells or to allow study of arborization patterns in the IPL. An additional severe limitation was that many of the radioligands employed had only limited specificity for individual subtypes of receptors. Thus, it was particularly difficult to study the distribution of receptor subtypes, such as the various subtypes of GABA, dopamine, or muscarinic acetylcholine receptors.

The application of molecular biological methods to the field of receptors has provided several new tools for the localization of specific receptors and their subtypes. As a result of such efforts, antibodies are available that recognize specific receptors including the nicotinic acetylcholine receptors, GABA-A receptors, muscarinic receptors, and glycine receptors. These highly specific antibodies can be used to stain retinal sections and thus permit the identification of the cells expressing each of these receptors. In the most successful instances, these methods may even permit detailed three-dimensional histological reconstruction of labeled cells and their identification as members of particular types of RGCs.

Several laboratories have employed these methods with considerable success in the bird retina (33,34), cat retina (35), and primate retina (36). An example of the application of such methods is shown in Fig. 7, a section of cat retina stained for the presence of nicotinic acetylcholine receptors. The somata of the large (α) cell is intensely stained for the presence of this receptor. The immunoreactivity can be found not only in the cell body but in distal dendrites and in the axon. The presence of nicotinic acetylcholine receptors in α cells implies that they receive significant input from the cholinergic amacrine cells. The lack of staining in some classes of cells must be interpreted with great caution, for we cannot exclude the possibility that these cells synthesize an alternate form of the receptor not recognized by the antibody.

One potentially important group of receptors for which a probe of this type is needed is the glutamate receptors. The major transmitter of bipolar cells is believed to be glutamate (29). There are various estimates as to the frequency of bipolar to ganglion cell contacts in different species, although it has been reported to be as many as 40% of the inputs to ganglion cells in cats, and as few as 15% to 20% in birds and ground squirrels. If suggestions that bipolar cells are uniformly glutamatergic is essentially correct, then we would assume that significant numbers of ganglion cells express one of the major types of glutamate receptors. However, at the present time methods for demonstrating

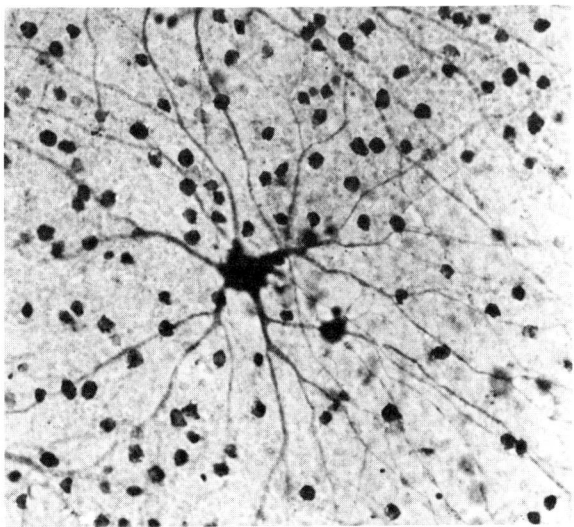

FIG. 7. An α cell in the retina of the cat. The cell displays nicotinic acetylcholine immunoreactivity.

glutamate receptor subtypes are limited to autoradiographic methods, with attendant drawbacks, particularly the lack of resolution. Thus, for now we have no evidence as to the numbers or types of ganglion cells that may express any one of the several types of glutamate receptors.

Unfortunately, we still do not have adequate methods for identifying the specific cells that express the various specific receptors for the individual neuropeptides.

RESPONSE TO AXOTOMY

Following damage to the axons of RGCs in warm-blooded vertebrates, ganglion cells generally fail to reestablish their central connections. In young animals there is often a rapid loss of ganglion cells, whereas in older mammals, there is a slower, but still irretrievable loss of ganglion cells. This failure to reestablish axonal connections with the brain has long puzzled students of the visual system, for it stands in sharp contrast to the seeming ease with which the optic fibers reconnect with the brain in amphibia and teleost fish. In frogs, the fibers not only reconnect, but the animal regains much of its original ability to track and capture small objects of prey. Thus, the assumption was that the axons of all ganglion cells regenerated. However, only recently has this regenerative ability been more carefully examined. Humphrey (37), for example, found that only approximately 50% of the fibers reestablish contact during the first year. The remaining ganglion cells apparently fail to establish central connections and presumably die.

There are several distinct types of ganglion cells in the frog retina (1), and if only 50% of all cells survive, does the loss of cells occur equally in each of the subtypes of ganglion cells? The studies of Kuljis and Karten (24) suggest that biochemically different subsets of ganglion cells differ in their potential for survival and reconnection with their appropriate central targets. Thus substance P-containing ganglion cells are more likely to survive and reestablish terminations in the appropriate tectal lamina than are bombesin-containing ganglion cells.

The realization that ganglion cells constitute a heterogeneous grouping not only in their three-dimensional morphology and responses to visual stimuli, but also in their biochemical content and differential response to injury, emphasizes the importance of knowing more about the biochemistry and other characteristics of each subgroup. It also implies that different pharmacological strategies may be required for encouraging the survival and regeneration of specific subgroups of ganglion cells. A major limitation in further characterizing the response of ganglion cells to injury is consequent to our lack of adequate simple methods to discriminate the various subgroups from each other.

RESPONSE TO GROWTH FACTORS

Many authors have hypothesized that the survival of ganglion cells depends on the availability of various trophic and growth factors retrogradely transported from the brain. Destruction of ganglion cell axons presumably results in the loss of the availability of these vital substances. Although the identity of these substances is still largely unknown, some studies demonstrate that neuronotrophic factors such as nerve growth factor (NGF) and fibroblast growth factor (FGF) may play a role. Sievers et al. (38), for example, showed that intraocular administration of FGF enhances the survival of RGCs. We do not know precisely which ganglion cells because the identity of the surviving populations was not reported. A more recent study (39) has demonstrated a significant enhancement of survival of substance P-containing ganglion cells in the chick as a result of the intraocular administration of NGF. Unlike our earlier studies in the frog, however, these were only short-term experiments, and there was no evidence of reestablishment of central connections. Further studies with both NGF and FGF and other growth factors are desirable and may eventually provide prospects of intraocular pharmacotherapy for the treatment of optic nerve damage.

GENERAL OBSERVATIONS

In this brief review we have attempted to emphasize our changing concepts of RGCs. Although there is still no unified view regarding their nature, recent research has indicated that ganglion cells are extremely heterogeneous in a variety of characteristics. We must emphasize that ganglion cells constitute a single class only in the sense that they all possess an axonal process directed into the optic nerve.

The traditional classification of ganglion cells was based exclusively on limited morphological and physiological distinctions. Although these features are still considered of major importance, the recent discovery that different types of ganglion cells vary in the transmitters used, the receptors elaborated, and responses to injury will profoundly modify our concepts of the nature of information transfer from ganglion cells to central brain structures.

The difficulties in characterizing RGCs apply equally to many of the other neuronal cell types in the retina. In spite of the confusing diversity of neurotransmitters, modulators, and hormones, we still cannot identify the particular transmitters employed by several major retinal cell types.

Several of the studies described here suggest that different categories of RGCs are more likely to survive damage to their axons. Further characterization of such determinants may prove of value in the development of pharmacotherapies for salvaging vision following optic nerve damage, as in trauma, glaucoma, multiple sclerosis, and diabetic retinopathy.

ACKNOWLEDGMENTS

We express our gratitude for the continuing support in this work provided by the National Institutes of Health: grants NEI-EY06890 and NINDS NS24560 to H.J.K.; NEI-EY07845 to K.T.K.; NEI-EY04067 to N.C.B. and by the Office of Naval Research: N00014-88-K-0504 to H.J.K. N.C.B. also acknowledges support from Veterans Administration Medical Research Funds.

REFERENCES

1. Ramón y Cajal S. *The structure of the retina*, Thorpe SA, Glickstein M., trans. Springfield, IL: Charles C. Thomas, 1972.
2. Famiglietti EV, Kolb H. Structural bases for the on and off center responses in retinal ganglion cells. *Science* 1976;194:193–195.
3. Famiglietti EV, Kaneko A, Tachibana M. Neuronal architecture of on and off pathways to ganglion cells of the carp retina. *Science* 1977;198:1267–1269.
4. Nelson RE, Famiglietti EV, Kolb H. Intracellular staining reveals different levels of stratification for on- and off-center ganglion cells in the cat retina. *J Neurophysiol* 1978;41:472–483.
5. Lettvin JY, Maturana HR, Pitts WH, McCulloch WS. Two remarks on the visual system of the frog. In: Rosenblith WA, ed. *Sensory communication*. Cambridge, MA: MIT Press, 1961;757–781.
6. Karten HJ, Fite KV, Brecha N. Specific projections of displaced retinal ganglion cells upon the accessory optic system in the pigeon (*Columba livia*). *Proc Natl Acad Sci USA* 1977;74:1753–1756.
7. Dogiel AS. Uber das Verhalten der nervosen Elemente in der Retina der Ganoiden, Reptilien, Vogel und Saugetiere. *Anat Anz* 1888;3:133–143.
8. Hartline HK. The response of single optic nerve fibers of the vertebrate eye to illumination of the retina. *Am J Physiol* 1938;121:400–415.
9. Barlow H. Summation and inhibition in the frog's retina. *J Physiol* 1953;119:69–88.
10. Kuffler SW. Discharge patterns and functional organization of mammalian retina. *J Neurophysiol* 1953;16:37–68.
11. Maturana HR, Lettvin JY, McCulloch WS, Pitts WH. Anatomy and physiology of vision in the frog (*Rana pipiens*). *J Gen Physiol* 1960;43:129–175.
12. Enroth-Cugell C. Robson JG. The contrast sensitivity of retinal ganglion cells of the cat. *J Physiol* 1966;187:517–552.
13. Cleland BG, Dubin MW, Levick WR. Sustained and transient neurons in the cat's retina and lateral geniculate nucleus. *J Physiol* 1971;217:473–496.
14. Stone J, Fukuda Y. Properties of cat retinal ganglion cells: a comparison of W-cells with X- and Y-cells. *J Neurophysiol* 1974;37:722–748.
15. Cleland BG, Levick WR. Brisk and sluggish concentrically organized ganglion cells in the cat's retina. *J Physiol* 1974;240:421–456.
16. Boycott BB, Wässle H. The morphological types of ganglion cells of the domestic cat's retina. *J Physiol* 1974;240:397–419.
17. Dowling JE. *The retina: an approachable part of the brain*. Cambridge, MA: Harvard University Press, 1987.
18. Yu BC, Watt CB, Lam DM, Fry KR. GABAergic ganglion cells in the rabbit retina. *Brain Res* 1988;439:376–382.
19. Britto LRG, Keyser KT, Hamassaki DE, Karten HJ. Catecholaminergic subpopulation of retinal displaced ganglion cells projects to the accessory optic nucleus in the pigeon (*Columba livia*). *J Comp Neurol* 1988;269:109–117.
20. Brunken WJ, Witkovsky P, Karten HJ. Retinal neurochemistry of three elasmobranch species: an immunohistochemical approach. *J Comp Neurol* 1986;243:1–12.
21. Hadjiconstantinou M, Mariani AP, Panula P, Joh TH, Neff NH. Immunohistochemical evidence for epinephrine-containing retinal amacrine cells. *Neuroscience* 1984;13:547–551.

22. Foster GA, Hökfelt T, Coyle JT, Goldstein M. Immunohistochemical evidence for phenylethanolamine-N-methyltransferase-positive/tyrosine hydroxylase-negative neurones in the retina and the posterior hypothalamus of the rat. *Brain Res* 1985;330:183-188.
23. Park DH, Teitelman G, Evinger MJ, et al. Phenylethanolamine N-methyltransferase-containing neurons in the rat retina: immunohistochemistry, immunochemistry and molecular biology. *J Neurosci* 1986;6:1108-1113.
24. Kuljis RO, Karten HJ. Regeneration of peptide-containing retinofugal axons into the optic tectum with reappearance of a substance P-containing lamina. *J Comp Neurol* 1985;240:1-15.
25. Kuljis RO, Krause JE, Karten HJ. Peptide-like immunoreactivity in anuran optic nerve fibers. *J Comp Neurol* 1984;226:222-237.
26. Ehrlich D, Keyser K, Karten HJ. Distribution of substance P-like immunoreactive retinal ganglion cells and their pattern of termination in the optic tectum of the chick (*Gallus gallus*). *J Comp Neurol* 1987;266:220-233.
27. Brecha N, Johnson D, Bolz J, Sharma S, Parnavelas JG, Lieberman AR. Substance P immunoreactive retinal ganglion cells and their central axon terminals in the rabbit. *Nature* 1987;327:155-158.
28. Eldred WD, Isayama T, Reiner A, Carraway R. Ganglion cells in the turtle retina contain the neuropeptide LANT-6. *J Neurosci* 1988;8:119-132.
29. Massey SC, Redburn D. Transmitter circuits in the vertebrate retina. *Prog Neurobiol* 1987;28:55-96.
30. Yazulla S, Schmidt J. Radioautographic localization of (^{125}I)-α-bungarotoxin binding sites in the retinas of goldfish and turtle. *Vision Res* 1976; 16:878-880.
31. Yazulla S, Schmidt J. Two types of receptors for bungarotoxin in the synaptic layers of the pigeon retina. *Brain Res* 1977;138:45-57.
32. Vogel Z, Maloney GJ, Ling A, Daniels MP. Identification of synaptic acetylcholine receptor sites in retina with peroxidase-labeled α-bungarotoxin. *Proc Natl Acad Sci USA* 1977;74:3268-3272.
33. Yazulla S, Studholme KM, Vitorica J, deBlas AL. Immunocytochemical localization of $GABA_A$ receptors in goldfish and chicken retinas. *J Comp Neurol* 1989;280:15-26.
34. Keyser KT, Hughes TE, Whiting PJ, Lindstrom JM, Karten HJ. Cholinoceptive neurons in the retina of the chick: an immunohistochemical study of the nicotinic acetylcholine receptors. *Visual Neuroscience* 1988;1:349-366.
35. Jäger J, Wässle H. Localization of glycine uptake and receptors in the carp retina. *Neurosci Lett* 1987;75:147-151.
36. Hughes TE, Carey RG, Victoria J, deBlas AL, Karten HJ. Immunohistochemical localization of $GABA_A$ receptors in the retina of the new world primate *Saimini sciureus*. *Visual Neuroscience* (*in press*).
37. Humphrey MF. Effect of different optic nerve lesions on retinal ganglion cell death in the frog *Rana pipiens*. *J Comp Neurol* 1987;266:209-219.
38. Sievers J, Hausmann B, Unsicker K, Berry M. Fibroblastic growth factors promote the survival of adult rat retinal ganglion cells after transection of the optic nerve. *Neurosci Lett* 1987;76:157-162.
39. Ehrlich D, Keyser K, Manthorpe M, Varon S, Karten HJ. Differential effects of axotomy on substance P-containing and nicotinic acetylcholine receptor-containing retinal ganglion cells: Time course of degeneration and effects of nerve growth factor. *Neuroscience* (*in press*).

Vision and the Brain,
edited by B. Cohen and I. Bodis-Wollner.
Raven Press, Ltd., New York © 1990.

The On and Off Channels of the Visual System

Peter H. Schiller

Department of Brain and Cognitive Sciences, Massachusetts Institute of Technology, Cambridge, Massachusetts 02139

In the late 1940s Stephen Kuffler (1) began a series of experiments in which he recorded from the retina of the optically intact cat eye. This work revealed two kinds of retinal ganglion cells: on-center cells, which were found to increase their discharge rate when light incremental stimuli were presented in their receptive field centers (bright stimuli), and off-center cells, which were found to increase their activity by light decremental stimuli (dark stimuli). Kuffler also found that the circular center of the receptive field of ganglion cells was surrounded by an inhibitory region that gave responses of the opposite polarity. As a result of this arrangement, ganglion cells were found to discharge more vigorously to small spots of light confined to the center of the receptive field than to large spots that stimulated both the center and the surround.

In the 1960s, as the result of the development of new techniques, it became possible to record intracellularly from the various cell types of the retina and to identify these cells anatomically by injecting them with dyes after the recording. This research established that receptors all hyperpolarize to light and that the on and off systems appear for the first time at the level of the bipolar cell (2). Sign-conserving synapses made on these cells by the receptor cells formed off bipolars, whereas sign inverting synapses made by the receptors formed on bipolar cells. Subsequent work has also suggested that photoreceptors all use glutamate as their neurotransmitter. It appears, therefore, that from the single-ended system of the receptors, nature has created a double-ended system at the bipolar cell level. It is likely that significant gains in visual information processing are reaped from this arrangement, although at this stage one can only conjecture what these gains might be. Throughout the years, several hypotheses have been advanced to attempt to explain why the on and off systems have evolved. Recently, as a result of an important discovery, it became possible to test some of these hypotheses. Slaughter and Miller (3) found that when they applied the glutamate neurotransmitter analogue 2-amino-4-phosphonobutyrate (APB) to the mudpuppy retina, the on bipolars, on amacrines, and on ganglion cells became unresponsive to light, whereas the off cells of the retina continued their light-related responses.

Subsequent to this discovery, a number of laboratories applied APB to the mammalian retina. Our studies have concentrated on the monkey. We began this work by developing a way of infusing APB into the retina so that the activity of single cells could be studied in various parts of the visual system before, during, and after APB application. Our physiological studies showed the following (4): (a) APB blocks the response of on-center ganglion cells and on-center lateral geniculate (LGN) cells while leaving the responses of off-center cells largely unaffected. An example of this, shown in Fig. 1, was obtained from multiple-unit recordings in magnocellular LGN. Following APB administration (center panel) the on response is eliminated. (b) The center-surround antagonism of off-center retinal ganglion cells and of off-center LGN cells is not significantly altered by APB administration. Figure 2 provides an example of this, showing the effect of center-surround stimulation for an on and off cell before and after the administration of APB. These findings suggest that the center-surround antagonism of retinal ganglion cells and LGN cells is not a product of the interaction between these two systems. The inhibitory surround mechanism is the product of the lateral systems of the retina comprised of the horizontal and amacrine cells. Our results suggest that the on and off systems in the geniculostriate pathway remain segregated up to cortex, a finding also supported by several other kinds of data. (c) In the visual cortex APB administration blocks the light edge responses of single cells but has little effect on the dark edge response (Fig. 3). This complex cell, which normally responds to both the light and dark edges of a moving bar (inset) discharges only to the dark edge following APB infusion. Other receptive field attributes, such as orientation and direction specificities, are unaffected by the administration of APB to the retina. These findings suggest that in the cortex the on and off systems converge on single cells but that this convergence is not responsible for the basic receptive field attributes of cortical cells, which are most likely the product of intracortical circuitry. Taken together, these findings suggest that the on and off systems did not evolve for the purposes of giving rise to the specific receptive field attributes of single cells in the visual system.

To gain further insight about the functions of the on and off system we next turned to psychophysical studies in which we examined the visual capacities of animals before, during, and after the on channel was blocked with APB. To accomplish this we briefly anesthetized the animals and injected concentrated APB into the vitreous humor. We trained animals in a variety of detection and discrimination tasks in which the task was to saccade to the correct target presented singly or in concert with other stimuli. Most commonly we used a color monitor, and eye movements were recorded with the scleral search coil method. This approach enabled us to obtain the percentage of both correct responses and response latencies. We examined a number of visual capacities, which included the detection of light incremental and decremental stimuli, the detection of movement, flicker, stereopsis, and the discrimination of color and pattern stimuli. We also assessed color and luminance contrast sensitivity

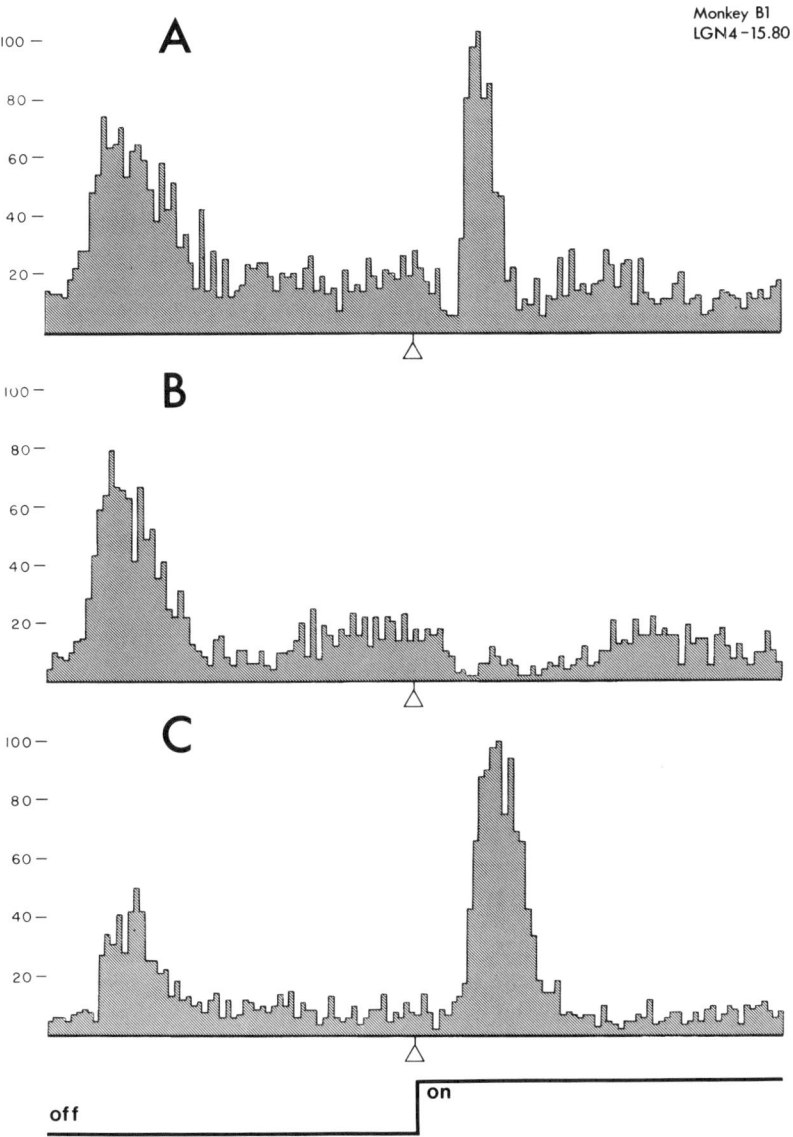

FIG. 1. Multiple-unit recordings from magnocellular LGN. Shown are stimulus histograms obtained before **(A)**, during **(B)**, and after **(C)** the effective administration of APB to the retina. The receptive field centers are stimulated with a small spot of light. The data are based on 30 trials.

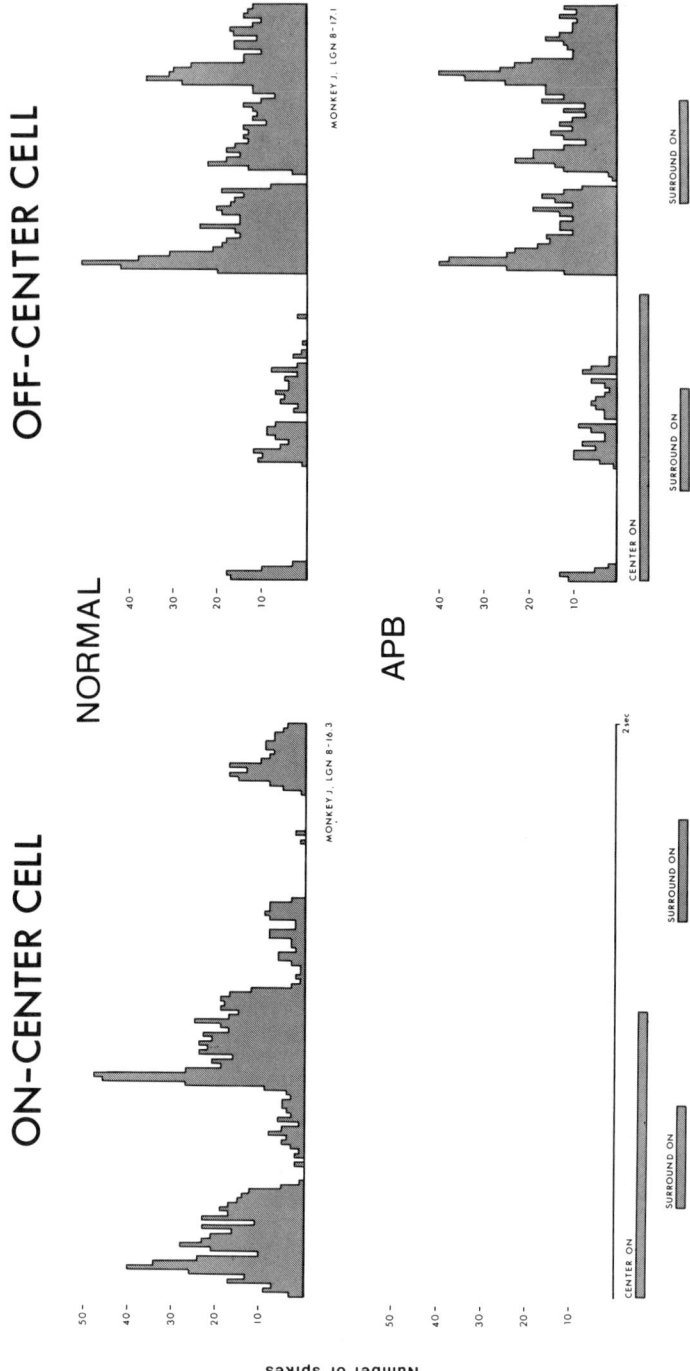

FIG. 2. The effect of retinal APB infusion on the center-surround responses of an on- and off-center red/green LGN cell. Following stimulation of the center of the receptive field with a small red spot, the surround is briefly stimulated with a large green spot. Surround stimulation is repeated during the off cycle. APB blocks all the responses of the on-center cell but does not dramatically alter the center-surround antagonism of the off-center cell suggesting the on and off systems do not interact significantly at the level of the LGN for the creation of the center-surround mechanism.

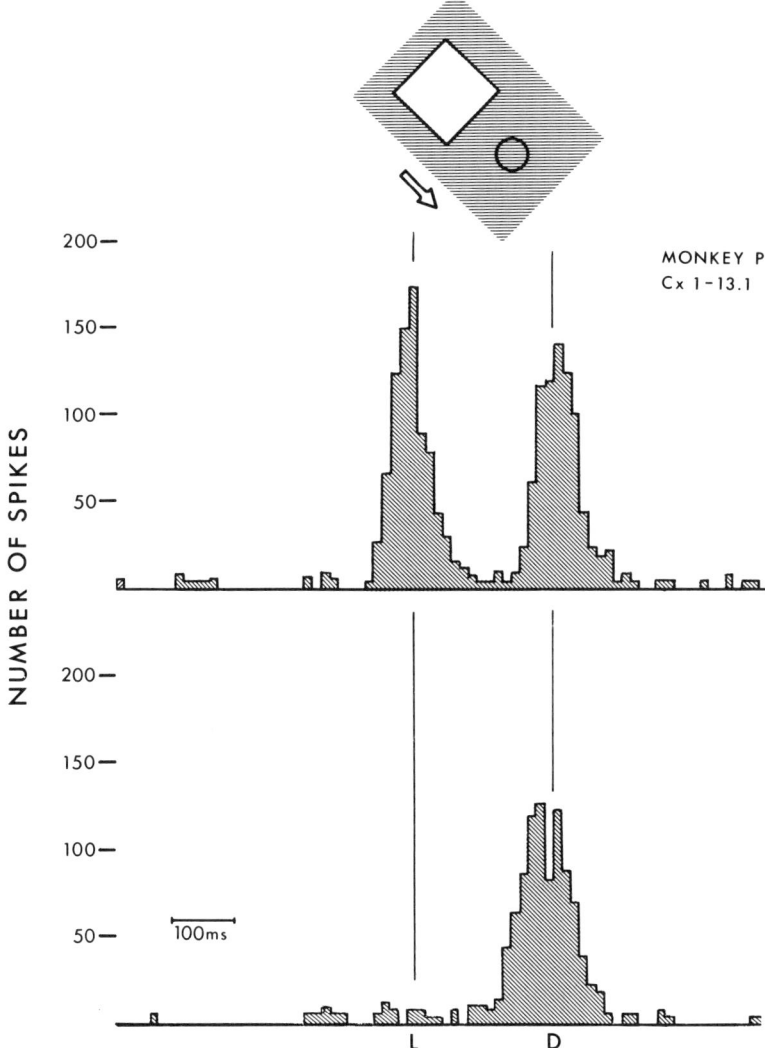

FIG. 3. The responses of a complex cell in the striate cortex to a light bar moving across the receptive field as shown on top. Under normal conditions, the cell discharges when the light and dark edges traverse the receptive field. Following retinal APB infusion, the light edge response disappears and the dark edge response is maintained, suggesting that the on and off channels converge on single cells in the cortex.

using a detection paradigm in which catch trials were used to minimize guessing. We studied visual capacities under both scotopic and photopic conditions. Our results can be summarized as follows (5): (a) There is a dramatic loss in the ability to detect light incremental but not light decremental stimuli. This is shown in Fig. 4; percentage of correct performance and the latency of the

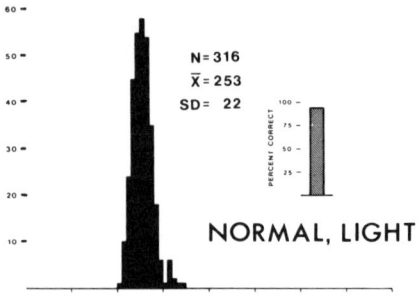
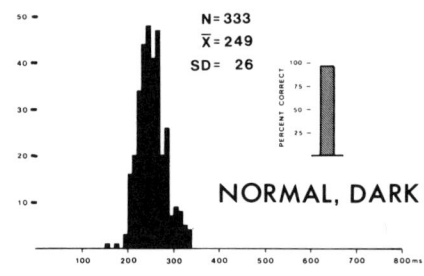
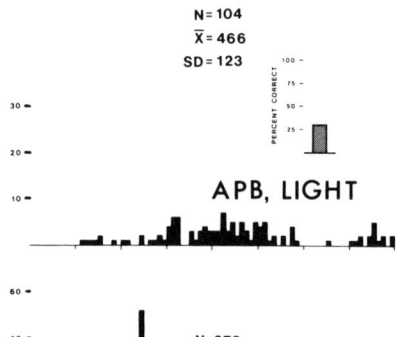
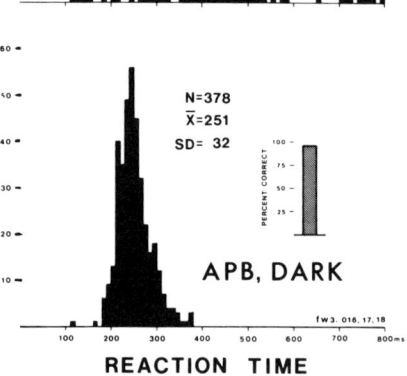

FIG. 4. The distribution of saccadic latencies and percentage of correct responses to light incremental (light) and light decremental (dark) stimuli obtained before and after APB injection into the vitreous humor of a rhesus monkey. Following on-channel blockage, the animal's ability to perceive and react to light stimuli is severely compromised. Insets show percentage of correct responses.

response is dramatically compromised for light incremental but not light decremental stimuli following the injection of APB into the vitreous. (b) There is a loss in luminance and color contrast sensitivity. (c) In agreement with recent data according to which the all rod bipolars depolarize to light (6), we found that in the dark-adapted animal perception is severely impaired for all stimuli (7). (d) There is little loss in the perception of movement, pattern, flicker, and stereopsis, but reaction times are increased by 30 to 60 msec.

The results of our psychophysical studies suggest two major reasons for the emergence of the on and off channels in vision: (a) to make possible the transmission of all cone-mediated information to the central nervous system with excitatory processes, thereby assuring rapid information transfer for stimuli seen both by virtue of light increment and light decrement and (b) to enhance contrast sensitivity.

REFERENCES

1. Kuffler SW. Discharge patterns and functional organization of mammalian retina. *J Neurophysiol* 1953;16:37–68.
2. Werblin FS, Dowling JE. Organization of the retina of the mudpuppy, *Nectorus maculosus*. II. Intracellular recording. *J Neurophysiol* 1969;32:339–355.
3. Slaughter MM, Miller RF. 2-amino-4-phosphonobutyric acid: a new pharmacological tool for retina research. *Science* 1981;211:182–184.
4. Schiller PH. Central connections of the retinal on and off pathways. *Nature* 1982;297:580–583.
5. Schiller PH, Sandell JH, Maunsell JHR. Functions of the on and off channels of the visual system. *Nature* 1986;322:824–825.
6. Mueller F, Waessle H, Voigt T. Pharmacological manipulation of the rod pathway in the cat retina. *J Neurophysiol* (*in press*).
7. Dolan RP, Schiller PH. Are there on and off bipolars in the primate retina? *Soc Neurosci Abstr* 1988;14:396.11.

Vision and the Brain,
edited by B. Cohen and I. Bodis-Wollner.
Raven Press, Ltd., New York © 1990.

Chemically Specified Systems in the Dorsal Lateral Geniculate Nucleus of Mammals

*[*][†]Pedro Pasik, [‡]Ricardo Molinar-Rode, and *Tauba Pasik

*Departments of *Neurology and †Anatomy, and the ‡Neurobiology Graduate Program, Mount Sinai School of Medicine, New York, New York 10029*

The lateral geniculate nucleus pars dorsalis (LGNd) has for many years been considered a rather enigmatic structure. Although it became known that it received most if not all the optic axons (1), it appeared that the physiologic characteristics of the LGNd neurons that project to the visual cortex (P-cells) did not differ to any great degree from those of the retinal ganglion cells. At present, however, a considerable amount of evidence has accumulated that points to the occurrence of many transformations of the visual input in the LGNd, stemming from the observation of an increase in surround inhibition in the receptive fields of geniculate cells as compared with ganglion cells (2). Important modulatory influences are exerted on the transmission properties of the LGNd, thus regulating the differential transfer of information according to the behavioral state. Indeed, there is a variety of other input sources to the LGNd, the terminal boutons of which are known to surpass by far the number of retinal endings (3). In addition, the local inhibitory interneurons (I-cells) are apparently critical for most of the functions that are being discovered at the geniculate level.

A promising line of investigation to probe the functional significance of the LGNd is to unravel the various chemically specified systems operating within the structure and their possible interactions. The following survey gives an account of the present state of knowledge regarding the various components of the LGNd circuitry. In assigning a neurotransmitter role to a substance, we have followed classically established criteria (4). Although one or another standard may be lacking in particular cases, the remaining features are compelling enough to warrant inclusion.

LGNd INPUTS

Retinal Source

The identification of the neurotransmitter(s) released by the terminals of the optic fibers was one of the oldest but least successful endeavors in neurochemistry. A first strategy involved measuring the contents of neuroactive substances in the LGNd and comparing them with those in the optic nerves. In this way, the initial possibility that acetylcholine (ACh), traditionally considered a prototype of an excitatory substance, might be the sought-after compound met with immediate objections. Thus, although the LGNd contains appreciable amounts of this substance (22 nmol/g in rat, recalculated from [5], representing 22% of the highest value found in the caudate nucleus), the optic nerve of several species is very low in ACh (6–8) as well as in its synthesizing enzyme (9,10). In fact, ACh increased in the LGNd after acute eye enucleation in the cat and rat (11,12), and its observed decrease 1 month after this procedure in the rabbit was interpreted as being due to transneuronal changes following deafferentation (13). Furthermore, choline acetyl transferase (ChAT) activity remained unchanged in the rat LGNd 1 to 6 weeks after eye enucleation (12,14). Although ACh has an excitatory effect on the cat LGNd neurons (15,16) and ACh antagonists clearly block this action, they fail to interfere with the response to visual as well as optic nerve or tract stimulation, or to the application of excitatory amino acids (15–18). Finally, no retinal terminals are labeled immunocytochemically by a ChAT antibody in the cat LGNd (19,20), and the few choline-accumulating neurons in the rabbit retinal ganglion cell layer are in fact displaced amacrine cells (21). It therefore seems clear that the source of LGNd ACh must be other than the retina.

Studies on the monoamines have led to a similar conclusion. Serotonin (5-HT) and norepinephrine (NE) are both present in the LGNd. Although the possibility that the retinogeniculate transmitter could be related to 5-HT was entertained (22), it was soon discarded because only traces were found in the optic nerve (8,23,24), and the levels in the LGNd remained unchanged after bilateral eye enucleation in the cat (11). Moreover, no serotoninergic retinal ganglion cells were ever detected (25). The amount of norepinephrine is also very low in the optic nerve (26). Finally, dopamine (DA) is barely measurable in the LGNd (27,28), and the ratio NE:DA is compatible with the presence of DA as a precursor of NE (29). Here again, evidence points to a nonretinal origin for the monoamine content of the LGNd.

The implication that the excitatory amino acids, glutamate (GLU) and aspartate (ASP), might be important in retinogeniculate transmission met with variable acceptance. The significance of their presence in central nervous system structures was diminished by the finding that the transmitter pool of these substances is considerably lower than the total amount of free amino acids (30), the remainder being a part of the metabolic pool for protein synthesis and breakdown. The amount of GLU is relatively low in the optic nerve of the cat (31) and the optic tract of the monkey (Molinar and Pasik, *unpublished data*). In the latter study, the LGNd had a higher content than the tract, and the amount was similar to that found in the LGNd of the rabbit (32,33) but lower than that in the rat (34). The effects of visual deafferentation on the LGNd varied. Unilateral eye enucleation in the rabbit (1–2 months survival) resulted in some decrease in the GLU and ASP content of the contralateral geniculate, but the difference with the ipsilateral counterpart was not significant (32). In the monkey, however, the section of one optic tract (1 week survival) yielded a significant decrease in GLU and ASP in the portion of the optic tract distal to the section and of GLU in the ipsilateral LGNd (35; *unpublished observations*). When determinations were made separately in magnocellular and parvocellular laminae, the significance level was maintained only in the latter (Fig. 1). The discrepancy between the reports in rabbits and monkeys may be more apparent than real. It is possible that the contribution of approximately 10% of noncrossing optic fibers in the rabbit may diminish the difference between the contralateral and ipsilateral geniculates, since their preservation in the contralateral side would tend to inflate the values, whereas their degeneration in the ipsilateral side would result in a lower level than that actually measured. In any event, it should be noted that the significant decreases found in the monkey are small (approximately 15%) and could still be due to secondary metabolic changes in other LGNd components caused by the optic deafferentation. In support of this interpretation is the finding of no change in the high affinity uptake for GLU in the rat geniculate 1 week after enucleation (34), which indicates a good preservation of glutamergic axon terminals in the

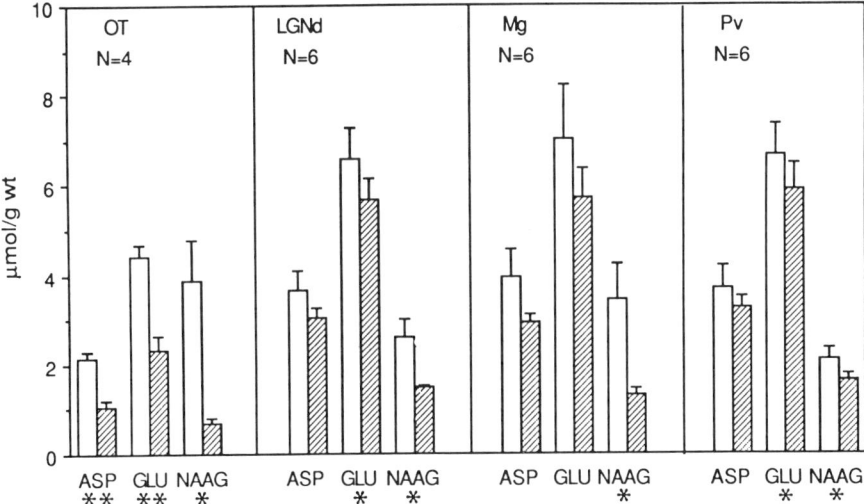

FIG. 1. HPLC measurements of micropunches from the monkey LGNd. Levels of aspartate (Asp), glutamate (Glu) and N-acetyl-aspartylglutamate (NAAG) in left- (*open bars*) and right- (*hatched bars*) sided structures 1 week after section of the right optic tract at its origin in the optic chiasm. Bars and segments represent means and standard errors, respectively. OT, optic tract distal to the section; LGN, lateral geniculate nucleus pars dorsalis; Mg, magnocellular laminae; Pv, parvocellular laminae. Significant differences between the means of normal left side and visually deafferented right side indicated by **, $p < 0.01$ and *, $p < 0.05$.

LGNd after section of the optic fibers. It is of interest that local electric stimulation of the LGNd in slices of rat brain produces a considerable increase in the release of GLU and ASP measured with an *in situ* dialysis probe (36). This result does not necessarily implicate the retinogeniculate terminals in such a release, since other elements in the geniculate neuropil could have been activated (see section on cortical source, p. 49).

The results of physiologic studies are also somewhat inconclusive. The excitatory properties of GLU and ASP on LGNd neurons have long been known (22), and the characteristics of their action, i.e., the very low threshold, quick response, and the almost immediate cessation of the effect, make them ideally suited as neurotransmitters. However, various tryptamines in concentrations that blocked LGNd transmissions were found to have little influence on the excitatory effect of GLU/ASP, thus making it unlikely that these substances are retinogeniculate transmitters (22). Yet, the same authors considered this possibility in the case in which 5-HT acted by suppressing the release of the transmitter. Favoring this viewpoint is a preliminary report in the cat showing a gradient of sensitivity of LGNd neurons to GLU and ASP, those receiving input from the central retina being more sensitive to the former, and those from the peripheral retina more sensitive to the latter compound (37).

Pharmacologic experiments have contributed significantly to this issue, but again the results have not been in strict agreement. Thus, in one study 1-hydroxy-3-amino-2-pyrrolidone (HA-966), a moderate antagonist at the *N*-methyl-D-aspartate- (NMDA) type receptor, and glutamate diethyl ester (GDEE), a selective antagonist at the quisqualate-type receptor, failed to depress the visually evoked firing of LGNd neurons in the cat (38). This led to the conclusion that GLU and ASP were not likely to be the transmitter released from optic nerve terminals. Although the lack of effect of GDEE was confirmed more recently (18), it was also reported that visual responses, as well as those elicited by NMDA and GLU, were blocked by HA-966 and α-aminoadipate, another moderate antagonist at NMDA-type receptors. These findings revived the idea that GLU, ASP, or a similar substance might be the retinogeniculate transmitter. In the latter study, the effects were the same on the responses of X and Y geniculate cells, both of the on and off types. A recent investigation, using rat brain slices, documented the effects of various antagonists on the excitatory postsynaptic potential (EPSP) elicited by electric stimulation of the optic tract (39). It was found that γ-D-glutamylglycine (DGG), an antagonist of responses to NMDA-receptor agonists and of kainate, reversibly inhibited the EPSP and the depolarization evoked by GLU and quisqualate. Contrariwise, D-2-amino-5-phosphonovalerate (APV), the most potent antagonist of NMDA, and 2-amino-4-phosphonobutyrate (APB), an antagonist apparently not acting on the NMDA-, quisqualate-, or kainate-type receptors, were inactive both in the presence or absence of Mg^{2+}. This lack of action was taken as indicating that the EPSP was not mediated by an

NMDA-type receptor but by a quisqualate/kainate type. These findings together with the similarity between the reversal potential of the EPSP and that produced by GLU gave "strong support in favor of a glutamate-like substance as the transmitter of the optic nerve in the rat." Interestingly, in rat LGNd slices, P-cells exhibited rhythmic depolarizations when in a Mg^{2+}-free medium. The addition of Mg^{2+} or APV, both blockers of NMDA receptors, abolished the depolarizations, which suggested the presence of these types of receptors in P-cells (40).

The presence and types of GLU receptors, as well as the action of antagonists and/or agonists in the LGNd also are controversial or at least different in the monkey and rat. In the monkey, no "appreciable concentrations" of receptors were demonstrated using tritiated L-GLU and α-amino-3-hydroxy-5-methyl-4-isoxazolepropionic acid (AMPA) (41). In the rat, however, AMPA, an agonist of the quisqualate-type receptor (for references on agonists and antagonists, see [42]), detected a Cl^-- and Na^+-independent site, although at levels only 15% of the maximum present in the CA1 region of the hippocampus (43). In a further study, Na^+-independent GLU binding sites were shown in amounts of 130 fmole/mg protein, representing 30% of the highest concentration found in the frontal cortex (44). A similar proportion of NMDA-sensitive GLU binding sites was observed in the LGNd at levels of 455 fmole/mg protein, equivalent to 30% of the maximum found in the CA1 hippocampal region (45). Finally, GLU binding was reported to be three to six times higher in the rat LGNd than in the visual cortex or the superior colliculus (46).

Immunocytochemistry has not contributed so far to the elucidation of the problem. In the only available study in the mouse and rat, GLU immunoreactivity was very weak in the LGNd where it was examined only at the light microscopy level (47). In any event, the antibody used was not considered to be a specific marker of glutamergic elements.

It is evident from this survey that the retinogeniculate transmitter is not known. However, there are indications that a substance related to excitatory amino acids may be the long sought-after compound. In recent years, attention has been focused on acetylated amino acids and acidic dipeptides as possible neurotransmitters (for review see [48]). In particular, N-acetyl-aspartyl-glutamate (NAAG) was found to have an uneven distribution in the central nervous system, decreasing from caudal to rostral levels. The concentration in rodent, horse, and monkey brains (0.4–0.7 μmol/g wet weight) is much lower than that of GLU and ASP (49–52). NAAG shows a high affinity for the Cl^--dependent specific binding sites of GLU, and its strong excitatory action on pyriform cortex neurons is antagonized by APB, and much less by APV, indicating that the recognition sites are similar to a GLU-receptor subtype different from those of the NMDA, quisqualate, or kainate types (48). Other investigators, however, found a strong antagonistic effect of APV on the NAAG-elicited excitation of spinal cord neurons in culture and concluded that the action of NAAG is due to the selective activation of NMDA-type receptors (53). Regarding the mechanism of action of NAAG it was proposed that its release from nerve terminals is followed by cleavage through an endopeptidase with the consequent local production of GLU/ ASP, which may in turn act on certain receptors as well as on sodium-dependent uptake processes (48). In spite of rather strong evidence for a possible role of NAAG in neurotransmission, it must be noted that its action is much less potent than that of GLU or NMDA (53) and also that it can be inactive in various *in vitro* and *in vivo* preparations (54). The latter study, however, did not include tests on specific sensory pathways, such as the terminal fields of the lateral olfactory stria, where NAAG was later shown to produce rapid onset and offset of excitation (55).

Recently, the levels of NAAG were determined in the optic tract and LGNd of the monkey (35). These structures contained higher amounts than those originally reported for brain (see above), of the order of 3.9 μmol/g in the tract and 2.6 μmol/g in the nucleus (Fig. 1). Similar values were also found in the LGNd of the rat (56). Most important, 1 week after optic tract section in the monkey, the concentrations had dropped significantly in the optic tract distal to the section (82%) and in the LGNd (43%). The larger decrease in the tract was interpreted as due to the homogeneous composition of the structure as opposed to the LGNd where the retinal terminals comprise a relatively small proportion of the total. Correlative immunocytochemical studies with a NAAG antibody have provided strong support for these biochemical findings. Thus, immunoreactivity was present in the majority of retinal ganglion cells of the rat, with intense fiber staining of the optic papilla, optic tract, and LGNd (56,57). In addition, the nucleus showed numerous puncta as well as small labeled cells in the medial portion. The fiber stain was almost absent in the tract and LGNd contralateral to an eye enucleation, but the immunoreactive cells persisted. Similar results were obtained in the cat and monkey, both for the retina and the LGNd (58,59). In the cat, it was reported that the location and size of the labeled retinal ganglion cells suggested that the on and off center, as well as X, Y, and W types were immunostained. The NAAG+ neurons in the LGNd, however, were less strongly immunoreactive, and the authors suggested that the antibody might be recognizing a related peptide since the reaction did not occur when the antiserum was preabsorbed with bovine serum albumin conjugated with either NAAG or aspartylglutamate (see section on LGNd intrinsic components, p. 64).

The possible role of various neuroactive peptides in retinogeniculate transmission should also be considered. Although the retina contains appreciable amounts of these compounds (for review see [25,60]), only substance P (SP) appears so far to be a likely candidate as suggested originally on the basis of measurements of SP activity in extracts of bovine optic nerve and retina (61). The concentrations of SP, however, vary widely in the optic nerve: 0.6 pmol/g wet tissue in the human (62), 4.5 pmol/g in rabbit (63); 64.5 pmol/g in rat (recalculated from [64]). Values are more comparable for the LGNd: 35.7

pmol/g in the human (62) and 81.6 to 90.0 pmol/g in rat (recalculated from [64,65]). Immunolabeling has helped to identify SP+ retinal cells. Following almost totally negative findings in the rat (66,67) and a suggestion of labeled ganglion cells in the monkey (68), a more definitive study was reported in the rabbit (69), which demonstrated 25% to 35% immunostained retinal ganglion cells, of which a high proportion could be filled by retrograde transport from the superior colliculi. Moreover, the immunoreactivity disappeared after optic nerve section. These neurons were present in all retinal regions and their dendrites arborized in the adjacent inner plexiform layer. The same study reported SP+ boutons of presumably retinal origin forming synapses in the LGNd with both P- and I-cell dendrites.

Regarding other neuropeptides, there is only one report describing the presence of large multipolar neurons in the ganglion cell layer immunoreactive for somatostatin (SS) (70). The occurrence of these cells decreased in frequency from the peripheral to the central retina. The significance of this finding, however, is not clear since no immunoreactivity was detected in the optic nerve or tract.

In summary, the data available to date suggest that the transmitters released in the LGNd by the majority of retinal terminals, including those of the X- and Y-types, are acetylated dipeptides related to NAAG acting on GLU receptors, either directly or through acidic amino acids derived from the dipeptide cleavage. It is possible that certain peptides may colocalize differentially with these compounds, giving rise to more than one type of chemically specified retinal input into the LGNd. Such could be the case of the SP+ cells reported in the rabbit. Double-labeling studies can easily test this possibility. Probably the most significant piece of evidence that is lacking at this time is direct physiologic evidence of the action of these proposed substances on the components of the LGNd circuitry.

Cortical Source

It is well-known that the striate cortex projects to the LGNd essentially through the pyramidal cells of layer 6 (71) and that their physiologic action is excitatory (72). The most likely candidate for the neurotransmitter in this pathway is GLU. Several lines of evidence point in this direction. Unilateral visual cortex ablation in the rabbit led to a significant drop in GLU levels in the ipsilateral LGNd when measured 1 to 2 months after surgery (32). This decrease was also seen in a similar experiment in the monkey in which a 70% drop in GLU was noted 3 months post-operatively (Molinar and Pasik, *unpublished data*). Although part of the loss could be attributed to retrograde degeneration of P-cells (see section on P-cells, p. 65) during the long survival period, a reduction of 32% was found in the rat only 1 week after the cortical resection (34). In addition, the latter study showed that the high-affinity uptake of L-GLU fell 75% in the LGNd and that this decrease predominated in the synaptosomal fraction. Furthermore, the postnatal development of the high-affinity GLU uptake correlated well with the formation of corticogeniculate endings (73). The high-affinity uptake of D-ASP, used as a marker for terminals utilizing GLU and/or ASP, also dropped 30% in similar experiments in the cat (74). Further support for the role of GLU in corticogeniculate transmission was the demonstration of a 14-fold increase in GLU released by K^+-induced stimulation of rat visual cortex slices and of the labeling of pyramidal neurons in layer 6 of the striate cortex following the injection of [^{3}H]-D-ASP locally or in the LGNd (75). The *in vivo* release of GLU and ASP was also obtained by local electric stimulation of the LGNd and, as mentioned in the survey of retinogeniculate transmission, this result could be due to the activation of corticogeniculate terminals (36).

There is evidence against the implication of other neuroactive substances in the corticogeniculate pathway. ACh can be ruled out on the basis that its concentration is not reduced in the rabbit LGNd 1 month after cortical ablation (13), and the ChAT activity is maintained in the rat LGNd after similar lesions (34). It is of interest that the deep acetyl cholinesterase (AChE) staining of parvocellular geniculate laminae in *Galago* and owl monkey was abolished by cortical ablation and that AChE+ cells appeared in layer 6 of the striate cortex (76), a result also obtained in the cat (77). The former authors, however, qualified their findings since the presence of AChE was not always considered a reliable index of cholinergic transmission. In fact, no ChAT+ cells were found in the cortex of the monkey (78) or cat (79). The evidence appears negative also for NAAG since the levels are very low in the striate cortex of the monkey (Molinar and Pasik, *unpublished data*), and NAAG immunoreactivity is present in pyramidal cells of layers 3 and 5 but not 6 of this cortical area (59).

In summary, strong evidence has accumulated suggesting that the corticogeniculate pathways utilize GLU as a neurotransmitter. (References have already been given for the existence of abundant GLU receptors in the LGNd [see section on retinal source, p. 43].)

Brain Stem Sources

The brain stem exerts a powerful and complex influence on geniculate transmission. At least three systems have been recognized, each utilizing a different neuroactive substance, namely ACh, 5-HT, and NE, in addition to several others of unknown nature.

Cholinergic System

A preceding section of this review led to the conclusion that ACh is not a neurotransmitter in the retinogeniculate pathway (see section on retinal source, p. 43) and may not participate in corticogeniculate transmission (see section on cortical source, p. 49). Yet, the LGNd contains an appreciable amount of ACh, which has been reported in the rat to be between 2 and 22 nmol/g wet tissue (recalculated from [5] and [80]), the discrepancy being due probably to procedural differences. In the search for the origin of cholinergic innervation of the LGNd, a study based on AChE staining in the rat has proposed the nucleus cuneiformis in the mesencephalic reticular formation (MRF) as the sole source (81). Lesions of this nucleus, which in fact extended also into the dorsal and ventral parabrachial nuclei and the marginal nucleus of the brachium conjunctivum, resulted in a marked decrease of AChE staining in the LGNd as well as a 40% to 50% reduction in ChAT activity (82). Recently, the use of retrograde tracers in combination with the immunocytochemical demonstration of ChAT, a more reliable marker for cholinergic elements, provided more definitive data. Injection of fluorescent tracers in the LGNd of the rat labeled neurons in the pontomesencephalotegmental complex, and these cells were also ChAT immunoreactive (83). Most of them were located in the pedunculopontine tegmental nucleus (PPTN) and the rostral portion of the dorsolateral tegmental nucleus (DLTN). Similar findings were obtained using horseradish peroxidase (HRP) as the tracer, but in this case the contribution to the LGNd came only from the PPTN (84). In the cat, double labeled cells for ChAT and rhodamine-latex microspheres deposited in the LGNd were numerous in what the authors designated as the central tegmental field, the marginal nucleus of the brachium conjunctivum and the locus ceruleus (85). The distribution of these neurons overlapped with that of cells containing the retrograde tracer and exhibiting immunoreactivity for dopamine β hydroxylase (DBH), a marker for NE.

The interpretation of some of the preceding findings has been somewhat hampered by problems of anatomic nomenclature of cholinergic tegmental nuclei. Thus, although the main group of ChAT-immunoreactive neurons was originally identified as the nucleus parabrachialis (86), it now appears that the central structures are the PPTN and the DLTN in both the rat and monkey. The presence of some immunostained cells extends from the PPTN rostrally into nucleus cuneiformis and caudally into nucleus parabrachialis, which in itself is devoid of such neurons (76,87). Another possible source of cholinergic innervation of the LGNd is the parabigeminal nucleus where numerous ChAT+ neurons have been recognized in mouse, cat, and monkey (88–90). Other investigators, however, have failed to detect ChAT-immunoreactive neurons in this structure (85,86). ChAT immunocytochemistry has also given information on the pattern of cholinergic innervation in the cat LGNd. Immunoreactive fibers form a dense plexus in laminae A and A_1 where no labeled cells are found (91). Ultrastructurally, there are ChAT+ boutons containing round vesicles and forming mostly symmetric synapses with both P-cell dendrites and I-cell presynaptic dendrites (19). It is noteworthy that a less reliable marker for cholinergic elements, i.e., AChE staining, has shown an uneven and different distribution in the LGNd of various species. The staining is more intense in the magnocellular laminae in the macaque (75,90,92), whereas it is stronger in the parvocellular subdivision in the bushbaby and owl monkey (74) as well as in the A and A_1 laminae in the cat (75).

Electrophysiologic and pharmacologic studies have clarified the role of ACh in LGNd transmission. The original finding in the barbiturate-anesthetized cat of a long-lasting facilitatory influence on the excitation of LGNd neurons by light or GLU (15) was superseded by the demonstration in the same species but without barbiturate anesthesia of a direct excitatory effect on most of these cells (16). Moreover, the action of ACh and GLU was enhanced by stimulation of the MRF. The application of benzoquinonium, an ACh antagonist, abolished the effects of both ACh and MRF stimulation. This was perhaps the first indication of a functional cholinergic pathway from the brain stem to the LGNd (see also [11]). The same study reported that a few geniculate cells were inhibited by ACh. Since no anatomic verification is available, the possibility that the recordings were obtained from perigeniculate nucleus (PGN) cells cannot be excluded (see section on diencephalic sources, p. 59). The strongly excitatory action of ACh applied equally well to all classes of LGNd neurons in the cat, i.e., the X- and Y-cells of either on- or off-center receptive fields (93).

The ACh receptors present in the LGNd have been considered mostly of the muscarinic type in the rat, guinea pig, and monkey. It was found that they bind to scopolamine (94–96), to quinuclidinyl benzylate (97,98), to both of these ligands (41), and to propylbenzilylcholine mustard (99). None of these substances, however, differentiates the various subtypes of muscarinic receptors, which have been implicated in the dual action of ACh, i.e., excitation of geniculate neurons and inhibition of PGN or thalamic reticular nucleus (TRN) cells (see section on diencephalic sources, p. 59). Recently, important species differences have been reported in the action of ACh on P cells of the LGNd when recorded in thalamic slices (100). Thus, the most common response present in rat, cat, and guinea pig was a slow depolarization via muscarinic receptors resulting from the suppression of K^+ conductance. In addition, an initial fast depolarization via nicotinic receptors occurred in the cat, whereas a hyperpolarizing response was characteristic of the guinea pig. Although nicotinic receptors, as labeled with α-bungarotoxin, were found in negligible amounts in the LGNd (101,102), recent studies in the rat have demonstrated a high density of receptors binding ACh and nicotine in the presence of atropine, which blocked those of muscarinic type (103). These results raise the possibility of yet another influence of ACh in the LGNd.

In summary, the LGNd is innervated by cholinergic pathways originating mostly in the PPTN complex. This subsystem, which is an important component of the "ascending reticular activating system," influences geniculate cells by direct excitation of P- and I-cells, the latter in turn inhibiting P-cells and thereby contributing to a sharpening of the tuning characteristics of geniculate neurons. In addition, ACh may disinhibit geniculate cells by its inhibitory action on PGN or TRN neurons (see section on diencephalic sources, p. 59).

Serotoninergic System

Serotonin (5-hydroxytryptamine [5-HT]) was the first substance considered to be a neurotransmitter candidate in the visual system following the demonstration of its depressant action on LGNd neurons in the cat when applied iontophoretically (22). The reported LGNd levels of 5-HT have varied greatly, probably because of methodological differences, going from nondetectable in the dog (24), to 0.27 to 0.35 μg/g in the cat (11) and 0.005 to 1 μg/g in the rat (recalculated from [104,105]). Having excluded the possibility that 5-HT could be the optic fiber transmitter (see section on retinal source, p. 43), the main origin of the serotoninergic innervation of the LGNd was found to be the midbrain dorsal raphe nuclei. These pathways were defined in the cat and rat by anterograde (106,107) and retrograde tracers (108,109), as well as by the specific uptake of [^{3}H]5-HT (110), and more recently by the double label of raphe neurons with a retrograde tracer injected into the LGNd and 5-HT immunoreactivity (85). The presence of serotoninergic fibers in the LGNd was shown in the rat by histofluorescence or immunofluorescence (111,112), and a more detailed analysis became possible by immunocytochemistry using an unlabeled serotonin antibody. Thus, several reports in the rat coincide in the description of a plexus of fine, varicose immunoreactive fibers of moderate density (67,113,114). A similar appearance was found in the cat, where the medial interlaminar nucleus and the C laminae received a heavier innervation than the A laminae (115–117), leading to the conclusion that the 5-HT system was influencing particularly the target neurons of the W-type retinal ganglion cells. One of these studies also gave information on the ultrastructural features of the 5-HT immunoreactive elements present in the A laminae (117). Fibers were described as exclusively unmyelinated, with varicosities filled with vesicles of mixed sizes and dark mitochondria. Only 4% of these profiles formed synaptic contacts that were of the asymmetric type. The illustrations of this study included at least three examples of postsynaptic elements with large mitochondria resembling P-cell dendrites. In no case was an immunostained bouton seen synapsing onto a profile containing synaptic vesicles, i.e., belonging to an I-cell presynaptic dendrite. Finally, in the monkey a plexus of fine-beaded fibers has been described as decreasing in density from the magnocellular to the parvocellular laminae and numerous puncta were present throughout (118–120). Electron microscopic observations included reaction products occasionally apparent in finely myelinated axons, but here again, most of the profiles followed in serial thin sections lacked morphologically defined synapses (119). The few synaptic contacts showed asymmetric thickenings, some with subjunctional dense bodies, and were located in the periphery of typical synaptic triadic arrangements (Fig. 2a).

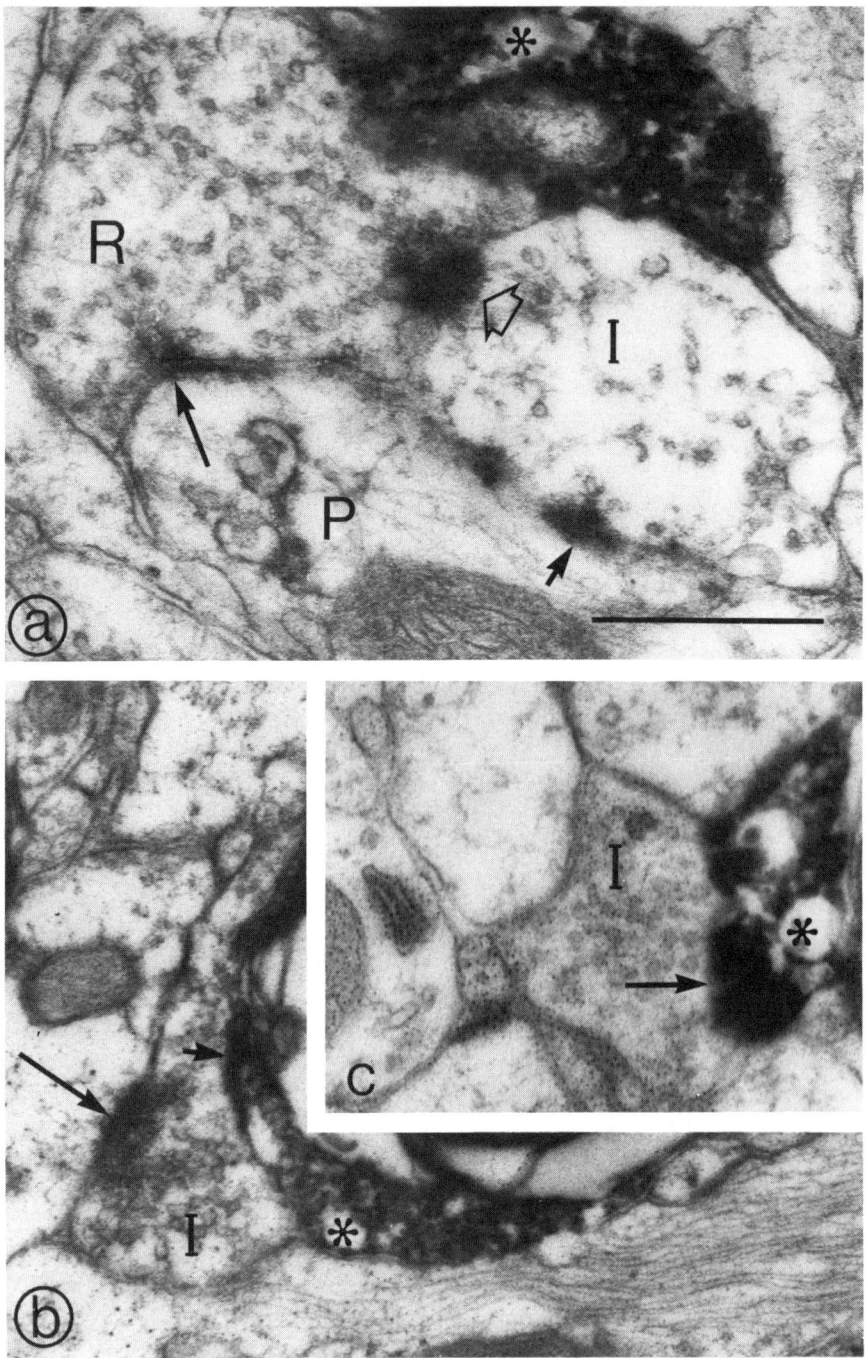

FIG. 2. Serotonin immunoreactive elements in the LGNd neuropil of the monkey. **a:** Triadic synaptic arrangement of a bouton with large ovoid or round vesicles, probably of retinal origin (R), presynaptic at *long arrow* to a P-cell dendrite (P), identified by the large mitochondrion and

Apparently at variance with the findings in the cat, in the majority of the serially reconstructed junctions the postsynaptic profiles contained synaptic vesicles and were interpreted as I-cell presynaptic dendrites (Fig. 2b).

The influence of 5-HT on LGNd neurons has been the subject of numerous reports, stimulated by the original findings of the effects of the intracarotid administration of lysergic acid diethylamide, a hallucinogenic drug known to interact with 5-HT (121–123). The initial demonstration that iontophoretic application of 5-HT suppressed the orthodromic response of cat LGNd neurons to optic nerve stimulation but not the response to GLU or the antidromic activation from stimulation of the optic radiations (22,124), led to the conclusion that 5-HT competed with the optic nerve transmitter for postsynaptic receptors. This view was challenged, however, when it was found that the depressant action was also extended to the excitatory influence of GLU and ACh and, at times, to antidromic stimulation as well (16), the difference in results being attributed to the use of barbiturate anesthesia in the earlier studies. The latter investigation also used visual stimulation in addition to electric shocks to the optic nerve. The possible mode of action was then changed to an altered excitability of the cell membrane (125). The argument continued with the report of a dose-dependent action of 5-HT, which at high levels acted as just stated and at low levels appeared to function presynaptically by blocking either the release of the excitatory transmitter from retinal terminals or the access to the receptors for that transmitter (126). In what appears to be a more definitive study, low doses of 5-HT did not affect the neuronal responses to spots of light covering the center of the receptive fields of X- and Y-cell types, as well as to the application of ACh or the excitatory amino acid homocysteic acid. High doses caused almost total depression of the spontaneous activity and that evoked by ACh and homocysteic acid, whereas the visual response remained almost unaffected (127). The latter effect was similar to that of γ-aminobutyric acid (GABA), a well-known inhibitory substance acting at postsynaptic sites. The authors concluded that 5-HT acts post-synaptically and interpreted the differences with previous results as due to the fact that responses to optic nerve or diffuse light stimulation were weaker and more susceptible to the depressive action of 5-HT than the powerful excitation evoked by spot targets. The inhibitory influence of 5-HT on LGNd neurons was also found in the rat where it mimicked the inhibitory action of dorsal raphe stimulation. Methysergide, a 5-HT receptor blocker, suppressed both of these effects (128).

---

the presence of cisterns, and to an I-cell presynaptic dendrite (I) at *open arrow*, the latter profile being presynaptic to the same P-cell dendrite at *short arrow*. An immunolabeled profile (*) is at the periphery of the complex. (From ref. 119.) **b,c:** Two immunoreactive profiles (**) that in serial sections were observed to form asymmetric synapses with elements containing synaptic vesicles, probably belonging to I-cell presynaptic dendrites (I) at regions close to the arrows (*short arrow* in [b]). The I profile in (b) is presynaptic to a dendrite at long arrow. Scale: 0.5 μm applies to all panels.

Although the depressive action of 5-HT seems to be well established, several reports have indicated that a certain proportion of cat LGNd neurons increase their firing frequency when exposed to this substance. In some cases the facilitated neurons were identified as I-cells or at least as cells of small size, whereas those that were depressed were the P-cells or larger neurons (129,130). Stimulation of the dorsal raphe nuclei also resulted in facilitation of some neurons and inhibition of others (131). The cells showing a decrease of their spontaneous firing rate as well as of the activity evoked by stimulation of the chiasm or light flashes were identified as P cells (132).

Serotonin receptors have been measured in the rat LGNd by quantitative autoradiography and found in quite different proportions with respect to their type. Moderate amounts of the $5-HT_1$ receptor(s), of approximately 30% of the concentration in the ventral pallidum, the richest area in this type, contrast with the low values for the $5-HT_2$ receptors, which reach only 5% of the highest concentration present in the frontal cortex (133,134). It is of interest that, at least in the rat hippocampus, the activation of $5-HT_1$ receptors increases K^+ conductance probably by direct coupling of a G protein to a K^+ channel (135).

Based on all these findings on the possible role of serotonin in LGNd transmission, it has been proposed (119) that this substance is released primarily from nonsynaptic varicosities, thereby acting on the P-cell membrane probably through $5-HT_1$ receptors, resulting in a decrease of the excitability of these neurons. In addition, serotonin released synaptically at asymmetric junctions with interneurons would excite these cells by way of $5-HT_2$ receptors. These I-cells would in turn inhibit P-cells through a GABA-mediated mechanism (see section on LGNd intrinsic components, p. 64). Similar inhibition of P-cells can be postulated for the heavy serotoninergic innervation of the cat PGN and the monkey TRN if indeed these neurons receive excitatory synapses from 5-HT boutons (see section on diencephalic sources, p. 59). The selective activation of the origin of serotoninergic afferents, i.e., the midbrain raphe nuclei during wakefulness, may result in the suppression of spontaneous background activity but not of that elicited by the visual stimulus, thus increasing the signal-to-noise ratio and consequently improving the attentive state toward the object of regard.

Noradrenergic System

The LGNd contains rather low amounts of NE, which have been variously reported, utilizing different methods, as 0.07 µg/g in the dog (26), 0.36 µg/g in the rat (28), and 1 µg/g in the same animal (27) where it represents 12% of the maximum found in the dorsomedial hypothalamic nucleus. The noradrenergic innervation of the LGNd was initially recognized in the rat by histofluorescence as a dense network of very fine varicose fibers originating in the brain stem (111, 136). The evenly distributed plexus was lost after bilateral destruction of the locus ceruleus (28,137). The latter studies succeeded in delineating the pathways for this bilateral innervation, the crossings occurring via the posterior and supraoptic commissures. Moreover, the system was found to be highly plastic since it increased markedly within 2 weeks after visual cortex removal (138). The origins of these pathways in the locus ceruleus were further recognized by the anterograde transport of tritiated amino acids (28,139) and the retrograde transport of HRP (28,140,141). Finally, an even clearer picture was suggested from immunofluorescence studies using an antibody against DBH. The description included a bundle originating in the locus ceruleus coursing toward the forebrain, with a component detaching at the level of the subthalamus, providing an extremely dense innervation to the LGNd (142). Observations in the cat are in essential agreement with those in the rat, although no information on the histofluorescence pattern is available. Here again, HRP-labeled neurons were observed in the locus ceruleus of both sides, ipsilateral more than contralateral, after injections restricted to the LGNd (143). A most dramatic demonstration was the double labeling of numerous locus ceruleus neurons with rhodamine-latex microspheres deposited into the LGNd and DBH immunoreactivity (85). These cells were higher in number on the side of the injection compared with those of the contralateral nucleus. The latter investigation also reported double labeled cells in the so-called central tegmental field, overlapping in general location with other retrogradely stained neurons exhibiting ChAT immunoreactivity (see section on cholinergic system, p. 50). Unfortunately, no results were given on DBH immunoreactivity within the LGNd. The data on primates are scanty. In the macaque, histofluorescence techniques have revealed a loose network of fine varicose fibers, somewhat denser in the LGNd than in the rest of the thalamus, with marked decreases after destruction of the locus ceruleus (144). More recently, however, DBH immunocytochemistry in the same species showed only a small number of fibers in the LGNd, some of which were seen coursing radially through the magnocellular layers. The paucity of immunoreactive fibers was even more striking in the LGNd of squirrel monkeys (120). The only information on ultrastructural features of NE terminals in the LGNd comes from the rat where treatment with 5-hydroxydopamine (5-OH-DA) apparently served to recognize degenerating boutons with dense core vesicles forming synapses with small, distal dendrites of P-cells (145).

Most of the early work on the physiologic action of NE in the LGNd was reported in the cat. Initial studies showed a weak depressant influence of similar characteristics but lesser magnitude than that of 5-HT (22). These findings were extended to include a strong depressant action on responses of many but not all LGNd neurons to optic nerve or visual stimulation, as well as to the excitatory effect of GLU, and even to the invasion of antidromically generated spikes (16). Soon afterward, however, it was reported that this effect applied to only 60% of the neurons tested, the remainder being excited either from the start or after an initial depression (126). Furthermore, NE was found to excite P-cells and depress what appeared to be I-cells (129). The latter findings were supported by the demonstration that the response to optic tract stimulation of physiologically identified P-cells was enhanced by a conditioning stimulus to the locus ceruleus (146). This enhancement did not occur in reserpinized animals but reappeared after intravenous administration of L-DOPA or intraventricular NE. These treatments did not succeed when the conditioned response was gradually eliminated by application of fusaric acid, a potent DBH inhibitor. Contrariwise, locus ceruleus stimulation depressed the responses of I-cells, and this action was equally abolished by reserpine and restored by L-DOPA and NE. The authors concluded that NE acted by inhibition of I-cells resulting in disinhibition of P-cells. Similar results were obtained in the rat with the additional supporting finding that the NE effect was markedly decreased in animals treated with α-methyl-p-tyrosine (147).

In a series of more recent studies in the rat, extracellular recordings showed that iontophoretically applied NE with low ejection currents and locus ceruleus stimulation had similar influences on the spontaneous activity of P-cells and on that evoked by optic chiasm stimulation or GLU deposits (132,148). In all cases the effect was a slowly developing facilitation of long duration. After sectioning the optic nerve, NE failed to excite "silent" cells but still facilitated their response to GLU. Since a GABA antagonist (picrotoxin) did not produce the latter effect, it was concluded that the action of NE might not be due to its influence on I-cells, which are most probably GABAergic (see section on LGNd intrinsic components, p. 64), but rather to a modulatory role, modifying the responses of target cells to other inputs. It was also found that the facilitatory effect of NE was blocked by phentolamine, an α-adrenergic receptor antagonist, and not by sotalol, a β-blocker (149). Moreover, the effects of both NE and locus ceruleus stimulation were blocked by prazosin, a selective α_1-receptor blocker (150), indicating that NE activated P-cells via this type of postsynaptic receptors. In fact, it has recently been shown that the rat LGNd is one of the richest structures in α_1-adrenergic receptors (151). The modulatory action of NE via this receptor type gained further support from the demonstration in LGN slices that NE stimulated the hydrolysis of phosphatidylinositol biphosphate leading to the activation of the second messengers diacylglycerol and inositol triphosphate. This process was not affected by propranolol (β-receptor antagonist) and was almost completely blocked by phentolamine (mixed α_1- and α_2-receptor blocker) and totally occluded by prazosin, a pure α_1-receptor antagonist (152). The NE effect was markedly reduced in the kainic acid lesioned LGNd, suggesting that a large proportion of the reaction occurred within LGNd neurons as opposed to afferent elements. It is also of interest that a certain amount of β-adrenergic receptors has been measured in the rat LGNd by their binding to dihydroalprenolol (98). Although these receptors may reside in nonneuronal components such as neuroglia and blood vessels, the possibility still exists that the depressant effect of NE on I-cells is mediated via a β receptor. A recent study on guinea pig and cat thalamic slices reported the main action of NE on P-cells to be a slow depolarization due to a decreased K^+ conductance (153). This action suppressed burst firing and promoted single-spike generation.

In summary, the noradrenergic ceruleogeniculate pathway exerts a powerful modulatory influence on LGNd transmission, which in many ways is opposite to the effects of 5-HT (see section on serotoninergic system, p. 53), at least in subprimate species. Since its effect is somewhat similar to that of ACh (see section on cholinergic system, p. 50), its functional significance may also be comparable. It has been adduced, for example, that the two agents may be instrumental in blocking the spike afterhyperpolarization, thereby decreasing the adaptation to excitatory inputs of long duration (154). Similarly, by moving the membrane potential away from the bursting firing range, and thereby favoring single-spike activity, these neuroactive substances would suppress thalamocortical rhythms and facilitate the transfer of sensory information to the cortex (153). One of the many questions that remains is whether the two systems differ in some way, accounting for their different morphologic substrata and pharmacologic properties.

Systems of Unknown Nature

In addition to the above reviewed brain stem inputs from known chemically specified systems, the LGNd receives afferents from the superior colliculus and certain pretectal nuclei, the existence of which has been ascertained in a variety of species: rat (141), cat (85,155,156), tree shrew and bushbaby (157), and monkey (158–160). The nature of the neuroactive substances in these pathways remains largely unknown.

Diencephalic Sources

Thalamic Reticular Nucleus

The main diencephalic afferents to the LGNd take origin in the "visual" segment of the thalamic reticular nucleus (vTRN), i.e., the portion of this structure that roughly lies in apposition to the LGNd. It is most probable that the PGN of the cat represents the visual sector of the TRN in this species, and the two structures will thus be considered as equivalent in the following survey. Anterograde and retrograde transport studies have shown in various monkey species as well as in the cat and rat that the vTRN projects exclusively to the LGNd and that both geniculocortical and corticogeniculate fibers, while passing through the vTRN, leave dense terminal plexuses in this structure (161). Furthermore, it has been demonstrated that axons of geniculate neurons collateralize in the PGN (162) and that this feature is more characteristic of Y-cells than of X-cells (163). The types of terminals originating in the vTRN of rat have been described in the LGNd after restrictive lesions of the former nucleus (164). The degenerated boutons include small profiles with round vesicles forming asymmetric synapses with small- and medium-size dendrites and large terminals containing flattened vesicles and establishing symmetric synapses with dendrites of various sizes and even with somata of what appear to be P-cells. The first type was interpreted as of cortical origin, the alterations of which resulted from interruption of cortical fibers passing through the vTRN, and the second type representing the endings of vTRN cells. Similar characteristics have been reported for the boutons labeled by injection of tritiated proline into the vTRN and transported anterogradely into the LGNd (165) with some additional features such as their being exclusively presynaptic and sometimes taking origin in myelinated axons. The reciprocal connectivity of the rat LGNd and vTRN have also been shown by retrograde transport techniques (166).

Given the intimate relationship between the vTRN and the LGNd, it is of additional interest to review the other inputs to the vTRN. Injection of tracers restricted to the vTRN in the rat resulted in retrogradely labeled cells in the midbrain reticular formation, periaqueductal gray matter, and the dorsal tegmental nucleus (DTN) (83,141). These authors did not find tagged cells in locus ceruleus and only an occasional one in the raphe nuclei. In two studies in the cat, however, the latter two structures were found to project to the PGN, but the results could have been confounded by the extension of the injection sites into the LGNd (85,167). It should be noted that several studies have failed to demonstrate brain stem afferents to the TRN (168,169). Immunocytochemistry, however, has helped to clarify this issue as well as the nature of the brain stem afferents to the vTRN and PGN. There is a consensus regarding the cholinergic innervation that originates in the DTN and PPTN in the rat (83,84). Although the latter investigation also reported a major input from nucleus basalis, this finding could be due to the rather anterior location of the tracer injection sites, which appears to be considerably more rostral than the visual segment of the TRN. In both the rat and cat, the vTRN and PGN contain a dense plexus of ChAT immunoreactive fine varicose fibers (19,91, 170). In the PGN, ChAT+ boutons with round vesicles and exclusively presynaptic make numerous en passant, mostly symmetrical synapses with dendrites, spines, and somata (19). The serotoninergic innervation is also very dense in the rat, cat, and monkey (113,117,120). In the PGN, most of the 5-HT+ varicosities do not form synapses, and when they do, the specializations of the membranes are asymmetric, i.e., in all similar to the observations in the LGNd (see section on serotoninergic system, p. 53). The NE innervation is also dense in the three species (85,120,137,142). The findings on 5-HT and NE stand in contrast to another investigation that found no such innervation of the vTRN in the rat (141). These authors attributed the discrepancy to the fact that their data applied strictly to the visually responsive TRN as opposed to more widely distributed regions of the TRN.

The nature of the vTRN or PGN neurons projecting to the LGNd has been discovered to be GABAergic on the basis of their immunoreactivity to glutamate decarboxylase (GAD). Following the original findings that the rat TRN contained a large proportion of GAD+ neurons as well as fibers and puncta, some of which appeared to contact the stained cells (171), it was shown that virtually all neurons in this nucleus are GAD immunoreactive in the rat, cat, and monkey (172–175). One of these studies succeeded in double labeling PGN neurons with HRP injected into the LGNd and GAD antiserum (173). Figure 3 illustrates the direct GABA immunoreactivity of the TRN in monkey material, a finding that had been reported earlier for the mouse (47). In addition, ultrastructural features of the PGN include the presence of at least two classes of GAD+ boutons (174). Large profiles, with dark mitochondria and pleomorphic vesicles forming symmetric synapses with other GAD+ dendrites and somata, were interpreted as belonging to axon collaterals of PGN neurons. Small boutons, also with pleomorphic vesicles, made

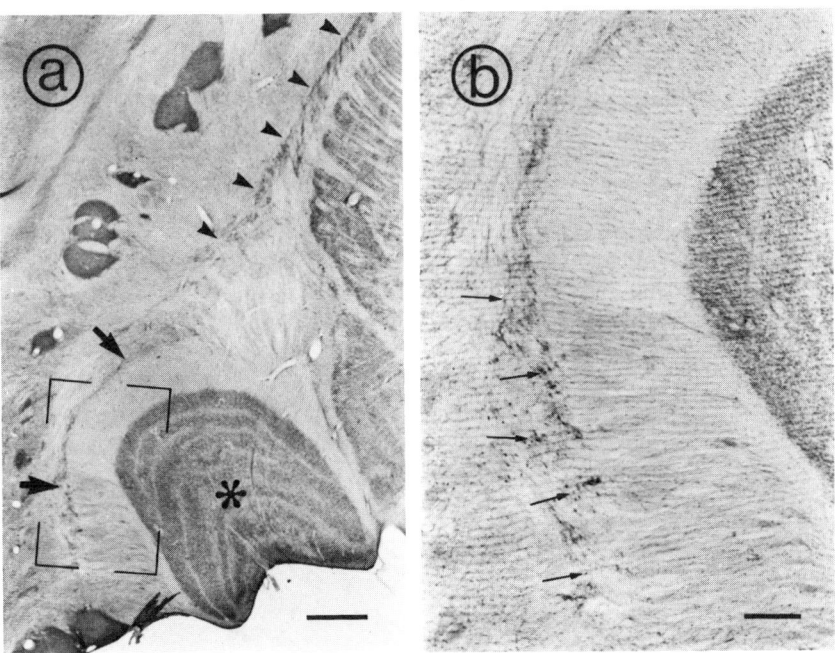

FIG. 3. GABA immunoreactivity present in monkey LGNd and surrounding structures. **a:** Panoramic view showing heavy labeling of LGNd (*), TRN (*arrow heads*), and its extension at the margin of the LGNd capsule probably representing the vTRN (*arrows*). Scale: 1 mm. **b:** Higher magnification of the area framed in (a) depicting the deeply stained neurons of the latter cell group (*arrows*). Scale: 300 μm.

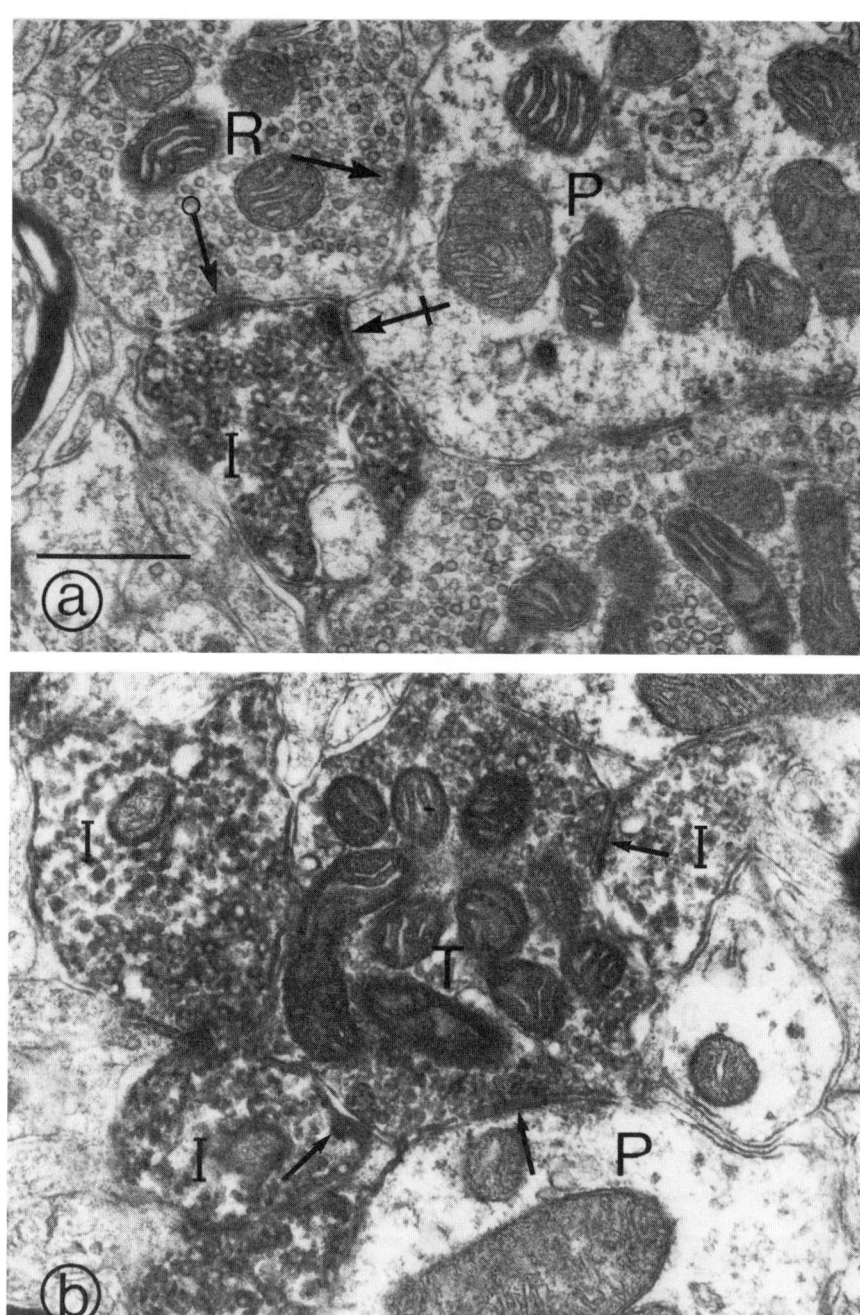

FIG. 4. GABA immunoreactivity in the monkey LGNd neuropil. **a:** Triadic synaptic arrangement of a retinal terminal (R), presynaptic to a P-cell dendrite (P) at *arrow* and to an intensely immunoreactive I-cell presynaptic dendrite (*) at *ringed arrow,* in turn presynaptic to the same P-cell profile at *crossed arrow.* (From ref. 215.) **b:** Immunoreactive axonal bouton (T), which in

serial symmetric synapses with other profiles of similar appearance and were considered as appendages of "presynaptic" dendrites of PGN cells. The former type corresponded well with terminals described in the extraglomerular neuropil of the rat LGNd, which were exclusively presynaptic and formed symmetric axodendritic synapses (172). These authors found only P-cell elements as the postsynaptic partners. However, an example of a similar type of terminal presynaptic to an I-cell dendrite in the monkey LGNd labeled with a direct GABA antibody is illustrated in Fig. 4b. The latter connectivity was also suggested for the cat LGNd (176). Developmental features of GABA immunoreactivity included intense labeling of the PGN in cat fetuses 2 weeks before term and a progressive decrease post-natally reaching the less dense adult pattern at 3 months (177).

The information on GABA receptors in the LGNd will be surveyed with reference to the intrinsic components of the structure (see section on LGNd intrinsic components, p. 64).

It is clear from the previous discussion that the main, if not the only, function of the vTRN or PGN is to inhibit LGNd neurons through a GABA-mediated mechanism. This action was demonstrated in the rat and cat in which stimulation of vTRN suppressed the responses of P-cells or the cortical evoked activity to optic chiasm or tract shocks (178,179). The effect has recently been confirmed and shown to be blocked by bicuculline (180). The major input to vTRN neurons from the LGNd derives from Y-cells in a rather discrete fashion since a small number of these cells converge onto single vTRN neurons (166). The latter elements project back to both Y- and W-cells. It is also known that PGN neurons have mutual inhibitory connections and that they project to both P- and I-geniculate cells (181). Although it appears that this is the basic mechanism giving rise to recurrent inhibition of LGNd neurons (182), at least four other systems influence this circuitry. One is the input from the visual cortex, most probably glutamergic, the inactivation of which has been shown in the rat to strongly depress all neurons in the vTRN (183). A second one is cholinergic which, as discussed earlier, is directly excitatory of LGNd neurons. This innervation, however, has been shown in the cat to be inhibitory of PGN cells (93,184) leading the latter authors to postulate that ACh exerts a dual influence on the LGNd: (a) enhancement of the stimulus-specific inhibition by excitation of both P- and I-cells, the latter in turn inhibiting P-cells, and (b) a nonspecific disinhibition of P-cells by inhibiting the PGN. The nonspecificity of the latter process was recently supported by the finding of an expanded area of inhibition beyond the receptive fields of LGNd cells, a phenomenon selectively canceled by ACh (185). The mechanism of action of

---

serial sections was found to be exclusively presynaptic, forms synapses (*arrows*) with GABA+ presynaptic dendrites (I) and an unlabeled P-cell dendrite (P). The density and size of mitochondria as well as the size and shape of the vesicles suggest that T is of a different nature than that of the I profiles and probably is of TRN origin. Scale: 0.5 μm applies to both panels.

ACh on TRN neurons was examined in guinea pig thalamic slices and found to be a hyperpolarization that was blocked by scopolamine but not pirenzepine (96). Since the latter compound exhibits a high affinity for the M_1 receptor (186), the process is probably due to activation of M_2 muscarinic receptors resulting in an increase of K^+ conductance.

The third system is noradrenergic. It was demonstrated in the rat that vTRN cells were activated by stimulation of, or GLU infusion in, the locus ceruleus as well as local application of NE. This process was blocked by α- but not β-adrenergic receptor antagonists (148). Finally, in the rat the serotoninergic system activated by stimulation of the dorsal raphe nuclei or by local application of 5-HT inhibited the responses of vTRN neurons elicited by cortical stimulation (128). These influences may be exerted over the LGNd and PGN by separate or the same brain stem neurons (187).

In summary, the TRN appears to be a crucial structure in the modulation of LGNd activity. The GABA-mediated recurrent inhibition of LGNd neurons exerted by its cells is in turn regulated by the influence of cortical and brain stem inputs on the TRN utilizing GLU, ACh, NE, and 5-HT. These inputs act similarly and directly on the LGNd as well, with the exception of the cholinergic one, which, while exciting LGNd neurons, inhibits the TRN. The influence of ACh and NE, directly and by way of the TRN, can account for changing the firing patterns of LGNd cells in the wakeful state, i.e., favoring the accurate transfer of information to the cortex. In fact, a role for ACh in the general increase of LGNd excitability during the waking condition is supported by recent findings in trained rats, where injection of atropine in the TRN altered the flash-evoked response of LGNd neurons in the thirsty-conditioned animal but not in the satiated relaxed state presumed to be of decreased vigilance (188). The role of the serotoninergic system, which also is activated in wakefulness, may relate more to the depression of spontaneous background activity during stimulus-specific responses thereby increasing the signal-to-noise ratio.

Hypothalamus

Another possible source of diencephalic input to the LGNd is the hypothalamus. HRP injected into the cat LGNd resulted in the labeling of cells bilaterally near the surface in the tuberal region, just lateral to the fornical columns (189). Apparently this finding was not pursued further, and no information on the chemical nature of this projection is available.

LGNd Intrinsic Components

It has been well established that the LGNd contains two major neuronal classes: the long-axoned principal cells projecting to the cortex (P cells) and the short-axoned interneurons that participate in local circuits (I-cells). The subcellular characteristics that differentiate the two types have recently been delineated in the monkey (190) and are illustrated in Fig. 5. A highly significant feature of I-cells is the ubiquitous presence of synaptic vesicles, so that any portion of the neuron, i.e., the soma, dendritic shaft and appendages, axon initial segment, and axon terminals may exhibit presynaptic sites. The existence of "presynaptic dendrites" gives origin to triadic, serial, and reciprocal synaptic arrangements (191–194), some of which include I-cell to I-cell synapses (195).

P-cells

The chemical specification of P-cells is still a matter of conjecture. There are some indications in the cat that GLU/ASP might be playing a role in geniculocortical transmission, mostly based on the suppressive effect of locally applied kynurenic acid on the responses of cortical neurons to visual stimuli or the application of GLU or ASP (196). The effect is maximal on cells with simple receptive fields that are located in layer IV and superficial VI and are known to receive the input from LGNd cells. These results have been confirmed and extended to include responses elicited by LGNd stimulation, particularly those of 1- to 2-msec latency, suggesting monosynaptic connectivity (197). Moreover, it appears that geniculocortical transmission is mediated by GLU/ASP acting on "non-NMDA" receptors because APV, a selective blocker of NMDA receptors (see section on retinal source, p. 43), suppressed only a few of the cortical cells tested. There is some evidence, however, against considering GLU/ASP as neurotransmitters in this pathway. It comes from the failure to label geniculate cells by retrograde transport of tritiated D-GLU or D-ASP injected into the cat visual cortex (79). When the injection is made into the LGNd, there is a diffuse labeling of cortical layer IV, the origin of which has been interpreted as collaterals of strongly labeled layer VI pyramidal cells. This opposing view has been questioned on the basis that the uptake and/or transport of tritiated putative neurotransmitters may not occur in some systems known to utilize the particular neuroactive substance (198).

The possibility has also been raised that NAAG may be an excitatory transmitter in the geniculocortical pathway (58). This view, however, is not supported by the proposed action of NAAG as a selective activator of NMDA receptors ([53], but see [48]) and the very low levels of NAAG in samples from monkey striate cortex centered on layer IV (Molinar and Pasik, *unpublished observations*).

Layer IV, the geniculorecipient site of the striate cortex, is strongly positive for AChE. The reaction does not reside in terminals from LGNd cells, however, because the stain persists after kainic acid lesions of the LGNd or after long survival eye enucleation (74). Only lesions of nucleus basalis succeed in

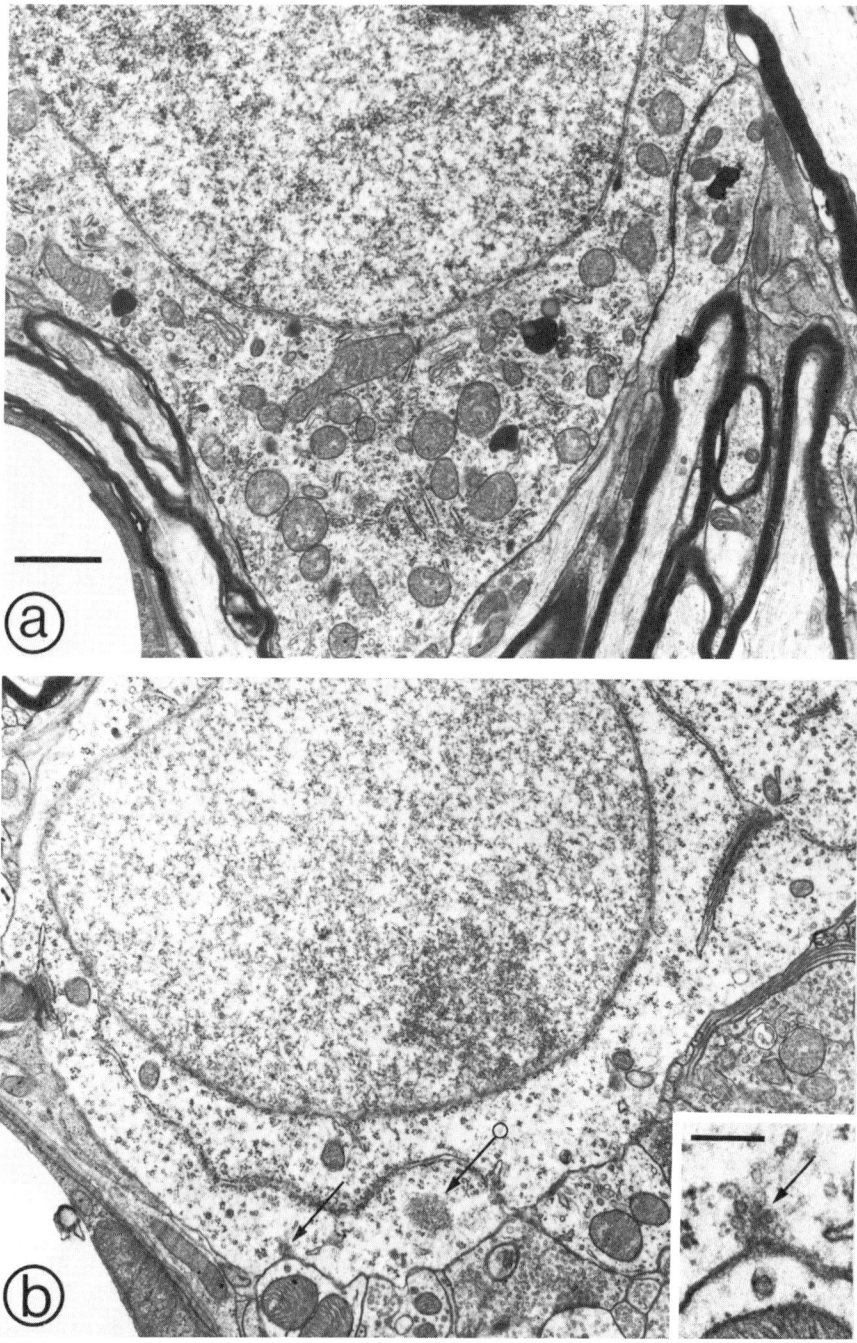

FIG. 5. Two neuronal types in the monkey LGNd. **a:** P-cell, rich in organelles including rough ER and large mitochondria; this is the cell type that shows signs of retrograde degeneration after ablation of striate cortex. **b:** I-cell with pale matrix, few scattered ER cisterns and polyribosomes, much smaller mitochondria than those of the P cells, a cluster of synaptic vesicles (*arrow*), better seen at higher magnification in the inset, and a finely granulated body (*ringed arrow*). Scales: 1 μm applies to (a) and (b); 0.25 μm in the inset. (From ref. 190.)

eliminating it (199), which pinpoints this nucleus as the sole source of cholinergic innervation of the visual cortex.

An intriguing new idea has recently arisen based on autoradiographic electron microscopic studies after injection of tritiated amino acids in the cat LGNd. There appear to be two types of LGNd P-cells: those with terminal boutons in layer IV containing round vesicles and forming asymmetric synapses and others with pleomorphic vesicles and establishing symmetric synaptic contacts (200). Since the latter boutons are very similar to those labeled for GABA in other studies, the authors argue that they may be inhibitory terminals of a certain class of small LGNd projecting neurons. Their very fine axons may fail to transport HRP retrogradely from the cortex, which could be the reason for their not being labeled after cortical injections of the enzyme (173,201,202). Leaving aside the issue of chemical specificity, the idea of another type of P-cell has been entertained earlier regarding the projection of the LGNd to prestriate cortex (203–205), and some of the possible morphologic features of these neurons have been recently reported (201,206).

Finally, it has been found in the rat that approximately 25% of retrogradely labeled LGNd cells from deposits of fluorescent tracers into the striate cortex also exhibit immunoreactivity to a cholecystokinin antibody (207). Although the finding argues in favor of some geniculocortical pathways containing this peptide, the authors considered the possibility that the antibody used recognized a product derived from the local colchicine treatment. In a subsequent study in the hamster and rat, only extraperikaryal immunostaining was reported (208) in the LGNd.

I-cells

Contrary to the uncertainty about the chemical specificity of P-cells, the I-cells are unequivocally GABAergic and responsible for the feedforward inhibition of P-cells. This long-suspected view found early support in the finding of small neurons in laminae A and A_1 of the cat LGNd, which accumulated tritiated GABA deposited less than 2 mm away (209). These cells did not contain laminar bodies, the presence of which was considered a property of P-cells. At the ultrastructural level, labeled terminals were observed to be postsynaptic to other unlabeled profiles of presumed retinal or cortical origin and presynaptic to P-cell dendrites and other labeled elements. Ample confirmation of this interpretation was obtained in several species by the immunocytochemical localization of GAD (rat [172], cat [173,174], monkey [175]). These authors described immunoreactive small, ovoid cells, some of bipolar appearance, with long dendrites bearing appendages, i.e., similar to the I-cells of Golgi preparations, as well as numerous puncta and fiber plexuses in all regions of the LGNd. In the cat, the clusters of terminals were more abundant in the A laminae and although most were of small size, 14% were of medium range, raising the possibility of two classes of I-cells related to the X- and Y-varieties. Moreover, the interneuronal nature of these cells was verified by the lack of double labeling with HRP injected into the visual cortex (173). In the monkey, the immunoreactivity was heaviest in the magnocellular laminae and some dendrites were seen crossing laminar boundaries. These same studies reported on the fine structure of labeled elements. GAD+ neurons had characteristically indented nuclei, and labeled boutons contained pleomorphic vesicles and were postsynaptic to presumably retinal and cortical terminals and presynaptic to P-cell dendrites. Some of these arrangements were triadic or serial in nature, and synaptic articulations between two labeled profiles were also seen. In the cat, an additional type of GAD+ terminal was described as being exclusively presynaptic and present only in the extraglomerular neuropil.

Possible problems involved in using the localization of the enzyme as opposed to the neuroactive substance itself (for discussion of this issue, see [210]) were superseded by the availability of antibodies recognizing GABA. Most of the findings of GAD immunoreactivity were confirmed with the use of direct GABA antibodies at the light microscopy level in the mouse and rat (47,211), cat (212,213), and monkey (202,214,215). In some of these studies, the use of postembedding immunocytochemistry made on 1-μm sections allowed the estimate of the proportion of GABA+ neurons, which was found to be 27% in the A laminae of the cat (213) and 22% in the rat (216). In the monkey, 35% and 25% of the neurons in magnocellular and parvocellular laminae, respectively, were immunostained (202). The latter figures, based on a single monkey, appear to be too high, particularly when compared with results using other methods of estimating the proportion of I-cells (190) and after considering the possible existence of some GABAergic P-cells (see section on P-cells, p. 65). Strong support for the interneuronal nature of most GABA+ cells is given by the findings in both the cat and monkey that these neurons do not contain HRP label in specimens with visual cortex injections of this enzyme (201,202). Furthermore, immunoreactivity was present in neurons previously identified in Golgi material as belonging to I-cells in both the rat (217) and cat (218). When silver was removed by gold-toning, the ultrastructural features of dendritic appendages and axon-like processes belonging to these cells were examined in the cat. They were found to contain pleomorphic vesicles and to be postsynaptic to terminals of the same nature plus others of presumably retinal, cortical, and PGN origin and presynaptic to dendrites of probably P- and I-cells. Although not illustrated, it was noted that the I-cell immunoreactive profiles entered into triadic synaptic arrangements. This feature can be clearly seen in Fig. 4a, taken from monkey material also processed with a direct GABA antibody (215).

Immunocytochemistry has also contributed to delineating some developmental aspects of the LGNd GABAergic systems. GAD+ cells appear in the fetal cat on embryonic day (E) 49 in the PGN and the C layers and only on

E56 in the A laminae. Post-natally, there is a progressive increase in the latter region coinciding with a decrease in the PGN and C laminae, reaching the adult pattern by the third month (177). It is of interest that GAD activity in the rat was found to increase from birth to 2 to 3 weeks but declined thereafter, stabilizing by 11 to 21 weeks (73,219). There are also physiologic and pharmacologic indications that the GABA inhibitory system in the cat begins to function only at 40 to 45 days after birth and reaches maturity by 100 days (220). In the human, GABA+ neurons are absent in 10- to 15-week fetuses and are observed for the first time at 21 weeks as scattered cells in the superficial regions, suggesting an early appearance in magnocellular segments, although no clear lamination is present at this stage (221). It should be noted that in the monkey, postsynaptic profiles containing synaptic vesicles, which presumably belong to GABAergic I-cells, are present at birth but become presynaptic only after 2 weeks (222).

Understanding GABA-mediated inhibitory processes in the LGNd has been greatly advanced by combined physiologic and pharmacologic studies, most of which have used the blocking action of bicuculline to identify GABA mechanisms. The role of the input from the vTRN and PGN, responsible for the recurrent type, has been discussed earlier (see section on diencephalic sources, p. 59). The relevant issue here is the participation of intrinsic interneurons as the source of the feedforward inhibition of P-cells, which is triggered by the retinal input. Initially, it was reported in the cat and rat that iontophoretically applied GABA suppressed the spontaneous discharge of P-cells as well as that evoked by excitatory amino acids and orthodromic and antidromic activation (223,224). As expected, these effects were blocked by bicuculline, which also suppressed the inhibition of P-cells elicited by stimulation of the contralateral eye (223,225). In the cat, GABA mediates visually elicited inhibitory processes in all types of geniculate cells, i.e., X- and Y-cells with on and off receptive field centers, since all are blocked by bicuculline (226). Furthermore, these authors demonstrated that application of this compound resulted in the persistence of the response of geniculate cells to a spot stimulus large enough to encompass the off surround of an on-center receptive field. Similarly, when the off surround was stimulated exclusively, bicuculline produced a strong excitation. Since these phenomena did not occur in retinal ganglion cells, they concluded that the GABA-mediated surround antagonism is generated in the LGNd resulting in much sharper attenuation of responses with increases in spot size. In fact, bicuculline made the geniculate cell responses resemble those of ganglion cells. Finally, by using annular stimuli it was shown that GABA inhibition sharpened the definition of the center-surround border of the receptive field. Another role for this mechanism is to increase the orientation bias of geniculate cells to slowly moving long lines with respect to their retinal counterparts, a phenomenon again abolished by bicuculline (227). In addition to the increases in the spontaneous and evoked discharges of X- and Y-geniculate cells, bicuculline augments the discharge frequency as a function of the contrast of stimulus gratings, an effect that does not occur under normal conditions (228). Moreover, it increases the slope of the contrast response curve of X- but not Y-cells and abolishes the low-frequency attenuation of the X-cell response leaving the function of the Y-cells intact. These results suggest that in the cat the X-cell system is more influenced by LGNd inhibitory mechanisms than the Y-cell system.

The molecular basis for the GABA role in the synaptic transactions at the LGNd are being clarified to some extent by recent studies on the existence and distribution of GABA receptors. At least two types have been considered: the $GABA_A$ and the $GABA_B$. Bicuculline blocks the former and is inactive on the latter (229). Therefore, all the GABA mechanisms reviewed in the previous paragraph must result from action on $GABA_A$ receptors, which leads to a Ca^{2+}-independent increase in Cl^- conductance. Indeed, studies in the rat have shown a high density of this receptor type in the LGNd as labeled with [^{3}H]muscimol, a potent GABA agonist acting on the $GABA_A$ but not the $GABA_B$ receptor (230), or with [^{3}H]GABA in the presence of baclofen and the absence of Ca^{2+}, conditions that only label the $GABA_A$ type (231). Moreover, the use of monoclonal antibodies raised against a purified $GABA_A$ receptor complex demonstrated a high receptor density in the "geniculate nuclei" (232). This technique overcomes some of the disadvantages of autoradiography such as poor resolution due to radiation scatter, ligand specificity, and ligand diffusion away from the binding site.

The mechanism of action of GABA in the LGNd is made more complex by the existence of $GABA_B$ receptors in this structure (231). In fact, the density of $GABA_B$ receptors labeled with [^{3}H]GABA in the presence of isoguvacine to block the $GABA_A$ receptors and of Ca^{2+} is somewhat higher than that of the $GABA_A$ type. The importance of $GABA_B$ receptor mechanisms is beginning to be understood on the basis of the discovery of a long-latency, long-lasting hyperpolarization in geniculate neurons elicited by optic tract stimulation in rat thalamic slices (233,234). This phenomenon, which occurs after the classic short-latency, brief hyperpolarization mediated by GABA acting on $GABA_A$ receptors, was shown to be a real IPSP generated also by I-cells since the preparation did not contain the vTRN. The late IPSP was not blocked by bicuculline and was enhanced by baclofen, a GABA agonist acting at $GABA_B$ sites. Therefore, it was considered the result of activation of the latter receptor type, in turn increasing K^+ conductance. This view was strongly supported by the results, in cat and rat slices, of the application of phaclofen, a new selective GABA antagonist at $GABA_B$ receptors, which inhibited the K^+-dependent, long-lasting IPSP, leaving intact the Cl^--dependent, early, brief response to GABA (235). These studies also showed an enhancing effect of bicuculline on the late inhibitory postsynaptic potential (IPSP), suggesting that the I-cells responsible for it are under the control of other I-cells through $GABA_A$ synapses. We have already noted the existence of synaptic contacts between I-cell dendrites in the monkey LGNd (195). Finally, it was also proposed that the late IPSP may be causing the rhythmic oscillations that characterize P-cell discharges through the action of vTRN GABAergic neurons on the I-cells mediating the $GABA_A$ early IPSP. Possible evidence for such synapses is provided in Fig. 4b. It is of additional interest that in rat hippocampal slices, $GABA_B$ receptors were found to increase K^+ conductance by coupling to the K^+ channel through linkage to a G protein (135), which may explain the long duration of the evoked response. Future immunocytochemical work may help to delineate the location of the $GABA_A$ and $GABA_B$ receptors in different elements of the LGNd neuropil. There are indeed various options for GABAergic synapses: I-cell to P-cell, I-cell to I-cell, vTRN to P-cell, vTRN to I-cell. The possibilities multiply if one considers that presynaptic I-cell elements may be axonic or dendritic, that the latter may participate in triadic, serial, or reciprocal arrangements, and that various receptor types may be present in different regions of the postsynaptic neuron, namely distal versus proximal dendrites, dendritic appendages, and even somata.

Last, it should be mentioned that intraventricular injection of 5,6-dihydroxytryptamine, a selective neurotoxin for serotoninergic neurons, caused extensive damage to a small population of cells in the LGNd of the cat (236). Because electron microscopy revealed only altered somata and dendrites with no signs of degeneration in axons or synaptic terminals, it was concluded that the damaged cells represented a class of interneurons of probably serotoninergic nature. A subsequent immunocytochemical investigation, however, provided only very weak evidence in favor of this view since only one immunoreactive neuron was recognized in the entire study (119).

In summary, there is firm evidence that GABA is the neurotransmitter of LGNd interneurons that mediates feedforward inhibition of P-cells. This type of inhibition imparts essential features to the transforms of visual information reaching the geniculate, such as sharpening of the center-surround antagonism in the receptive fields, increasing the orientation bias of geniculate cells, maintaining the constancy of responses to varying contrasts, and narrowing the tuning characteristics of X-type cells. In addition, the GABAergic interneurons are responsible for the binocular inhibition occurring on stimulation of the contralateral eye. It should be recalled that GABA also mediates the recurrent type of inhibition through the input originating in the PGN and vTRN (see section on diencephalic sources, p. 59).

CONCLUDING REMARKS

The preceding survey allows the formulation of a synthetic view of the functional significance of the LGNd, which can no longer be considered an enigmatic structure. Although some components of this formulation are highly speculative, it is hoped that they will serve as challenges for future research.

The neuronal circuits of the LGNd are activated by the retinal terminals, the majority of which may release acidic dipeptides related to NAAG, acting on some type of GLU receptor. Substance P may coexist in some of these terminals, and this raises the possibility that there may be different classes of retinal endings based on other neuropeptides colocalizing with an acidic dipeptide common to all.

The visual input is transformed in the LGNd, particularly through feedforward inhibitory processes mediated by the I-cells, which utilize GABA acting on $GABA_A$ receptors. These stimulus-specific functions of the LGNd include the generation of a strong surround antagonism in the receptive fields with sharpening of the center-surround border, the increase in the orientation bias to slowly moving long lines, and the maintenance of constancy in the discharge rate to changing contrasts. This type of inhibition contributes also to the fine spatial tuning of the X-cell types and the inhibitory responses occurring on stimulation of the opposite eye, which predominates in the Y-cell system. It is possible that these functions are influenced as well by corticogeniculate pathways, which are glutamergic and contact more distal regions of the P-cell dendritic trees.

In addition to the stimulus-specific transforms, the LGNd networks are under the control of at least three types of input from the brain stem that are activated during wakefulness and exert a more diffuse (nonspecific?) influence on the entire structure, reminiscent of that attributed to the "ascending reticular activating system." (a) A serotoninergic input, originating in the midbrain raphe nuclei, depresses LGNd excitability possibly through direct action on P-cells via $5-HT_1$ receptors and indirectly by exciting GABAergic I-cells via $5-HT_2$ receptors to result in an increase in signal-to-noise ratio while attending to specific stimuli. (b) A cholinergic input from neurons in the PPTN, and perhaps the parabigeminal nucleus, acts mostly on muscarinic receptors to move the membrane potential of geniculate cells away from the bursting firing range, thereby favoring single-spike activity, which increases the precision of information transfer to the cortex during the waking state. (c) A noradrenergic input from the locus ceruleus binding to α_1-receptors has an action similar to the cholinergic one. Finally, these three systems have yet another important nonspecific influence on the LGNd through their action on the TRN/PGN. The neurons of the latter structures, which also receive excitatory inputs from the geniculocortical and corticogeniculate pathways, are responsible for the GABA-mediated recurrent inhibition of geniculate cells and the long-range inhibition extending beyond the receptive fields.

Finally, the majority of the LGNd pathways to the cortex most probably utilize excitatory amino acids, although the existence of GABAergic P-cells has also been proposed. Peptides, such as cholecystokinin, may be present in some of these projections as well.

Many questions still remain unanswered, such as the precise geometry of the inputs onto different regions of the dendritic trees with the consequent interactions of the various neuroactive substances, the function of possible GABAergic cells projecting to the cortex, the significance of the late and prolonged IPSP generated at $GABA_B$ receptor sites, the role of nicotinic receptors, and possible distinctions between the actions of cholinergic and noradrenergic inputs.

ACKNOWLEDGMENTS

The original work of the present survey was supported in part by NIH grants EY-01926, NS-18657, NS-22953, P50 NS-11631, and P30 EY-01867. The skillful assistance of Rosemary Lang and Victor Rodriguez is gratefully acknowledged.

DEDICATION

The authors wish to dedicate this chapter to the memory of Professor Eduardo De Robertis (1913–1988), pioneer in the discovery of the morphologic and chemical bases of neural transmission, inspiring teacher, and beloved friend.

REFERENCES

1. Bunt AH, Hendrickson AE, Lund JS, Lund RD, Fuchs AF. Monkey retinal ganglion cells: morphometric analysis and tracing of axonal projections, with a consideration of the peroxidase technique. *J Comp Neurol* 1975;164:265–285.
2. Hubel DH, Wiesel TN. Integrative action in the cat's lateral geniculate body. *J Physiol (Lond)* 1961;155:385–398.
3. Guillery RN. Patterns of synaptic interconnections in the dorsal lateral geniculate nucleus of cat and monkey: a brief review. *Vision Res* 1971;3(suppl):211–227.
4. Werman R. Criteria for identification of central nervous system transmitter. *Comp Biochem Physiol* 1966;18:743–766.
5. Hoover DB, Muth EA, Jacobowitz DM. A mapping of the distribution of acetylcholine, choline acetyltransferase and acetylcholinesterase in discrete areas of rat brain. *Brain Res* 1978;153:295–306.
6. Loewi O, Hellauer H. Über das Acetylcholin in peripheren Nerven. *Pflugers Arch* 1938; 240:768–775.
7. MacIntosh FC. The distribution of acetylcholine in the peripheral and the central nervous system. *J Physiol (Lond)* 1941;99:436–442.
8. Cobbin LB, Leeder S, Pollard J. Smooth muscle stimulants in extracts of optic nerve and lateral geniculate bodies of sheep. *Br J Pharmacol* 1965;25:295–306.
9. Feldberg W, Vogt M. Acetylcholine synthesis in different regions of the central nervous system. *J Physiol (Lond)* 1948;107:372–381.
10. Hebb CO, Silver A. Choline acetylase in the central nervous system of man and some other mammals. *J Physiol (Lond)* 1956;134:718–728.
11. Deffenu G, Bertaccini G, Pepeu G. Acetylcholine and 5-hydroxytryptamine levels of the lateral geniculate bodies and superior colliculus of cats after visual deafferentation. *Exp Neurol* 1967;17:203–209.
12. Bigl V, Schober W. Cholinergic transmission in subcortical and cortical visual centers of rats: no evidence for the involvement of primary optic system. *Exp Brain Res* 1977;27:211–219.

13. Miller E, Heller A, Moore RY. Acetylcholine in rabbit visual system nuclei after enucleation and visual cortex ablations. *J Pharmacol Exp Ther* 1969;165:117–125.
14. Lund Karlsen R. Neurotransmitters of the mammalian visual system. In: Fonnum F, ed. *Amino acids as chemical transmitters.* New York: Plenum Press, NATO Advance Study Institute Series: Series A, Life Sciences, 1978;16:241–256.
15. Curtis DR, Davis R. The excitation of lateral geniculate neurons by quaternary ammonium derivatives. *J Physiol (Lond)* 1963;165:62–82.
16. Phillis JW, Tebecis AK, York DH. The inhibitory action of monoamines on lateral geniculate neurons. *J Physiol (Lond)* 1967;190:563–581.
17. Matsuoka I, Domino EF. Cholinergic modulation of single lateral geniculate neurons in the cat. *Neuropharmacology* 1972;11:241–251.
18. Kemp JA, Sillito SM. The nature of the excitatory transmitter mediating X- and Y-cell inputs to the cat dorsal lateral geniculate nucleus. *J Physiol (Lond)* 1982;323:377–391.
19. De Lima AD, Montero VM. The cholinergic innervation of the visual thalamus: an EM immunocytochemical study. *Exp Brain Res* 1985;59:206–212.
20. Fitzpatrick D, Raczkowski D. Distribution and morphology of cholinergic axons in the lateral geniculate nucleus and other thalamic nuclei in the cat. *Soc Neurosci Abstr* 1987;13:861.
21. Hayden SA, Mills JW, Masland RM. Acetylcholine synthesis by displaced amacrine cells. *Science* 1980;210:435–437.
22. Curtis DR, Davis R. Pharmacological studies upon neurones of the lateral geniculate nucleus of the cat. *Br J Pharmacol Chemother* 1962;18:217–246.
23. Amin AH, Crawford TBB, Gaddum JH. The distribution of substance P and 5-hydroxytryptamine in the central nervous system of the dog. *J Physiol (Lond)* 1954;126:596–618.
24. Bogdanski DF, Weissbach H, Udenfriend S. The distribution of serotonin, 5-hydroxytryptophan decarboxylase and monoamine oxidase in brain. *J Neurochem* 1957; 1:272–278.
25. Karten HJ, Keyser KT, Brecha NC. Biochemical and morphological heterogeneity of retinal ganglion cells. In: Cohen B, Bodis-Wollner I, eds. *Vision and the brain: the organization of the central visual system.* New York: Raven Press, 1989;19-33.
26. Vogt M. The concentration of sympathin in different parts of the central nervous system under normal conditions and after the administration of drugs. *J Physiol (Lond)* 1954;123:451–481.
27. Versteeg DHG, Van Der Gugten J, De Jong W, Palkovits M. Regional concentrations of noradrenaline and dopamine in rat brain. *Brain Res* 1976;113:563–574.
28. Kromer LF, Moore RY. A study of the organization of the locus coeruleus projections to the lateral geniculate nuclei in the albino rat. *Neuroscience* 1980;5:255–271.
29. Costa E, Green AR, Koslow SH, LeFevre HF, Revuelta AV, Wang C. Dopamine and norepinephrine in noradrenergic axons: a study in vivo of their precursor product relationship by mass fragmentography and radiochemistry. *Pharmacol Rev* 1972;34:167–190.
30. Fonnum F. Glutamate: a neurotransmitter in mammalian brain. *J Neurochem* 1984;42:1–11.
31. Johnson JL, Aprison MH. The distribution of glutamate and total free amino acids in thirteen specific regions of the cat central nervous system. *Brain Res* 1971;26:141–148.
32. Margolis RK, Heller A, Moore RY. Effects of changes in cellular composition following neuronal degeneration on amino acids in brain. *Brain Res* 1968;11:19–31.
33. Davis JM, Himwich JA, Agrawal HC. Some amino acids in the developing visual system. *Dev Psychobiol* 1969;2:34–39.
34. Lund Karlsen R, Fonnum F. Evidence for glutamate as neurotransmitter in the corticofugal fibers to the dorsal lateral geniculate body and the superior colliculus in rats. *Brain Res* 1978;151:457–467.
35. Molinar-Rode R, Pasik P. Possible neurotransmitters in the monkey retinogeniculate pathways. *Soc Neurosci Abstr* 1987;13:1434.
36. Sandberg M, Lindström S. Amino acids in the dorsal lateral geniculate nucleus of the cat: collection in vivo. *J Neurosci Methods* 1983;9:65–74.
37. Morgan R, Vrbova G, Wolstencroft JH. Correlations between the retinal input to lateral geniculate neurons and their relative response to glutamate and aspartate. *J Physiol (Lond)* 1972;224:41P–42P.
38. Tebecis AK. Studies on the identity of the optic nerve transmitter. *Brain Res* 1973;63:31–42.
39. Crunelli V, Kelly JS, Leresche N, Prichio M. On the excitatory post-synaptic potential

evoked by stimulation of the optic tract in the rat lateral geniculate nucleus. *J Physiol (Lond)* 1987;384:603–618.
40. Haby M, Leresche N, Jassik-Gerschenfeld D, Soltesz I, Crunelli V. Dépolarisations rythmiques spontanées dans les cellules principales du corps genouillé latéral in vitro: rôle des récepteurs NMDA. *C R Acad Sci [III]* 1988;306:195–199.
41. Shaw C, Cynader M. Laminar distribution of receptors in monkey (Macaca fascicularis) geniculostriate system. *J Comp Neurol* 1986;248:301–312.
42. Foster AC, Fagg GC. Acidic amino acid binding sites in mammalian neuronal membranes: their characteristics and relationship to synaptic receptors. *Brain Res Rev* 1984;7:103–164.
43. Rainbow TC, Wieczorek CM, Halpain S. Quantitative autoradiography of binding sites for [^{3}H]AMPA, a structural analog of glutamic acid. *Brain Res* 1984;309:173–177.
44. Halpain S, Wieczorek CM, Rainbow TC. Localization of L-glutamate receptors in rat brain by quantitative autoradiography. *J Neurosci* 1984;4:2247–2258.
45. Monaghan DT, Cotman CW. Distribution of N-methyl-D-aspartate-sensitive L-[^{3}H]glutamate binding sites in rat brain. *J Neurosci* 1985;5:2909–2919.
46. Schliebs R, Kullman E, Bigl V. Development of glutamate binding sites in the visual structures of the rat brain. Effect of visual pattern deprivation. *Biomed Biochim Acta* 1986;45:495–506.
47. Ottersen OP, Storm-Mathisen J. Glutamate- and GABA-containing neurons in the mouse and rat brain, as demonstrated with a new immunocytochemical technique. *J Comp Neurol* 1984;229:374–392.
48. Coyle JT, Blakely R, Zaczek R, et al. Acidic peptides in brain: do they act at putative glutamergic synapses? In: Ben-Ari Y, Schwarcz R, eds. *Excitatory amino acids and epilepsy.* New York: Plenum Press, 1986;11:375–384.
49. Curatolo A, d'Arcangelo P, Lino A, Brancati A. Distribution of N-acetyl-aspartic and N-acetyl-aspartyl-glutamic acids in nervous tissue. *J Neurochem* 1965;12:339–342.
50. Reichelt KL, Kvamme E. Acetylated and peptide bound glutamate and aspartate in brain. *J Neurochem* 1967;14:987–996.
51. Reichelt KL, Fonnum F. Subcellular localization of N-acetyl-aspartyl-glutamate, N-acetyl-glutamate and glutathione in brain. *J Neurochem* 1969;16:1409–1416.
52. Koller KJ, Zaczek R, Coyle JT. N-acetyl-aspartyl-glutamate: regional levels in rat brain and the effects of brain lesions as determined by a new HPLC method. *J Neurochem* 1984;43:1136–1142.
53. Westbrook GL, Mayer ML, Namboodiri MAA, Neale JH. High concentrations of N-acetylaspartyl-glutamate (NAAG) selectively activate NMDA receptors on mouse spinal cord neurons in cell culture. *J Neurosci* 1986;6:3385–3392.
54. Riveros N, Orrego F. A study of possible excitatory effects of N-acetylaspartylglutamate in different in vivo and in vitro brain preparations. *Brain Res* 1984;299:393–395.
55. ffrench-Mullen JMH, Koller K, Zaczek R, Coyle JT, Hori N, Carpenter DO. N-acetylaspartylglutamate: possible role as the neurotransmitter of the lateral olfactory tract. *Proc Natl Acad Sci USA* 1985;82:3897–3900.
56. Anderson KJ, Borja MA, Cotman CW, Moffett JR, Namboodiri MAA, Neale JH. N-acetyl-aspartylglutamate identified in the rat retinal ganglion cells and their projections in the brain. *Brain Res* 1987;411:172–177.
57. Anderson KJ, Monaghan DT, Cangro CB, Namboodiri MAA, Neale JH, Cotman CW. Localization of N-acetylaspartylglutamate-like immunoreactivity in selected areas of the rat brain. *Neurosci Lett* 1986;72:14–20.
58. Tieman SB, Cangro CB, Neale JH. N-acetylaspartylglutamate immunoreactivity in neurons of the cat's visual system. *Brain Res* 1987;420:188–193.
59. Tieman SB, Hamilton CR, Vermeire BA, Namboodiri MAA, Neale JH. N-acetylaspartyl-glutamate immunoreactivity in neurons of the monkey's visual pathway. *Soc Neurosci Abstr* 1987;13:992.
60. Brecha N. Retinal neurotransmitters: histochemical and biochemical studies. In: Emson PC, ed. *Chemical neuroanatomy.* New York: Raven Press, 1983;85–129.
61. Winder AF, Patsalos PN. Substance P and retinal neurotransmission. *Biochem Soc Trans* 1974;2:1260–1261.
62. Cooper PE, Fernstrom MH, Rorstad SE, Leeman SE, Martin JB. The regional distribution of somatostatin, substance P and neurotensin in human brain. *Brain Res* 1981;218:219–232.

63. Unger WG, Butler JM, Cole DF, Bloom SR, McGregor GP. Substance P, vasoactive intestinal polypeptide (VIP) and somatostatin levels in ocular tissue of normal and sensorily denervated rabbit eye. *Exp Eye Res* 1981;32:797–801.
64. Kanazawa I, Jessell T. Post mortem changes and regional distribution of substance P in the rat and mouse nervous system. *Brain Res* 1976;117:362–367.
65. Brownstein MJ, Mroz EA, Kizer JS, Palkovits M, Leeman SE. Regional distribution of substance P in the brain of the rat. *Brain Res* 1976;116:299–305.
66. Ljungdahl Å, Hökfelt T, Nilsson G. Distribution of substance P-like immunoreactivity in the central nervous system of the rat. I. Cell bodies and nerve terminals. *Neuroscience* 1978; 3:861–943.
67. Mantyh PW, Kemp JA. The distribution of putative neurotransmitters in the lateral geniculate nucleus of the rat. *Brain Res* 1983;288:344–348.
68. Brecha N, Hendrickson A, Florén I, Karten HJ. Localization of substance P-like immunoreactivity within the monkey retina. *Invest Ophthalmol Vis Sci* 1982;23:147–153.
69. Brecha N, Johnson D, Bolz J, Sharma S, Parnavelas JG, Lieberman AR. Substance P-immunoreactive retinal ganglion cells and their axon terminals in the rabbit. *Nature* 1987; 327:155–158.
70. Krisch B, Leonhardt H. Demonstration of a somatostatin-like activity in retinal cells of the rat. *Cell Tissue Res* 1979;204:127–140.
71. Lund JD, Lund RD, Hendrickson AE, Bunt AH, Fuchs AF. The origin of efferent pathways from the primary visual cortex, Area 17, of the macaque monkey as shown by retrograde transport of horseradish peroxidase. *J Comp Neurol* 1975;164:287–304.
72. Ahlsén G, Grant K, Lindström S. Monosynaptic excitation of principal cells in the lateral geniculate nucleus by corticofugal fibers. *Brain Res* 1982;234:454–548.
73. Kvale I, Fosse VM, Fonnum F. Development of neurotransmitter parameters in the lateral geniculate body, superior colliculus and visual cortex of the albino rat. *Dev Brain Res* 1983;7:137–145.
74. Fosse VM, Heggelund P, Iversen E, Fonnum F. Effects of area 17 ablation on neurotransmitter parameters in efferents to area 18, the lateral geniculate body, pulvinar and superior colliculus in the cat. *Neurosci Lett* 1984;52:323–328.
75. Baughman RW, Gilbert CD. Aspartate and glutamate as possible neurotransmitters in the visual cortex. *Neuroscience* 1981;1:427–439.
76. Fitzpatrick D, Diamond IT. Distribution of acetylcholinesterase in the geniculo-striate system of Galago senegalensis and Aotus trivirgatus: evidence for the origin of the reaction product in the lateral geniculate body. *J Comp Neurol* 1980;194:703–720.
77. Dean AF, Bunch ST, Tolhurst DJ, Lewis PR. The distribution of acetylcholinesterase in the lateral geniculate nucleus of the cat and monkey. *Brain Res* 1982;244:123–134.
78. Mesulam M-M, Mufson EJ, Levey AI, Wainer BH. Atlas of cholinergic neurons in the forebrain and upper brain stem of the macaque based on monoclonal choline acetyltransferase immunohistochemistry and acetylcholinesterase histochemistry. *Neuroscience* 1984;12:669–686.
79. De Lima AD, Singer W. Cholinergic innervation of the cat striate cortex: a choline acetyltransferase immunocytochemical analysis. *J Comp Neurol* 1986;250:824–888.
80. Vizi SE, Palkovits M. Acetylcholine content in different regions of the rat brain. *Brain Res Bull* 1978;3:93–96.
81. Shute CCD, Lewis PR. The ascending cholinergic reticular system: neocortical, olfactory and subcortical projections. *Brain* 1967;90:497–520.
82. Hoover DB, Jacobowitz DM. Neurochemical and histochemical studies of the effect of a lesion of the nucleus cuneiformis on the cholinergic innervation of discrete areas of the rat brain. *Brain Res* 1979;170:113–122.
83. Woolf NJ, Butcher LL. Cholinergic systems in the rat brain: III. Projections from the pontomesencephalic tegmentum of the thalamus, tectum, basal ganglia and basal forebrain. *Brain Res Bull* 1986;16:603–637.
84. Hallanger AE, Levey AI, Lee HJ, Rye DB, Wainer BH. The origin of cholinergic and other subcortical afferents to the thalamus in the rat. *J Comp Neurol* 1987;262:105–124.
85. De Lima AD, Singer W. The brain stem projection to the lateral geniculate nucleus in the cat: identification of cholinergic and monoaminergic elements. *J Comp Neurol* 1987;259:92–121.

86. Kimura H, McGeer PL, Peng JH, McGeer EG. The central cholinergic system studied by choline acetyltransferase immunohistochemistry in the cat. *J Comp Neurol* 1981;200:151–201.
87. Mesulam MM, Mufson EJ, Wainer BH, Levey AI. Central cholinergic pathways in the rat: an overview based on an alternative nomenclature (Ch1–Ch6). *Neuroscience* 1983;10:1185–1201.
88. Mufson EJ, Martin TL, Mash DC, Wainer BH, Mesulam M. Cholinergic projections from the parabigeminal nucleus (Ch8) to the superior colliculus in the mouse: a combined analysis of horseradish peroxidase transport and choline acetyltransferase immunohistochemistry. *Brain Res* 1986;370:144–148.
89. Vincent SR, Reiner PB. The immunohistochemical localization of choline acetyltransferase in the cat brain. *Brain Res* 1987;18:371–415.
90. Lysakowski A, Standage GP, Benevento LA. Histochemical and architectonic differentiation of zones of pretectal and collicular inputs to the pulvinar and dorsal lateral geniculate nuclei in the macaque. *J Comp Neurol* 1986;250:431–448.
91. Stichel CC, Singer W. Organization and morphological characteristics of choline acetyltransferase-containing fibers in the visual thalamus and striate cortex of the cat. *Neuroscience* 1985;53:155–160.
92. Graybiel AM, Ragsdale CW. Pseudocholinesterase staining in the primary visual pathway of the macaque monkey. *Nature* 1982;229:439–442.
93. Sillito AM, Kemp JA, Berardi N. The cholinergic influence on the function of the cat dorsal lateral geniculate nucleus (DLGN). *Brain Res* 1983;280:299–307.
94. Wamsley JK, Zarbin M, Birdsall N, Kuhar MJ. Muscarinic cholinergic receptors: autoradiographic localization of high and low affinity agonist binding sites. *Brain Res* 1980;200:1–12.
95. Dohanich GP, Johnson AE, Nock B, McEwen BS, Feder HH. Distribution of cholinergic muscarinic binding sites in guinea-pig brain as determined by in vitro autoradiography of 3H-N-methylscopolamine binding. *Eur J Pharmacol* 1985;119:9–16.
96. McCormick DA, Prince DA. Acetylcholine induces burst firing in thalamic reticular neurones by activating a potassium conductance. *Nature* 1986;319:402–405.
97. Kobayashi RM, Brownstein M, Saavedra JM, Palkovits M. Choline acetyltransferase content in discrete regions of the rat brain stem. *J Neurochem* 1975;24:637–640.
98. Schliebs R, Bigl V, Biesold D. Development of muscarinic cholinergic receptor binding in the visual system of monocularly deprived and dark reared rats. *Neurochem Res* 1982;7:1181–1198.
99. Rotter A, Birdsall NJM, Burgen ASV, Field PM, Hulme EC, Raisman G. Muscarinic receptors in the central nervous system of the rat. I. Technique for autoradiographic localization of the binding of {3H} propylbenzilylcholine mustard and its distribution in the forebrain. *Brain Res Rev* 1979;1:141–166.
100. McCormick DA, Prince DA. Actions of acetylcholine in the guinea-pig and cat medial and lateral geniculate nuclei, in vitro. *J Physiol (Lond)* 1987;392:147–165.
101. Segal M, Dudai Y, Amsterdam A. Distribution of an alpha-bungarotoxin-binding cholinergic nicotinic receptor in rat brain. *Brain Res* 1978;148:105–119.
102. Hunt S, Schmidt J. Some observations on the binding patterns of alpha-bungarotoxin in the central nervous system of the rat. *Brain Res* 1978;157:213–232.
103. Clarke PBS, Schwartz RD, Paul SM, Pert CB, Pert A. Nicotinic binding in rat brain: autoradiographic comparison of [^{3}H]acetylcholine, [^{3}H]nicotine, and [^{125}I]-α-bungarotoxin. *J Neurosci* 1985;5:1307–1315.
104. Cano J, Reinoso-Suárez F. Postnatal development in the serotonin content of brain visual structures. *Dev Brain Res* 1982;5:199–201.
105. Palkovits M, Brownstein M, Saavedra JM. Serotonin content of the brain stem nuclei in the rat. *Brain Res* 1974;80:237–249.
106. Bobillier P, Petitjean F, Salvert D, Ligier M, Seguin S. Differential projections of the nucleus raphe dorsalis and nucleus raphe centralis as revealed by autoradiography. *Brain Res* 1975;85:205–210.
107. Moore RY, Halaris AE, Jones BE. Serotonin neurons of the midbrain raphe: ascending projections. *J Comp Neurol* 1978;180:417–438.
108. Leger L, Salvert D, Touret M, Jouvet M. Delineation of dorsal lateral geniculate afferents

from the cat brain stem as visualized by the horseradish peroxidase technique. *Brain Res* 1975;93:490-496.
109. Pasquier DA, Villar MJ. Specific serotonergic projections to the lateral geniculate body from the lateral cell groups of the dorsal raphe nucleus. *Brain Res* 1982;249:142-146.
110. Chan-Palay V. Indoleamine neurons and their processes in the normal rat brain and in chronic diet-induced thiamine deficiency demonstrated by uptake of 3H-serotonin. *J Comp Neurol* 1977;176:467-494.
111. Fuxe K. The distribution of monoamine terminals in the central nervous system. *Acta Physiol Scand* 1965;64(suppl 247):38-85.
112. Steinbuch HWM. Distribution of serotonin immunoreactivity in the central nervous system of the rat—cell bodies and terminals. *Neuroscience* 1981;6:557-618.
113. Cropper EC, Eisenman JS, Azmitia EC. An immunocytochemical study of the serotonergic innervation of the thalamus of the rat. *J Comp Neurol* 1984;224:38-50.
114. Luth H-J, Seidel I. Immunohistochemische Charakterisierung serotoninerger Afferenzen im visuellen System der Ratte. *J Hirnforsch* 1987;28:591-600.
115. Ueda S, Sano Y. Distributional pattern of serotonin-immunoreactive nerve fibers in the lateral geniculate nucleus of the rat, cat and monkey (Macaca fuscata). *Cell Tissue Res* 1986;243:249-253.
116. Mize RR, Payne MP. The innervation density of serotonergic (5-HT) fibers varies in different subdivisions of the cat lateral geniculate nucleus complex. *Neuroscience* 1987;82:133-139.
117. De Lima AD, Singer W. The serotoninergic fibers in the dorsal lateral geniculate nucleus of the cat: distribution and synaptic connections demonstrated with immunocytochemistry. *J Comp Neurol* 1987;258:339-351.
118. Pasik T, Pasik P, Holstein GR. Serotonin immunoreactivity in the monkey dorsal lateral geniculate nucleus. *Soc Neurosci Abstr* 1983;9:1047.
119. Pasik P, Pasik T, Holstein GR. Serotonin-immunoreactivity in the monkey lateral geniculate nucleus. *Exp Brain Res* 1988;69:662-666.
120. Morrison JH, Foote SL. Noradrenergic and serotoninergic innervation of cortical, thalamic and tectal visual structures in Old and New World monkeys. *J Comp Neurol* 1986;243:117-138.
121. Evarts EV, Landau W, Freygang W, Marshall WH. Some effects of lysergic acid diethylamide and bufotenine on electrical activity in the cat's visual system. *Am J Physiol* 1955;181:594-598.
122. Bishop PO, Field G, Hennessy BL, Smith JR. Action of D-lysergic acid diethylamide on lateral geniculate synapses. *J Neurophysiol* 1958;21:529-549.
123. Bishop PO, Burke W, Hayhow WR. Lysergic acid diethylamide block of lateral geniculate synapses and relief by repetitive stimulation. *Exp Neurol* 1959;1:556-568.
124. Curtis DR, Davis R. A central action of 5-hydroxytryptamine and noradrenaline. *Nature* 1961;192:1083-1084.
125. Phillis JW. The pharmacology of thalamic and geniculate neurons. *Int Rev Neurobiol* 1971;14:1-48.
126. Tebecis AK, Di Maria A. A re-evaluation of the mode of action of 5-hydroxy-tryptamine on lateral geniculate neurons: comparison with catecholamines and LSD. *Exp Brain Res* 1972;14:480-493.
127. Kemp JA, Roberts HC, Sillito AM. Further studies on the action of 5-hydroxytryptamine in the dorsal lateral geniculate nucleus of the cat. *Brain Res* 1982;246:334-337.
128. Yoshida M, Sasa M, Takori S. Serotonin-mediated inhibition from dorsal raphe nucleus neurons in dorsal lateral geniculate and thalamic reticular nuclei. *Brain Res* 1984;290:95-105.
129. Satinsky D. Pharmacological responsiveness of lateral geniculate nucleus neurons. *Int J Neuropharmacol* 1967;6:387-397.
130. Rinaldi P, Sutko M, Mahnke JH, Verzeano M. Serotonin in the lateral geniculate. *Physiol Behav* 1975;14:95-102.
131. Foote WE, Maciewicz RJ, Mordes JP. Effect of midbrain raphe and lateral mesencephalic stimulation on spontaneous and evoked activity in the lateral geniculate of the cat. *Exp Brain Res* 1974;18:124-130.
132. Rogawski MA, Aghajanian GK. Norepinephrine and serotonin: opposite effects on the

activity of lateral geniculate nucleus evoked by optic pathway stimulation. *Exp Neurol* 1980;69:678–694.
133. Pazos A, Cortéz R, Palacios JM. Quantitative autoradiographic mapping of serotonin receptors in the rat brain. II. Serotonin-2 receptors. *Brain Res* 1985;346:231–249.
134. Pazos A, Palacios JM. Quantitative autoradiographic mapping of serotonin receptors in the rat brain. I. Serotonin-1 receptors. *Brain Res* 1985;346:205–230.
135. Andrade R, Malenka RC, Nicoll RA. A G protein couples serotonin and GABAb receptors to the same channels in hippocampus. *Science* 1986;234:1261–1265.
136. Andén NE, Dahlstrom A, Fuxe K, Larsson K, Olson L, Ungerstedt U. Ascending monoamine neurons to the telencephalon and diencephalon. *Acta Physiol Scand* 1966; 67:313–326.
137. Lindvall O, Björklund A, Nobin A, Stenevi U. The adrenergic innervation of the rat thalamus as revealed by the glyoxilic acid fluorescence method. *J Comp Neurol* 1974; 154:317–348.
138. Stenevi U, Björkland A, Moore RY. Growth of intact central adrenergic axons in the denervated lateral geniculate body. *Exp Neurol* 1972;35:290–299.
139. Jones BE, Moore RY. Ascending projections of the locus ceruleus in the rat. II. Autoradiographic study. *Brain Res* 1977;127:23–53.
140. Luth H-J, Schober W, Winkelmann E, Berger U. Die catecholaminergen Verbindungen im visuellen System der Albinoratte. *Acta Histochem* 1978;63:114–126.
141. Mackay-Sim A, Sefton AJ, Martin PR. Subcortical projections to lateral geniculate and thalamic reticular nuclei in the hooded rat. *J Comp Neurol* 1983;213:24–35.
142. Swanson LW, Hartman BK. The central adrenergic system: an immunofluorescence study of the location of cell bodies and their efferent connections in the rat utilizing dopamine-beta-hydroxylase as a marker. *J Comp Neurol* 1975;163:467–506.
143. Hughes HC, Mullikin WH. Brain afferents to the lateral geniculate nucleus of the cat. *Exp Brain Res* 1984;54:253–258.
144. Ishikawa M, Tanaka C. Morphological organization of catecholamine terminals in the diencephalon of the rhesus monkey. *Brain Res* 1977;119:43–55.
145. Luth HJ, Brauer K, Winkelmann E. Ultrastrukturelle und histochemische Untersuchungen zur Afferenztopistik der Geniculo-corticalen Relaiszelle (GCR-zelle). *J Hirnforsch* 1980; 21:39–51.
146. Nakai Y, Takaori S. Influence of norepinephrine-containing neurons derived from the locus coeruleus on lateral geniculate neuronal activities of cats. *Brain Res* 1974;71:47–60.
147. Kayama T, Negi T, Sugitani M, Iwama K. Effects of locus coeruleus stimulation on neuronal activities of dorsal lateral geniculate nucleus and perigeniculate reticular nucleus of the rat. *Neuroscience* 1982;7:655–666.
148. Rogawski MA, Aghajanian GK. Modulation of lateral geniculate neurone excitability by noradrenaline microiontophoresis or locus coeruleus stimulation. *Nature* 1980;287:731–734.
149. Rogawski MA, Aghajanian GK. Activation of lateral geniculate neurons by norepinephrine: mediation by an alpha-adrenergic receptor. *Brain Res* 1980;182:345–359.
150. Rogawski MA, Aghajanian GK. Activation of lateral geniculate neurons by locus coeruleus or dorsal noradrenergic bundle stimulation: selective blockade by the α_1 adrenoceptor antagonist prazosin. *Brain Res* 1982;250:31–39.
151. Jones LS, Gauger LL, Davis JN. Anatomy of brain α_1 adrenergic receptors: in vitro autoradiography with [125I]-HEAT. *J Comp Neurol* 1985;231:190–208.
152. Kemp JA, Downes CP. Noradrenaline-stimulated inositol phospholipid breakdown in rat dorsal lateral geniculate nucleus neurones. *Brain Res* 1986;371:314–318.
153. McCormick DA, Prince DA. Noradrenergic modulation of firing pattern in guinea pig and cat thalamic neurons, in vitro. *J Neurophysiol* 1986;59:978–996.
154. Sherman SM, Koch C. The control of retinogeniculate transmission in the mammalian lateral geniculate nucleus. *Exp Brain Res* 1986;63:1–20.
155. Graybiel AM, Berson DM. Autoradiographic evidence for a projection from the pretectal nucleus of the optic tract to the dorsal lateral geniculate complex in the cat. *Brain Res* 1980;195:1–12.
156. Torrealba F, Partlow GD, Guillery RW. Organization of the projection from the superior colliculus to the dorsal lateral geniculate nucleus of the cat. *Neuroscience* 1981;7: 1341–1360.

157. Fitzpatrick D, Carey RG, Diamond LT. The projection of the superior colliculus upon the lateral geniculate body in Tupaia glis and Galago senegalensis. *Brain Res* 1980;194:494-499.
158. Benevento LA, Fallon JH. The ascending projections of the superior colliculus in the rhesus monkey (Macaca mulatta). *J Comp Neurol* 1975;160:339-362.
159. Harting JK, Casagrande VA, Weber JT. The projection of the primate superior colliculus upon the dorsal lateral geniculate nucleus: autoradiographic demonstration of interlaminar distribution of tectogeniculate axons. *Brain Res* 1987;150:593-599.
160. Harting JK, Huerta MF, Frankfurter AJ, Strominger NL, Royce JG. Ascending pathways from the monkey superior colliculus: an autoradiographic analysis. *J Comp Neurol* 1980; 192:853-862.
161. Jones EG. Some aspects of the organization of the thalamic reticular complex. *J Comp Neurol* 1975;162:285-308.
162. Ahlsén G, Lindström S, Sybirska E. Subcortical axon collaterals of principal cells in the lateral geniculate body of the cat. *Brain Res* 1978;156:106-109.
163. Friedlander MJ, Lin CS, Stanford LR, Sherman MS. Morphology of functionally identified neurons in lateral geniculate nucleus of the cat. *J Neurophysiol* 1981;46:80-129.
164. Ohara PT, Sefton AJ, Lieberman AR. Mode of termination of afferents from the thalamic reticular nucleus in the dorsal lateral geniculate nucleus of the rat. *Brain Res* 1980;197: 503-506.
165. Montero VM, Scott GL. Synaptic terminals in the dorsal lateral geniculate nucleus from neurons of the thalamic reticular nucleus: a light and electron microscope autoradiographic study. *Neuroscience* 1981;6:2561-2577.
166. Hale PT, Sefton JA, Baur LA, Cottee LJ. Interrelations of the rat's thalamic reticular and dorsal lateral geniculate nuclei. *Exp Brain Res* 1982;45:217-229.
167. Ahlsén G, Lo F-S. Projection of brain stem neurons to the perigeniculate nucleus and the lateral geniculate nucleus in the cat. *Brain Res* 1982;238:433-438.
168. Sotgiu ML, Marini G, Esposti D, Fava E. A horseradish peroxidase study of afferent projections to nucleus reticularis thalami in the cat. *Arch Ital Biol* 1981;119:151-159.
169. Berry DJ, Ohara PT, Jeffery G, Lieberman AR. Are there connections between the thalamic reticular nucleus and the brain stem reticular formation? *J Comp Neurol* 1986; 243:347-362.
170. Levey AI, Hallanger AE, Wainer BH. Choline acetyltransferase immunoreactivity in the rat thalamus. *J Comp Neurol* 1987;257:317-332.
171. Houser CR, Vaughn JE. GABA neurons are the major cell type of the nucleus reticularis thalami. *Brain Res* 1980;200:341-354.
172. Ohara PT, Lieberman AR, Hunt SP, Wu J-Y. Neuronal elements containing glutamic acid decarboxylase (GAD) in the dorsal lateral geniculate nucleus of the rat: immunohistochemical studies by light and electron microscopy. *Neuroscience* 1983;8:189-211.
173. Fitzpatrick GR, Penny GR, Schmechel DE. Glutamic acid decarboxylase-immunoreactive neurons and terminals in the lateral geniculate nucleus of the cat. *J Neurosci* 1984;4:1809-1829.
174. Montero VM, Singer W. Ultrastructure and synaptic relations of neural elements containing glutamic acid decarboxylase (GAD) in the perigeniculate nucleus of the cat. *Exp Brain Res* 1984;56:115-125.
175. Hendrickson AE, Ogren MP, Vaughn JE, Barber RP, Wu J-Y. Light and electron microscopic immunocytochemical localization of glutamic acid decarboxylase in monkey geniculate complex: evidence for gabaergic neurons and synapses. *J Neurosci* 1983;3:1245-1262.
176. Montero VM, Singer W. Ultrastructural identification of somata and neural processes immunoreactive to antibodies against glutamic acid decarboxylase (GAD) in the dorsal lateral geniculate nucleus of the cat. *Exp Brain Res* 1985;59:151-165.
177. Shotwell SL, Shatz CJ, Luskin ML. Development of glutamic acid decarboxylase immunoreactivity in the cat's lateral geniculate nucleus. *J Neurosci* 1986;6:1410-1423.
178. Sumitomo I, Nakamura M, Iwama K. Location and function of the so-called interneurons of rat lateral geniculate body. *Exp Neurol* 1976;51:110-123.
179. Yingling CD, Skinner JE. Selective regulation of thalamic sensory relay nuclei by nucleus reticularis thalami. *Electroencephalogr Clin Neurophysiol* 1976;41:476-482.
180. Kayama Y. Ascending, descending and local control of neuronal activity in the rat lateral geniculate nucleus. *Vision Res* 1985;25:339-347.

181. Ahlsén G, Lindström S, Lo F-S. Interaction between inhibitory pathways to principal cells in the lateral geniculate nucleus of the cat. *Exp Brain Res* 1985;58:134–143.
182. Dubin MW, Cleland BG. Organization of visual inputs to interneurons of lateral geniculate nucleus of the cat. *J Neurophysiol* 1977;40:410–427.
183. Kayama Y, Shosaku A, Doty RW. Cryogenic blockage of the visual cortico-thalamic projection in the rat. *Exp Brain Res* 1984;54:157–165.
184. Godfraind JM. Acetylcholine and somatically evoked inhibition on perigeniculate neurones in the cat. *Br J Pharmacol* 1978;63:295–302.
185. Eysel UT, Pape H-C, Van Schayck R. Excitatory and differentially disinhibitory actions of acetylcholine in the lateral geniculate nucleus of the cat. *J Physiol (Lond)* 1986;370:233–254.
186. Hammer R, Berrie CP, Birdsall NJM, Burgen ASV, Hulme EC. Pirenzepine distinguishes between different subclasses of muscarinic receptors. *Nature* 1980;283:90–92.
187. Ahlsén G. Brain stem neurones with differential projection to functional subregions of the dorsal lateral geniculate complex in the cat. *Neuroscience* 1984;12:817–838.
188. Albrecht D, Davidowa H, Gabriel HJ. Influence of atropine microinjection into nucleus reticularis thalami on activity of lateral geniculate nucleus neurones in freely moving rats. *Behav Brain Res* 1986;19:49–57.
189. Sakai K, Leger L, Salvert D, Touret M, Jouvet M. Mise en évidence d'une projection directe des aires hypothalamiques vers le corps genouillé latéral et le cortext visuel chez le chat par la technique de peroxydase. *Experientia* 1975;31:1350–1352.
190. Hámori J, Pasik P, Pasik T. Differential frequency of P-cells and I-cells in the magnocellular and parvocellular laminae of monkey lateral geniculate nucleus. An ultrastructural study. *Exp Brain Res* 1983;52:57–66.
191. Famiglietti Jr EV, Peters A. The synaptic glomerulus and the intrinsic neuron in the dorsal lateral geniculate nucleus of the cat. *J Comp Neurol* 1972;144:285–334.
192. Lieberman AR. Neurons with presynaptic perikarya and presynaptic dendrites in the rat lateral geniculate nucleus. *Brain Res* 1973;59:35–59.
193. Hámori J, Pasik T, Pasik P, Szentágothai J. Triadic synaptic arrangements and their possible significance in the lateral geniculate nucleus of the monkey. *Brain Res* 1974;80:379–393.
194. Hámori J, Pasik T, Pasik P. Electron-microscopic identification of axonal initial segments belonging to interneurons in the dorsal lateral geniculate nucleus of the monkey. *Neuroscience* 1978;3:403–412.
195. Pasik P, Pasik T, Hámori J. Synapses between interneurons in the lateral geniculate nucleus of monkeys. *Exp Brain Res* 1976;25:1–13.
196. Tsumoto T, Masui H, Sato H. Excitatory amino acid transmitters in neuronal circuits of the cat visual cortex. *J Neurophysiol* 1986;55:469–483.
197. Hagihara K, Tsumoto T, Sato H, Hata Y. Actions of excitatory amino acid antagonists on geniculo-cortical transmission in the cat's visual cortex. *Exp Brain Res* 1988;69:407–416.
198. Wiklund L, Künzle H, Cuénod M. Failure to demonstrate retrograde labelling of cerebellar Purkinje cells after injection of [^{3}H]GABA in Deiters' nucleus. *Neurosci Lett* 1983;38:23–28.
199. Bear MF, Carnes KM, Ebner FF. An investigation of cholinergic circuitry in cat striate cortex using acetylcholinesterase histochemistry. *J Comp Neurol* 1985;234:411–430.
200. Einstein G, Davis LT, Sterling P. Ultrastructure of synapses from the A-laminae of the lateral geniculate nucleus in layer IV of the cat striate cortex. *J Comp Neurol* 1987;260:63–75.
201. Montero VM. The interneuronal nature of GABAergic neurons in the lateral geniculate nucleus of the rhesus monkey: a combined HRP and GABA-immunocytochemical study. *Exp Brain Res* 1986;64:615–622.
202. Montero VM, Zempel J. The proportion and size of GABA-immunoreactive neurons in the magnocellular and parvocellular layers of the lateral geniculate nucleus of the rhesus monkey. *Exp Brain Res* 1986;62:215–223.
203. Wong-Riley MTT. Projections from the dorsal lateral geniculate nucleus to prestriate cortex in the squirrel monkey as demonstrated by retrograde transport of horseradish peroxidase. *Brain Res* 1976;109:595–600.
204. Yukie M, Iwai E. Direct projection from the dorsal lateral geniculate nucleus to the prestriate cortex in macaque monkeys. *J Comp Neurol* 1981;201:81–97.
205. Yoshida K, Benevento LA. The projection from the dorsal lateral geniculate nucleus of the

thalamus to extrastriate visual association cortex in the macaque monkey. *Neurosci Lett* 1981;22:103–108.
206. Pasik P, Pasik T, Hámori J. A newly recognized element in the monkey dorsal lateral geniculate nucleus exhibiting both presynaptic and postsynaptic sites. *J Neurocytol* 1986; 15:177–186.
207. Fallon JH, Seroogy KB. Visual and auditory pathways contain cholecystokinin: evidence from immunofluorescence and retrograde tracing. *Neurosci Lett* 1984;45:81–87.
208. Miceli MO, Van-der-Kooy D, Post CA, Della-Fera MA, Baile CA. Differential distributions of cholecystokinin in hamster and rat forebrain. *Brain Res* 1987;402:318–330.
209. Sterling P, Davis TL. Neurons in cat geniculate nucleus that concentrate exogenous [^{3}H]-gamma-aminobutyric acid (GABA). *J Comp Neurol* 1980;192:737–749.
210. Hodgson AJ, Penke B, Erdei A, Chubb WI, Somogyi P. Antisera to γ-aminobutyric acid. I. Production and characterization using a new model system. *J Histochem Cytochem* 1985;33:229–239.
211. Gabbott PLA, Somogyi J, Stewart MG, Hámori J. GABA-immunoreactive neurons in the rat dorsal lateral geniculate nucleus: light microscopical observations. *Brain Res* 1985; 346:171–175.
212. Montero VM, Zempel J. Evidence for two types of GABA-containing interneurons in the A-laminae of the cat lateral geniculate nucleus: a double-label HRP and GABA-immunocytochemical study. *Exp Brain Res* 1985;60:603–609.
213. Madarász M, Somogyi G, Somogyi J, Hámori J. Numerical estimation of gamma-aminobutyric acid (GABA)-containing neurons in three thalamic nuclei of the cat: direct GABA immunocytochemistry. *Neurosci Lett* 1985;61:73–78.
214. Pasik P, Pasik T, Hámori J, Holstein G. GABA-immunoreactivity in monkey lateral geniculate nucleus (LGN) at light and electron microscopic levels. *Soc Neurosci Abstr* 1985;11:317.
215. Pasik P, Pasik T, Hámori J, Holstein GR. Light and electron microscopic visualization of GABAergic elements in the monkey brain by means of a direct GABA antibody. In: Racagni G, Donoso AO, eds. *GABA in endocrine function*. New York: Raven Press, *Adv Biochem Psychopharm* 1986;42:13–24.
216. Gabbott PLA, Somogyi J, Stewart MG, Hámori J. A quantitative investigation of the neuronal composition of the rat dorsal lateral geniculate nucleus using GABA-immunocytochemistry. *Neuroscience* 1986;19:101–111.
217. Gabbott PLA, Somogyi J, Stewart MG, Hámori J. GABA-immunoreactive neurons in the dorsal lateral geniculate nucleus of the rat: characterization by combined Golgi-impregnation and immunocytochemistry. *Exp Brain Res* 1986;61:311–322.
218. Montero VM. Localization of γ-aminobutyric acid (GABA) in type 3 cells and demonstration of their source to F2 terminals in the cat lateral geniculate nucleus: a Golgi-electron-microscopic GABA-immunocytochemical study. *J Comp Neurol* 1986;254:228–245.
219. McDonald JK, Speciale SG, Parnavelas JG. The development of glutamic acid decarboxylase in the visual cortex and the dorsal lateral geniculate nucleus of the rat. *Brain Res* 1981;217:364–367.
220. Berardi N, Morrone CM. Development of γ-aminobutyric acid mediated inhibition of X cells in the cat lateral geniculate nucleus. *J Physiol (Lond)* 1984;357:525–537.
221. Wadhwa S, Hámori J, Bijlani V. Immunohistochemical localization of GABAergic cells in the developing human dorsal lateral geniculate nucleus. *Neurosci Lett* 1985;61:97–101.
222. Hámori J, Pasik P, Pasik T. Postnatal differentiation of "presynaptic dendrites" in the lateral geniculate nucleus of the rhesus monkey. In: Kreutzberg GW, ed. *Physiology and pathology of dendrites*. New York: Raven Press, *Adv Neurol* 1975;12:149–161.
223. Curtis DR, Tebecis KA. Bicuculline and thalamic inhibition. *Exp Brain Res* 1972;16:210–218.
224. Kayama Y, Hsiao C-F, Fukuda Y, Iwama K. Sensitivity to GABA of neurons of the dorsal and ventral lateral geniculate nuclei in the rat. *Brain Res* 1981;211:202–205.
225. Pape H-C, Eysel UT. Binocular interactions in the lateral geniculate nucleus of the cat: GABAergic inhibition reduced by dominant afferent activity. *Exp Brain Res* 1986;61:265–271.
226. Sillito AM, Kemp JA. The influence of GABAergic inhibitory processes of the receptive field structure of X and Y cells in the cat dorsal lateral geniculate nucleus (DLGN). *Brain Res* 1983;277:63–77.

227. Vidyasagar TR. Contribution of inhibitory mechanisms to the orientation sensitivity of cat dLGN neurones. *Exp Brain Res* 1984;55:192–195.
228. Berardi N, Morrone MD. The role of gamma-aminobutyric acid mediated inhibition in the response properties of cat lateral geniculate nucleus neurones. *J Physiol (Lond)* 1984; 357:505–524.
229. Bowery GP, Price GW, Hudson AL, Hill DR, Wilkin GP, Turnbull MJ. GABA receptor multiplicity. Visualization of different receptor types in the mammalian CNS. *Neuropharmacol* 1984;23:219–232.
230. Palacios JM, Wamsley JK, Kuhar MJ. High affinity GABA receptors—autoradiographic localization. *Brain Res* 1981;222:285–307.
231. Bowery NG, Hudson AL, Price GW. GABAa and GABAb receptor site distribution in the rat central nervous system. *Neuroscience* 1987;20:365–383.
232. Richards JG, Schoch P, Haring PL, Takacs B, Mohler H. Resolving GABAa/benzodiazepine receptors: cellular and subcellular localization in the CNS with monoclonal antibodies. *J Neurosci* 1987;7:1866–1886.
233. Hirsch JC, Burnod Y. A synaptically evoked late hyperpolarization in the rat dorsolateral geniculate neurons *in vitro*. *Neuroscience* 1987;23:457–468.
234. Crunelli V, Haby M, Jassik-Gerschenfeld D, Leresche N, Pirchio M. Cl⁻- and K⁺-dependent inhibitory postsynaptic potentials evoked by interneurons of the rat lateral geniculate nucleus. *J Physiol (Lond)* 1988;399:153–176.
235. Soltesz I, Haby M, Leresche N, Crunelli V. The $GABA_B$ antagonist phaclofen inhibits the late K⁺-dependent IPSP in cat and rat thalamic and hippocampal neurones. *Brain Res* 1988;448:351–354.
236. Pecci Saavedra J, Pérez Lloret I. Degeneration of interneurons in the lateral geniculate nucleus after 5,6-dihydroxytryptamine treatment. *Int J Neurosci* 1979;10:15–19.

Note added in proofs. Several articles relevant to the preceding review have appeared in the literature since submission of this chapter. Cholinergic influences on LGNd transmission were reexamined in the cat and found to be in agreement with previous findings of enhancing the excitability of P-cells and inhibiting both the I-cells and PGN neurons. The effects, mostly mediated through muscarinic receptors, appeared to be more marked on X- than on Y-cells (Francesconi et al., *J Neurophysiol* 1988;59:1690–1718). Moreover, the action of ACh on physiologically and morphologically characterized I-cells in slices of cat LGNd was defined as a hyperpolarization through an increase in K⁺ conductance of a muscarinic receptor (McCormick and Pape, *Nature* 1988;334:246–248). The distribution of GABA immunoreactivity in the LGNd of the tree shrew was reported to exhibit a medial to lateral density gradient, suggesting differential inhibitory processes in the on, off, and W pathways (Holdefer et al., *Visual Neurosci* 1988;1:189–204). Finally, another article on the serotoninergic innervation of the monkey LGNd appeared with similar conclusions as those reviewed above, except that no ventral to dorsal density gradient in 5-HT immunoreactivity was observed (Wilson and Hendrickson, *Visual Neurosci* 1988;1:517–539).

Neural Mechanisms Underlying Modifiability of Response Properties in Developing Cat Visual Cortex

M. Cynader, C. Shaw, G. Prusky, and F. Van Huizen

Department of Ophthalmology, University of British Columbia, Vancouver, British Columbia, Canada V5Z 3N9

The past two decades have witnessed a tremendous increase in our understanding of the development of visual processing mechanisms. The pioneering efforts of Hubel and Wiesel (1) established that visual cortex neurons in young animals display only a rudimentary form of the precise selectivity for stimulus orientation, direction, and binocular combination that is present in the mature organism. The rough selectivity of the neonatal kitten cortex increases even without visual exposure for a short period of time (2), but unless appropriate visual exposure is provided, visual capacities do not develop appropriately in animals subjected to prolonged dark rearing or binocular lid suture. In such animals, most visual cortex units are unresponsive or only weakly responsive to visual stimuli. In addition, they lack orientation, direction, and stereoselectivity as well as the other feature-specific properties that distinguish cortical cells from neurons earlier on in the visual pathways (3–6). The effects of atypical visual exposure can be highly specific, depending on the visual deprivation regime that is imposed. Thus, rearing animals in a stroboscopically illuminated environment, in which continuous retinal motion is prevented throughout early development, results in a specific loss of direction selectivity in cortical neurons of these animals (7). Tested later in life under conditions of normal illumination, strobe-reared animals show a selective deficit in motion perception (8). In the same animals, the development of other cortical unit properties such as orientation selectivity appears to be unaffected by the stroboscopic rearing procedure. A wide variety of selective deprivations have been imposed. For example, animals have been reared with restricted exposure to stimuli of one orientation (9–12) or to stimuli moving in one direction (13,14). In these selective deprivation procedures, neurons fail to develop selective preferences for the stimuli that were absent throughout early postnatal development. In general the selective deprivation experiments lead to the conclusion that the feature-specific properties of cortical cells become appropriate to the artificially created environment rather than the naturally occurring one.

The most common form of selective deprivation occurring in humans results from an abnormality in the visual media of one or both eyes during early development. It is common for young children to have peripheral visual disorders such as cataract, myopia or hyperopia, or some other disorder that results in a degradation of visual images through the affected eye. If the optical defect is not corrected early in life, the affected eye rarely regains normal visual capabilities, even if the peripheral optical defect is treated satisfactorily in adulthood. The long-term debilitating consequences of reduced early vision through one eye led to the development of an animal model for this set of clinical conditions by Wiesel and Hubel (15,16). They showed that rearing kittens with one eyelid sutured resulted in a series of changes throughout the visual pathways and in reduced visual capabilities of the eye that had been prevented from seeing during early development. In the lateral geniculate nucleus (LGN), neurons connected to the deprived eye were shrunken by more than 40% relative to neurons connected to the other eye (17). In addition, examination of the terminal fields of the shrunken LGN cells in the cortex showed that LGN axons connected to the deprived eye occupied less than 20% of the area of the cortex, whereas the other nonsutured eye had an expanded representation covering more than 80% of the thalamic recipient zone in cortical layer IV (18). Single-unit recording studies showed that stimuli presented through the sutured eye failed to influence the vast majority of cortical cells. Instead, the nonsutured eye became the sole effective route for visual stimuli. Figure 1 illustrates the distribution of cortical ocular dominance in normal cats (19) and in kittens in which vision in one eye was blurred during early development by rearing with a negative lens over one eye (20). Similar observations have been made in primates (21). The loss of cortical unit responsivity to stimulation of the deprived eye is almost certainly the basis for the behavioral observation that kittens (and humans) reared under conditions in which input to one eye is degraded are unable to use the deprived eye for vision when both eyes are allowed to view normally (22,23).

THE DETERMINANTS OF AMBLYOPIA

The Locus of the Effects of Reduced Vision in One Eye

There is evidence that the loss of visual capacities and the associated alterations in the visual system are due to competitive interactions between the two eyes, rather than being the simple result of disuse. The behavioral effects of monocular eyelid suture are considerably less severe for the deprived eye if the *other* eye is sutured as well (16). In addition, Guillery (24) showed that a

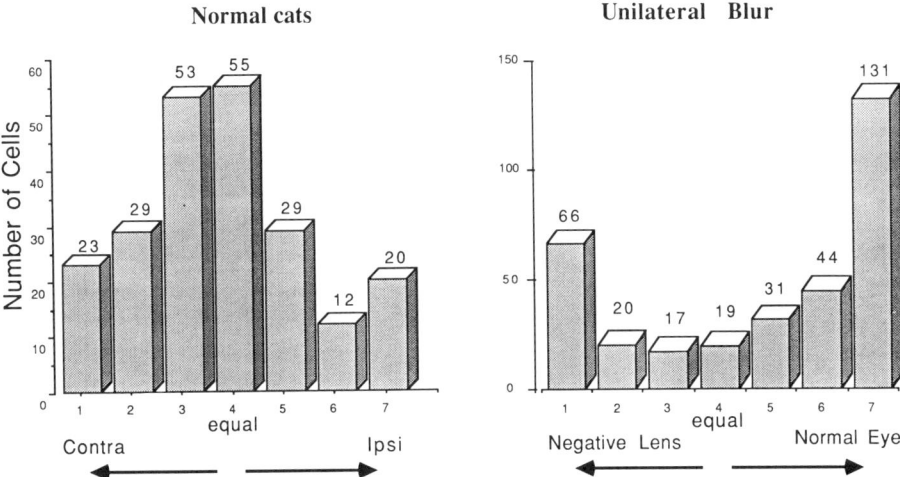

FIG. 1. The **left panel** illustrates the distribution of cortical ocular dominance for neurons in the cat visual cortex (19). On the abscissa, the numbers from 1 to 7 represent a contralateral to ipsilateral trend, with cells in group 1 driven exclusively via the contralateral eye, cells in group 4 driven equally via either eye, and cells in group 7 driven exclusively via the ipsilateral eye. The **right panel** indicates the effect of rearing with one eye viewing through a negative lens while the other eye views normally. Here, the numbers from 1 to 7 represent a trend from neurons driven exclusively via the negative lens eye to the normal eye. Note that few neurons are binocularly driven and that many more neurons are influenced by the normal eye than by the deprived eye.

partial lesion in the retina of the nondeprived eye prevented geniculate cell shrinkage at the corresponding locus in the LGN lamina connected to the deprived eye. Although changes associated with monocular deprivation have been demonstrated at the level of retinogeniculate terminals, lateral geniculate body somata, in LGN terminals, and in cortical cell responses, the evidence indicates that the primary site of binocular competition is cortical, and that the other changes in soma size and terminal fields are secondary to this primary cortical competition. Several sources of evidence that support this conclusion are detailed below.

Cynader and Mitchell (25) showed that it is possible to make binocular competition completely orientation dependent by raising kittens with goggles so that one eye viewed normally and the other looked through a cylindrical lens that defocused contours of vertical orientation selectively. The basic argument is that, since visual cortex is the first site in the visual pathways at which fine-grained orientation selectivity occurs, an orientation-dependent binocular competition can only occur at the level of visual cortical cells. The results of this investigation showed that the loss of visual responsivity by the deprived eye could be made completely dependent on the orientation of the neuron under study, supporting the hypothesis that the site of binocular competition is cortical.

This suggestion has been further strengthened by a series of experiments that showed that modification of neuromodulator and neurotransmitter functions in the cortex could prevent the normal effects of monocular deprivation (26–30). Infusion of amino acids and their agonists further implicates the postsynaptic cortical cell in the plasticity process and sheds an interesting light on the required relationship between pre- and postsynaptic activity in cortical modifiability. Shaw and Cynader (29) infused glutamate into the cortex for a 2-week period during monocular exposure of young kittens and found that this largely prevented the ocular dominance shift that normally occurred. Control recordings during the infusion period showed that cortical neurons, in general, failed to respond well to visual stimuli from either eye during the infusion period. The lack of ocular dominance modification was attributed to the reduced ability of the cortical cells to respond to the unbalanced LGN afferent input. The implication is that effective postsynaptic responses to the unequal presynaptic inputs representing the two eyes is necessary for ocular dominance modification to occur.

An even more striking result was obtained by Reiter and Stryker (30). They infused muscimol, an agonist of the inhibitory neurotransmitter gamma-aminobutyric acid (GABA), during a period of monocular exposure in young kittens. Recordings during the infusion period revealed virtually no activity at all among postsynaptic cortical elements during the infusion period. Recordings after the infusion period showed that the deprived eye subsequently *increased* its effectiveness in cortical cells compared to the normally viewing eye. Reiter and Stryker suggest that inputs that fail to evoke postsynaptic responses are disconnected from the cortical cell. Since the exposed eye carried stronger input to the unresponsive cortical cells, the strength of its disconnection is greater than that of the deprived eye.

The Critical Period

A second determinant of competitive binocular interactions is the age of the animal. It is now well established that competitive binocular interactions occur within a critical period (31,32) that peaks in kittens at approximately 4 weeks of age. At this time, eyelid closure for as brief a period as a few hours produces prolonged and profound effects on both visual capacities and cortical unit responses. Progressively smaller effects of monocular deprivation result as the animals age. A search for the mechanisms underlying visual cortical plasticity must take this time dependence into account. Yet there is evidence that the critical period itself is not necessarily immutable. We and others have found that the sensitivity of the organism to monocular deprivation depends on the animal's rearing history (33–35).

Using an experimental paradigm in which cats were reared in the dark until long after the end of the chronologically defined critical period, and only then brought into the light for monocular deprivation, we found that monocular deprivation can produce marked effects on cortical ocular dominance no matter how long an animal is kept in the dark (Fig. 2). Further experiments (34) demonstrated that dark-reared cats undergo a new critical period in the first few weeks after they are brought into the light. This was shown by dark rearing animals throughout the naturally occurring critical period and then bringing them into a normally illuminated environment for 3 months of monocular deprivation. If the monocular deprivation is started immediately or after only a few weeks of light exposure, strong deprivation effects result. However, waiting 6 weeks to start monocular deprivation results in a much smaller loss of cortical responsivity by the deprived eye, and an 8 to 12 week wait before monocular deprivation results in little or no effect. Therefore, when animals are brought out of the dark, they seem to undergo a new critical period that lasts on the order of 2 months (Fig. 3). The time dependence of the effectiveness of binocular competition in normal animals, its prolongation in dark-reared animals, and the "new" critical period induced after a dark-reared animal is exposed to a normally illuminated environment all set a series of constraints that a cellular mechanism for binocular competition must explain.

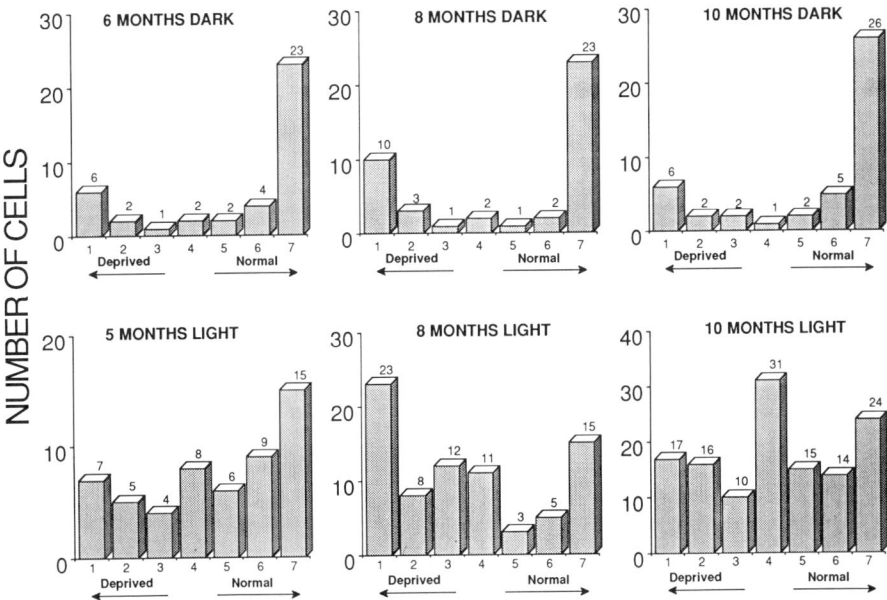

FIG. 2. The effects of 3 months of monocular suture on the distribution of cortical ocular dominance in dark-reared and light-reared cats of comparable ages. Conventions for this figure are similar to those for Fig. 1 with cells in group 1 driven by the previously deprived eye and those of group 7 driven by the normal eye. In the dark-reared cats, most cells encountered prefer inputs presented via the normal eye regardless of the animal's age at the onset of monocular suture. In the normal cats (lower three panels), the effects of monocular deprivation become less pronounced as older animals are sutured.

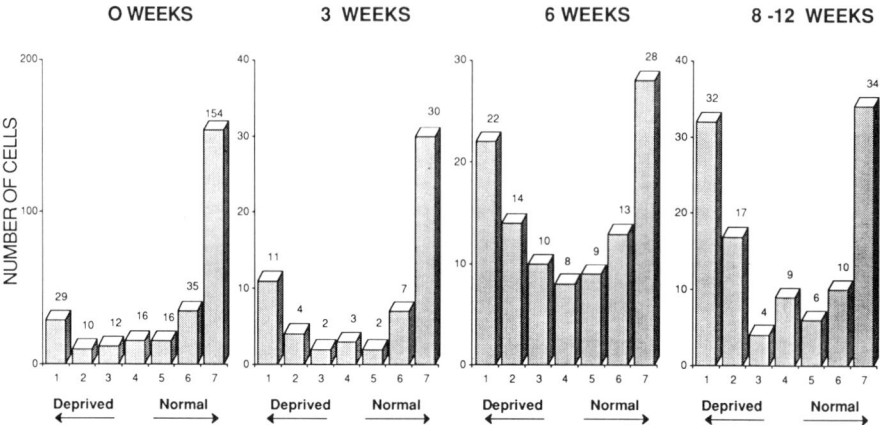

FIG. 3. The effects of 2 months of monocular deprivation on cortical ocular dominance in animals allowed various durations of binocular visual exposure following 4 months of dark rearing. Conventions are as for Fig. 1. The nondeprived eye controls a substantial majority of the neurons encountered in the animals allowed 0 to 3 weeks of light exposure before monocular deprivation was instituted. The effects are less pronounced in animals allowed 6 or more weeks of binocular visual exposure before monocular deprivation. In all cases, binocular excitatory convergence (cells in group 3–5) is considerably reduced relative to the normal cats of Fig. 1.

Extravisual Factors

A third determinant of the binocular competition that underlies amblyopia is the requirement for nonvisual modulatory inputs. After the first demonstrations by Hubel and Wiesel (31) that it was possible to modify cortical ocular dominance in young kittens by closing one eye for very brief periods, several different investigators attempted to record from the visual cortex of lightly anesthetized paralyzed kittens to monitor the alterations of cortical ocular dominance in individual cells during and following brief periods of monocular deprivation. In general, these experiments failed to demonstrate effective modification of neuronal responses, despite the fact that neurons responded effectively to the visual stimuli presented through the nondeprived eye at the time of recording. The reasons for the inability of visual stimuli to modify cortical neuronal organization in acute conditioning experiments remain unclear. It has been suggested (32,33) that signals from ocular proprioception are necessary and that it is essential that the eyes move about in order for unequal visual exposure in the two eyes to alter cortical ocular dominance. This finding may be related to suggestions that modifiability of cortical ocular dominance requires attentional mechanisms mediated by monoaminergic and/or cholinergic systems that terminate heavily within the visual cortex (26,27). Perhaps the most neutral statement we can make in the face of our current ignorance is that some sort of enabling input seems to be important to allow cortical modifiability to occur during the critical period. The nature of this enabling signal remains unknown, but it may well be linked to the substantial innervation of neocortex by neuromodulatory substances.

TOWARD CELLULAR MECHANISMS OF VISUAL CORTEX PLASTICITY: DEVELOPMENTAL ALTERATIONS OF NEUROTRANSMITTER RECEPTORS

Localization of Receptors

Neurotransmitter receptors are protein moieties, usually located on the surfaces of neurons or glial elements, that bind specific hormones or neurotransmitters and hence evoke cellular responses. In recent years, the development of *in vitro* autoradiographic methods has made it possible to localize and characterize receptors associated with a wide variety of neurotransmitters and neuromodulators in the central nervous system. In view of the importance of chemical communication in visual cortex for the modification of neuronal responses, we have undertaken a systematic study of the development, location, and characteristics (number and affinity) of neurotransmitter receptors within the developing kitten visual cortex. An example of the sort of data obtainable with receptor autoradiography methods is shown in Fig. 4. The

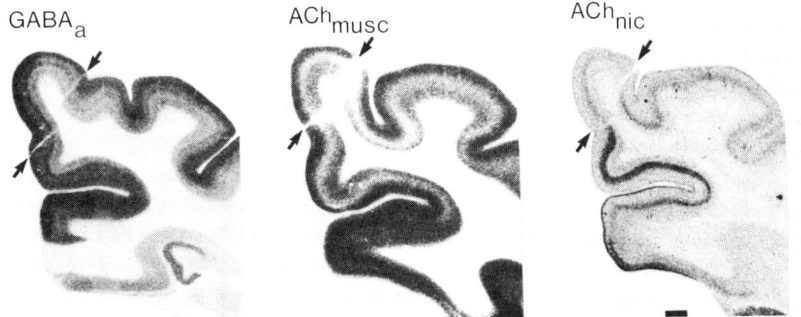

FIG. 4. Illustrates the distribution of binding sites for GABA$_A$ receptors (labeled with [^{3}H]muscimol), muscarinic acetylcholine receptors (labeled with [^{3}H]QNB), and nicotinic acetylcholine receptors (labeled with [^{3}H]nicotine). GABA$_A$ receptors (**left panel**) show some concentration in the superficial cortical layers (layers I–III) but exhibit densest binding in layer IV. The deeper cortical layers (layers V and VI) show the lowest level of binding. The muscarinic acetylcholine receptors (**middle panel**) are concentrated in layers I through III, with a prominent gap in layers IV and V and increased density again in layer VI. The nicotinic receptors (**right panel**) are specifically located in cortical layer IV with little binding in other layers. In all panels *arrows* demarcate the zone of cortex that was surgically undercut. The undercutting procedure has little effect on the GABA$_A$ and muscarinic acetylcholine receptors but eliminates the nicotinic binding sites in the undercut zone. In this and subsequent receptor autoadiography figures, increasing darkness in the photograph indicates increasing density of receptors. Scale bar: 1 mm.

figure illustrates coronal sections through the visual cortex and the distribution of three populations of receptors that we have studied. The left panel of the figure shows the laminar and regional distribution of $GABA_A$-receptor binding sites within the cortex, as assessed using [^{3}H]muscimol (36). Increased levels of darkness represent increased binding. Although there is substantial binding in the superficial cortical layers, the highest concentration of binding sites appears to be in layer IV; the lowest concentrations appear in layers V and VI, the deepest cortical layers. The white matter is unlabeled.

The center panel of Fig. 4 illustrates the distribution of muscarinic acetylcholinergic receptors as labeled with [^{3}H]quinuclidinylbenzilate (QNB) (37). The panel shows that binding is densest (darkest) in the outermost layers of the cortex, layers I through III, with a conspicuous gap in layer IV and an increase in binding in the deepest cortical layers, layers V and VI. The white matter is again unlabeled. The right panel of Fig. 4 illustrates the distribution and density of nicotinic acetylcholinergic receptors, as labeled with [^{3}H]nicotine (38). These binding sites are specifically located within layer IV of the cortex.

Note in Fig. 4 the arrows demarcating a zone of discontinuity in the visual cortex tissue. The animals whose autoradiograms are illustrated in Fig. 4 were in fact not normal animals, but animals in which a portion of the visual cortex was surgically isolated from the rest of the brain several weeks before sacrifice. This was performed by making three 1-cm deep scalpel cuts: two cuts extended from the midline to the lateral edge of the marginal gyrus; the third cut ran parallel to the midline but was angled at 45° from the lateral edge of the marginal gyrus toward the medial bank. This procedure produced triangular blocks of isolated cortex that included the crown of the gyrus and portions of the medial bank of the visual cortex. The arrows demarcate the isolated zone in each of the coronal sections.

Following this surgical isolation of a part of the visual cortex, the tissue survives rather well (39). The $GABA_A$ receptors, labeled with [^{3}H]muscimol, and the muscarinic receptors, labeled with [^{3}H]QNB, appear to be completely unaffected by the undercut procedure. The nicotine binding sites in the right-hand panel of Fig. 4, however, essentially disappear within the undercut zone. These data support the notion that nicotinic binding sites are not intrinsic to cortical elements, but rather that they are located on the axons of extracortical inputs. In other experiments we have localized them to terminals of LGN afferents within the cortex (38,40). The muscarinic and GABAergic sites, by contrast, must be associated with intrinsic cortical elements rather than with cortical afferentation. The methods of receptor autoradiography have enabled us to define the laminar distribution of nearly 20 different binding sites in the cortex. By using surgical techniques, such as undercutting, and neuron-specific toxins, we have been able to infer cellular location as well. These efforts are reviewed in Prusky et al. (38), Shaw et al. (41), and Cynader and Shaw (42).

Neurotransmitter Receptor Development

The development of neurotransmitter receptors within the cortex follows idiosyncratic patterns for the different receptors that we have studied. In all cases, the overall number of receptors increases during postnatal development to a peak that occurs within the critical period. Thereafter, one observes either an overall loss of receptor number into adulthood or, for other receptors, a maintenance of the level achieved during the critical period. Figure 5 illustrates the distribution and density of two classes of acetylcholine-linked

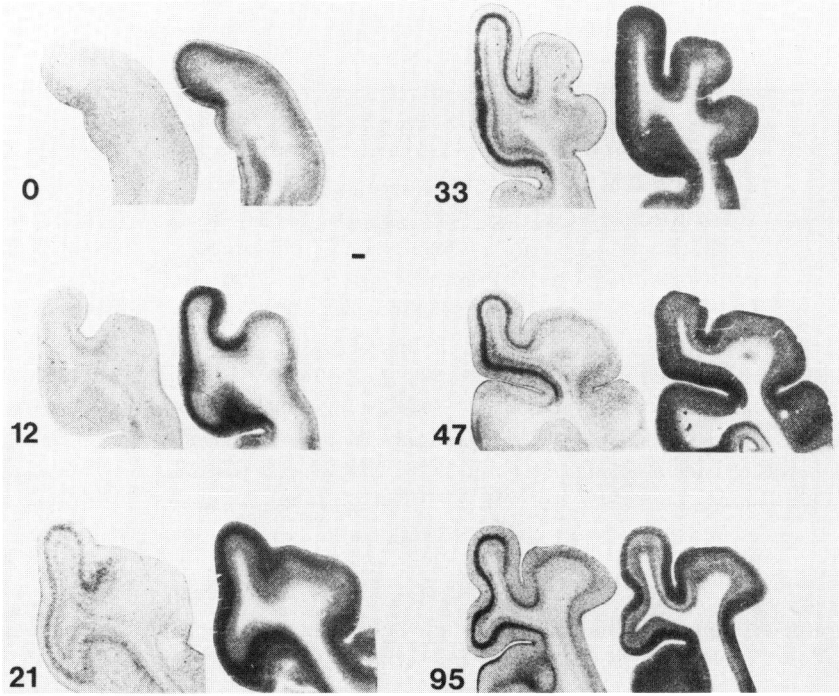

FIG. 5. The distribution of [^{3}H]nicotine and [^{3}H]QNB (muscarinic) binding sites in the visual cortex of kittens of different ages. The photographs represent kittens of ages 0, 12, 21, 33, 47, and 95 days. The number to the left of each pair of sections represents the ages of the kittens. The left-hand member of each pair of sections illustrates nicotine binding sites. Note the age-related increase in the binding in layer IV and to a lesser extent in layers I and VI in the primary visual cortex. There are few laminar-specific binding sites in young animals but binding sites begin to concentrate in layer IV at 21 days and reach their full adult density by postnatal day 47. The right-hand member of each pair of sections represents [^{3}H]QNB binding. Note the high density in layer IV in 0- and 12-day-old kittens. By 21 days of age, muscarinic receptors are also found in superficial layers and in the 33-day-old kittens, layers I through IV are a zone of concentration. At 47 days of age, the middle layers of the cortex show lower levels of binding than the superficial and deep layers, and this trend continues and becomes more pronounced in the 95-day-old kitten. The pattern of binding in adult cats (Fig. 4) is very similar to that observed in the 95-day-old kitten. Scale bar: 1 mm.

receptors during postnatal development of the visual cortex. The left-hand member of each pair represents nicotinic binding sites, and the right-hand member of each pair represents muscarinic binding sites studied in an adjacent section of the same kitten. The nicotinic sites show a gradual increase during development, with low concentrations in the 0- and 12-day-old animals, and high levels of binding in layer IV by 33 and 47 days of age. Note the remarkable concentration in the 33- and 47-day-old animals of receptors in the *visual* cortex as opposed to the subadjacent cingulate cortex or the extravisual cortex of the lateral suprasylvian area. In the 95-day-old animal, receptors have spread outside of the primary striate cortex to the adjacent cortical fields. Note that regardless of the animal's age, the greatest concentration of nicotine receptors is found in layer IV of the cortex.

The constancy of laminar distribution for the nicotinic binding sites contrasts with the developmental pattern observed for the muscarinic binding sites (the right-hand member of each pair in Fig. 5). In the neonatal animal (day 0) muscarinic binding sites are concentrated in the middle layers of the cortex and are present in far greater numbers than are nicotinic receptors. Note the concentration within the visual cortex and near absence in neighboring cortical fields. At 12 days of age, the increased preponderance of muscarinic receptors is still observed, and they are still located in layer IV, but by 21 days of age, as *nicotinic* receptors begin to appear in layer IV, one begins to notice muscarinic receptors located in the superficial cortical layers as well. This trend is even more pronounced at 33 days of age, by which time muscarinic receptors appear to be located in nearly all of the superficial (layers I–IV) cortical layers. At 47 days of age, muscarinic receptors are concentrated in layers I to III and VI. This pattern is retained, with some further thinning out of muscarinic receptors in layer IV, during the next several weeks, and the 95-day-old pattern is similar to that observed in adults. The adult pattern, as seen in Fig. 4, emphasizes inner and outer cortical layers, whereas layer IV is sparsely labeled. Thus, the muscarinic acetylcholine receptors, unlike their nicotinic counterparts, appear to change their *laminar distribution* during the critical period. From an initial concentration in layer IV (the input layer), these binding sites essentially *reverse* in distribution to favor all cortical layers except layer IV by adulthood.

We have examined more than 20 different binding sites in the kitten visual cortex as a function of the animal's age. We find, in fact, that the type of receptor redistribution illustrated by the muscarinic binding sites is a common pattern. Nearly two-thirds of all receptor populations show some form of redistribution in visual cortex during postnatal development (43). Figure 6 is a summary diagram illustrating the distribution of neurotransmitter receptors of various types in the cortex of neonatal versus adult animals. (For references, see [42,43]). At the top of each column the name of the particular neurotransmitter-neuromodulator and the associated ligand is displayed. The layers of the cortex are illustrated on the left of each figure. The density

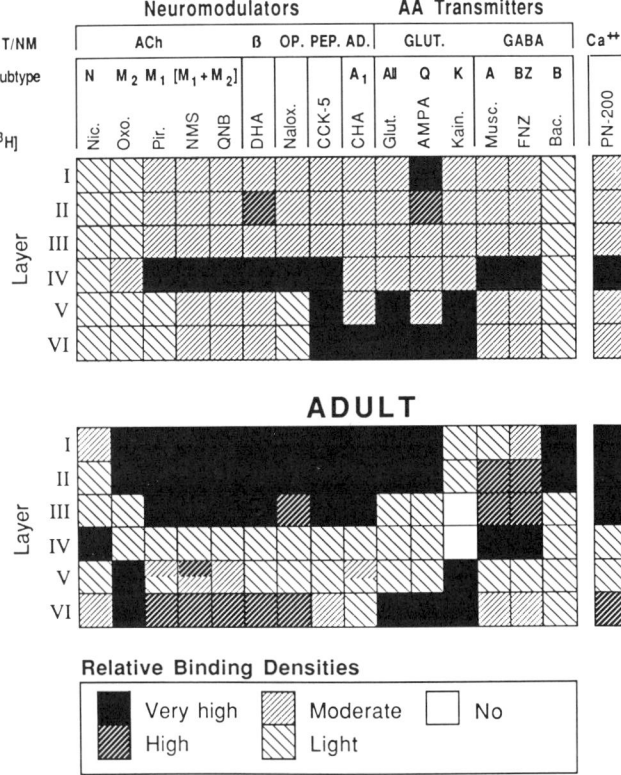

FIG. 6. A schematic distribution of the laminar binding patterns for 16 binding sites studied in neonatal (1–3-day-old) kittens and in adult cats. The top row of the figure lists the neurotransmitters (NT) and neuromodulators (NM) whose receptors have been examined. These include those for acetylcholine (ACH), β-adrenergic (BETA), opiates (OP), peptides (PEP), and for A_1-adenosine (AD) within the broad class of neuromodulatory substances. Binding sites for glutamate and GABA represent the amino acid transmitters. The various receptor subtypes are illustrated on the row below. The tritiated ligand employed is illustrated in the subsequent row. The cortex is divided into six layers and the density of binding is illustrated using the shading scale given at the bottom of the figure. In neonatal kittens the most common patterns of binding observed are either little or no discernible binding (nicotine, oxytremorine, baclofen), or a pronounced peak in layer IV. The glutamate-related binding sites appear concentrated in layer VI in the neonatal kitten. In adult animals, the pattern is very different, with relatively few binding sites (nicotine, muscimol, and flunitrazepam) concentrated in layer IV. Most receptors show a distribution emphasizing layers I through III and VI.

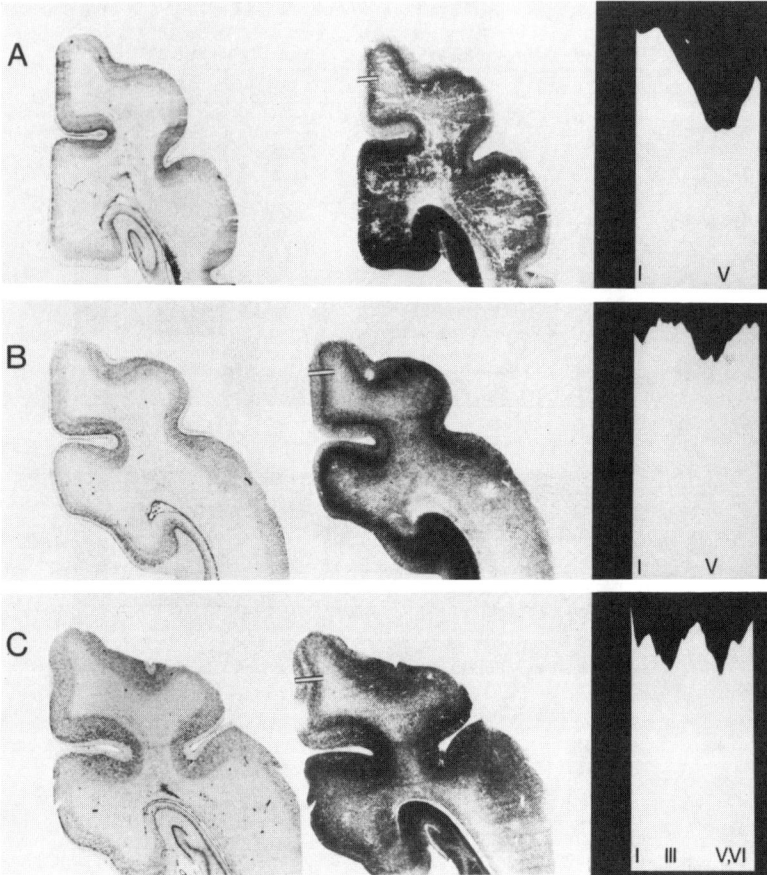

FIG. 7. The ontogeny of phorbol ester binding sites in kitten visual cortex. The left column shows Nissl-stained coronal sections of kittens of various ages, the middle column autoradiograms obtained from the same sections, and the right column optical density profiles measured across the indicated regions of area 17. Note that increasing elevation on the vertical axis of the profile denotes increasing levels of binding. The numbers on the profiles' horizontal axis indicate the laminar location of the optical density measurements. The six panels of the binding patterns were obtained in newborn (**A**), 3-day-old (**B**), 15-day-old (**C**), 31-day-old (**D**), 40-day-old (**E**), and

of receptors within each layer relative to other cortical layers is indicated by the density of shading in each cell of Fig. 6. Darker shading indicates greater receptor density. For some neurotransmitter receptors, including $GABA_A$, and some of the subsets of glutamate receptors, the relative distribution of binding sites appears to remain constant throughout postnatal development with the former sites concentrated in layer IV throughout development, and the latter favoring superficial and deep layers throughout. Other binding sites, including muscarinic receptors, β-adrenergic receptors, calcium channel binding sites, opiate receptors, and cholecystokinin-5 receptors, show a

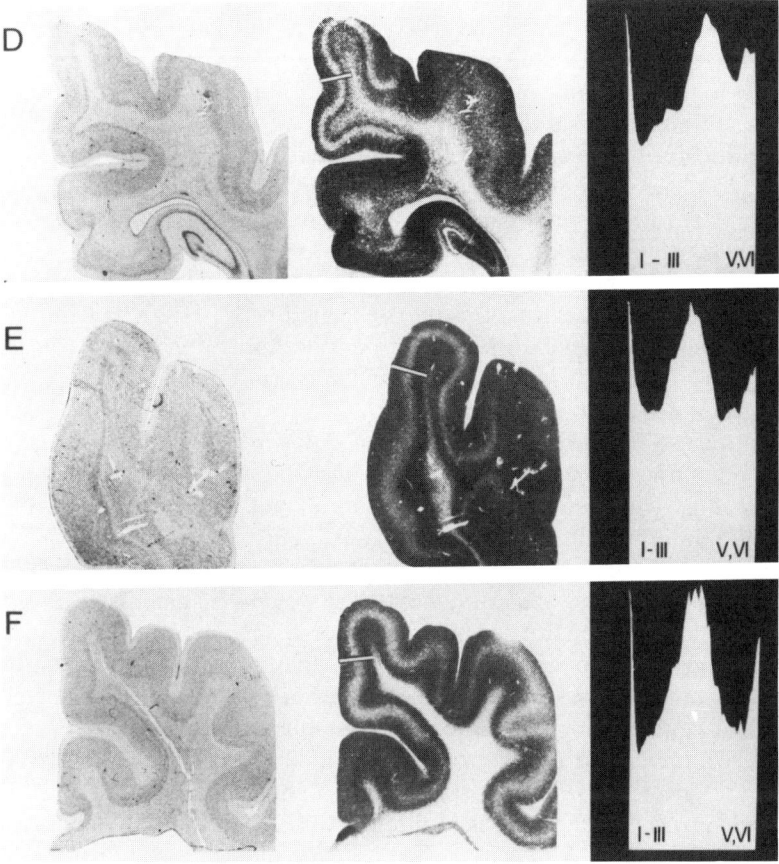

60-day-old (**F**) kittens. Note that layer V contains the highest level of binding sites in the young kittens with layer III first illustrating substantial binding in 15-day-old kittens and the binding increasing dramatically in layers I and II in still older kittens. The adult pattern is similar to that observed in 60-day-old kittens, with dense binding in all layers except layer IV. Note that this final pattern of binding is very similar to that observed with QNB (Fig. 5). The detailed developmental pattern is, however, very different.

pattern in which layer IV has the densest binding early in life, with this pattern reversing to involve a preferential distribution within superficial and deep layers later in development. Individual receptors may show highly individual and idiosyncratic patterns. The A_1-adenosine receptor (labeled with [^{3}H]CHA) favors the deep cortical layers early in life and superficial and deep layers in adulthood. Other receptors, including those for nicotine and baclofen, are not observed at birth, but are clearly present in adulthood. Certain patterns are notable by their absence. We have yet to find any binding sites that concentrate in superficial cortical layers early in life and then favor deeper layers in adulthood. This may reflect the ontogenetic history of the cortex, with cells of the superficial layers being generated later in life than those of the deep layers. It would be far too simple, however, to suggest that any or all of the receptor redistributions that are depicted in Fig. 6 simply follow the ontogenetic history of cortical neurons.

Thus, different transmitter receptors appear to undergo specific changes in distribution during postnatal development. In all cases the receptor redistributions take place during the physiologically defined critical period for alteration of cortical unit responses. The ontogenetic time courses of the alterations in distribution also vary from receptor to receptor. This may even apply to receptors that show the same neonatal and adult pattern of distribution. For example, the muscarinic receptors (labeled with [^{3}H]QNB) and the calcium binding sites (labeled with PN200) are both found in layer IV in young animals and in superficial and deep layers in old animals, but the calcium binding sites appear to vacate layer IV by 20 days of age, whereas muscarinic receptors can still be found in this layer at 30 days of age. In some cases, pairs of receptors may show the same laminar distribution in both young and old animals (e.g., pirenzepine and oxotremorine) but may show very different patterns at intermediate ages.

Activation of receptors frequently leads to intracellular responses via coupling to G proteins and to second messenger systems that mediate transmembrane signaling. One major second messenger system involves the turnover of inositol lipids in the plasma membrane and the consequent activation of intracellular protein kinase C (PKC). PKC has been shown to participate in a myriad of cellular functions and can phosphorylate a wide variety of substrates. We have used *in vitro* autoradiographic techniques to localize PKC within the developing visual cortex. Figure 7 shows the distribution of PKC (as labeled with [^{3}H]phorbol-12,13-dibutyrate [PDBU]) within the visual cortex of the developing kitten (44). The left side of each panel displays Nissl-stained coronal sections of kitten visual cortex. The middle column shows autoradiograms of the same sections, and the right column contains an optical density profile obtained across the medial bank of area 17 of each autoradiogram from layers I to VI. It is clear that even the newborn kitten exhibits a specific binding pattern within area 17 with the highest concentration of binding sites in layer V. The adult pattern of binding is characterized by high levels of binding in all cortical layers except layer IV. Thus, the redistribution of binding sites that has been found for neurotransmitter receptors on the surface of cortical elements appears to be paralleled by a redistribution during postnatal development of second messenger systems within the cortex.

Effects of Input on Postnatal Development of Neurotransmitter Receptors

We noted earlier that the critical period for cortical plasticity can itself be altered by preventing the visual system from obtaining a normal pattern of input during postnatal development. We found that the redistribution of neurotransmitter receptors normally observed during the critical period also depends on normal input to the cortex. Figure 8 illustrates the effects of surgically undercutting a portion of the visual cortex in a young animal, 23 days of age, and allowing the animal to survive throughout the period during which muscarinic acetylcholine receptors would normally have altered their laminar distribution (until 49 days of age). Figure 8 is comprised of several panels illustrating: (a) The effect of the surgical undercut on Nissl staining in the

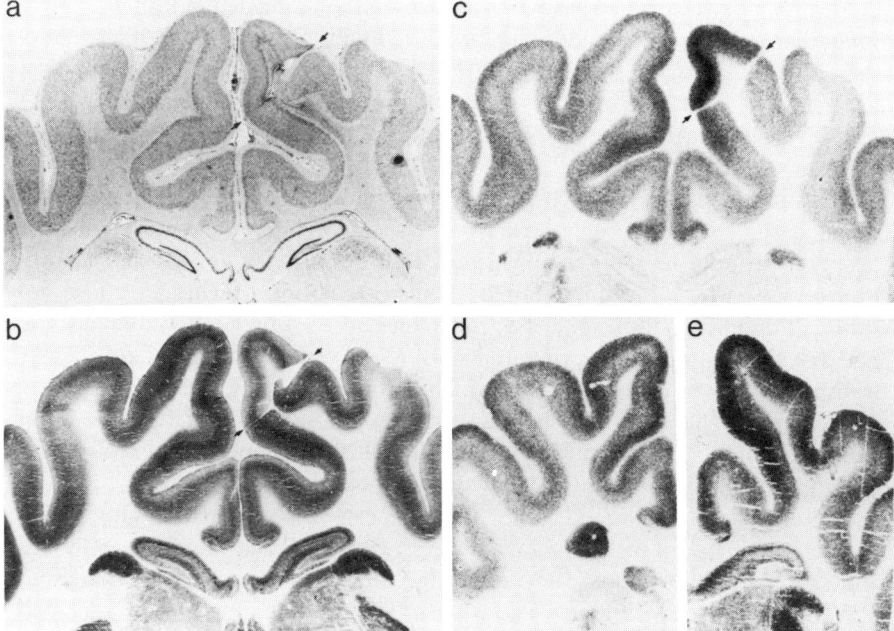

FIG. 8. a: A section of the control and undercut cortex was stained for Nissl substance with cresyl violet. The undercut cortex appears normal except for gliosis along the cut. Control cortex is on the left. **b:** Alternate sections of both cortices were processed for cytochrome C oxidase histochemistry (48). The reaction products, especially the dense band in layer IV, are less well defined but still present in the undercut zone as in the normal cortex. This difference from normal cortex may reflect maturational differences in the undercut zone. **c–e:** Autoradiograms illustrate the distribution of muscarinic ACh receptors (left). An adjacent section to those of a and b was incubated with [^{3}H]QNB to visualize the distribution of muscarinic cholinergic receptors. The resulting autoradiogram shows that receptors in the control hemisphere (left side of c) are concentrated in layers I–III and VI. In the undercut zone of the opposite hemisphere (right side of c), receptors are instead concentrated in cortical layer IV. This pattern closely resembles that of a normal 27-day-old kitten shown in e for comparison. Muscarinic receptor binding in an unoperated kitten of 46 days of age is illustrated in d. Note the similarity to the pattern observed in the control hemisphere of 8c. Muscarinic ACh receptors were labeled with 5–7 nM [^{3}H]QNB for 60 min at 20°C. Nonspecific binding was determined by coincubation of alternate sections with 10^{-4} M atropine sulfate. Ultrafilm exposure: c, 14 days; d, 12 days; e, 16 days. All autoradiograms have been photographed for highest contrast. For all panels, calibration bar = 1 mm.

cortex; little effect is observed indicating the normality of the tissue; (b) This conclusion is reinforced by the relative lack of alteration of cytochrome oxidase activity in the undercut zone; (c) The distribution of muscarinic receptors in the undercut zone is compared with that outside the undercut zone. In the control cortex (Fig. 8c, left) muscarinic acetylcholine-receptor distribution is typical of that for an animal of this postnatal age (49 days) (37), i.e., layers I to III and VI show the densest binding. These results are in marked contrast to the binding observed in the undercut zone of the opposite cortex, which more closely resembles that typically seen in the cortex of a much younger kitten (i.e., the age of this kitten at the time of surgery). Within the isolated zone, the binding is densest in layer IV and appears denser overall than outside the undercut area. Immediately outside the undercut zone, the binding pattern resembles that of the control cortex. Figure 8d illustrates [^{3}H]QNB binding in a normal 46-day-old kitten for comparison to the control cortex in Fig. 8c. Figure 8e illustrates [^{3}H]QNB binding in a normal 27-day-old kitten for comparison with the undercut zone of Fig. 8c.

The failure of receptors to redistribute following isolation of part of the visual cortex early in life appears to be a general phenomenon. We have observed effects like those illustrated in Fig. 8 for several other neurotransmitter receptors that change their distribution (including those for cholecystokinin, adenosine, and various muscarinic subtypes). We have yet to observe the normal developmental pattern of redistribution of any neurotransmitter receptor in animals in which the surgical isolation was performed early in life. The data thus lend support to the notion that basic receptor characteristics in cat visual cortex are under the influence of extracortical factors. The mechanisms by which external inputs regulate the receptor redistribution normally observed as the animal ages remain uncertain. Our undercutting procedure removes many sources of extracortical input from the affected zone, including those representing visual influences from the thalamus and also modulatory influences conveyed via cholinergic, noradrenergic, and serotonergic inputs. The role of alterations in cortical *electrical* activity, which may be especially disrupted in layer IV, the major input, layer in the failure of the receptors to redistribute, remains uncertain as well. In addition, a trophic factor or factors released by one or more of the cortical afferent systems may play an important role in receptor redistribution, and this may be affected by the undercut procedure.

We have also begun to examine the effects of less severe restrictions of input than those produced by undercutting the cortex early in life on receptor binding parameters. Figure 9 illustrates the distribution of binding sites for [^{3}H]cyclohexyladenosine (CHA), an A_1-adenosine receptor agonist, in normal and dark-reared cats. In normal animals, layers I to III are heavily labeled as is a thin zone in the upper part of layer V. Binding in dark-reared cats, illustrated on the right of Fig. 9 is quite different from that of the normal animals, with a failure to achieve the normal pattern involving layers I, II, III,

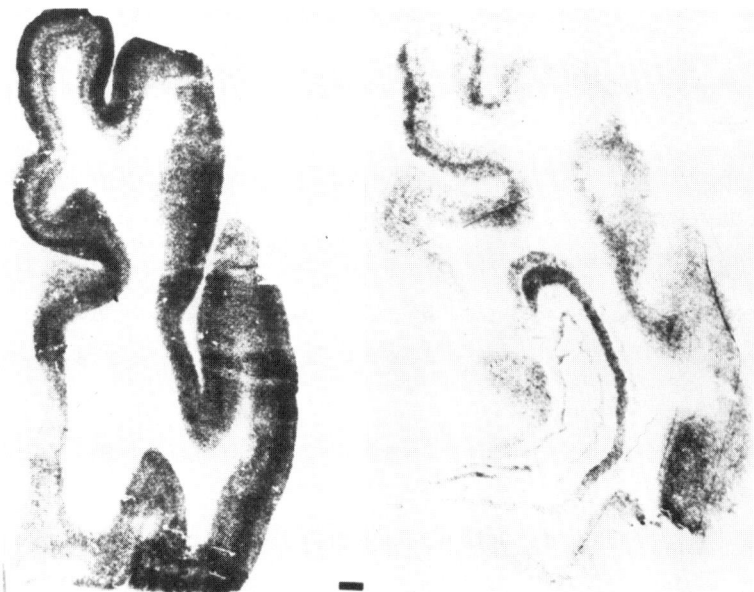

FIG. 9. The distribution of A_1-adenosine binding sites in normal (**left**) and dark-reared (**right**) cat visual cortex. In normal cats, A_1-adenosine receptors are densest in layers I–III and in a narrow zone at the top of layer V. In dark-reared animals only layer III is heavily labeled, and the overall number of receptors is reduced by more than 50%.

and V. Instead one sees many fewer binding sites than normal cats with a concentration only in layer III.

We are currently exploring the effects of dark rearing on the distribution of a variety of neurotransmitter receptors. It is clear that some receptors follow their normal developmental course regardless of dark rearing. Others, such as the adenosinergic receptors previously described, appear to be vulnerable to this manipulation. In still other receptors that we have studied, such as those for acetylcholine and GABA, the normal adult *distribution* of receptors is achieved despite the deprivation, but one sees alterations in other basic parameters such as number and affinity (45).

We have naturally been interested in examining the effects of various durations of selective *monocular* exposure on receptor distributions and number. We were initially disappointed by our findings indicating that monocular deprivation seems to have little or no effect on the pattern of laminar distribution of any receptor population that we have studied during postnatal development. Receptors appear to go through their normal redistribution patterns at about the same time regardless of the pattern of monocular deprivation (short-term, long-term, starting at various ages) that we have imposed. Nor have these manipulations caused receptors to aggregate into columns representing one eye or another. The most striking effect on receptors that we have observed thus far is a marked increase in the number of GABAergic receptors in visual cortex of monocularly deprived cats (39). However, a failure to find alterations in the developmental pattern of any particular receptor system with monocular deprivation does not imply that this receptor system plays no role in the cortical plasticity process. There is good evidence that binocular competition and synaptic plasticity is going on in the cortex during the critical period *whether or not* one eye is at a competitive disadvantage during the critical period. Monocular deprivation and its variants simply shift the balance of the competitive process, enabling us to discern a victor and hence that the competition has taken place. In retrospect, it is thus perhaps not surprising that most receptors appear to be unperturbed by monocular visual exposure.

Cellular Mechanisms Underlying Redistribution of Neurotransmitter Receptors

The striking alteration in the distribution of neurotransmitter receptors during development could have several causes: (a) Receptor redistribution occurs because of migration of neurons or glia with which the receptors are associated. (b) Receptor redistribution occurs because receptors are located on axons or dendrites, and these processes are continuing to extend during postnatal development. The receptors are simply carried along by the extending processes and thus attain different distributions as a function of age. (c) Receptors are transiently expressed by certain populations of neurons or glial cells at certain stages of cortical development and are then eliminated and proliferate *de novo* in other neuronal populations in later stages. Receptor autoradiography is in general unable to distinguish between these outlined possibilities. Although the method is reliable and quantifiable, its spatial resolution is insufficient to visualize the individual somata or neuronal processes on which the receptors in question are located.

To obtain higher resolution information on this issue, we have used monoclonal antibodies against receptor binding sites to visualize neurotransmitter receptors and their alterations during postnatal development. Figure 10 illustrates binding of muscarinic receptors using a monoclonal antibody M35 (46). The top panels of Fig. 10 are low-power views comparing the binding of receptors in 28-day-old and adult cats. In the young kitten, whose binding pattern is illustrated at the top left of Fig. 10, receptors are concentrated in layer IV with some binding at the top of layer II, a pattern similar to, but not exactly the same as, that observed with [^{3}H]QNB binding (Fig. 5). In the adult animal illustrated on the top right panel of Fig. 10, the distribution favors superficial and deep layers, as is observed with [^{3}H]QNB autoradiography in normal adult animals. The lower panels of Fig. 10 show that the binding in layer IV of the young kitten cortex is concentrated around the somata of

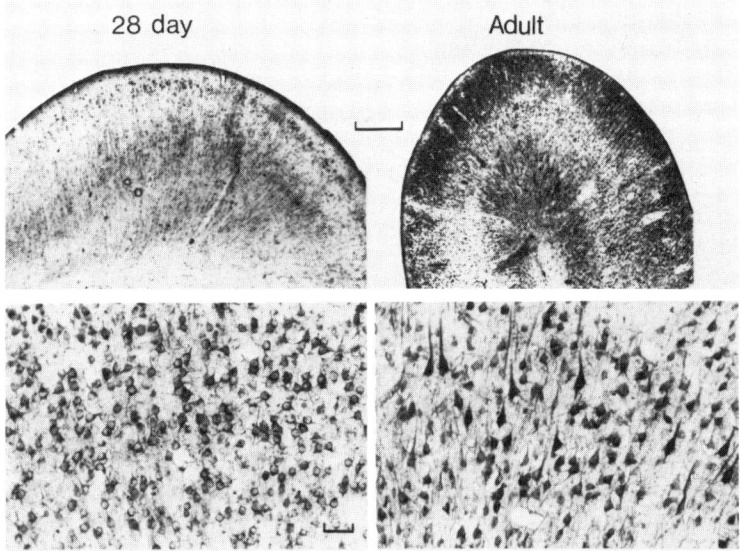

FIG. 10. Immunocytochemical labeling of the muscarinic receptor in 28-day-old (**left**) and adult (**right**) cat visual cortex using a monoclonal antibody. The upper panels represent low-magnification views of the pattern of binding in the crown of the visual cortex. Note that the immunostained cells are densest in layer IV in the young animal and least dense in this layer of the adult animal. Scale bar = 0.5 mm. The lower two panels illustrate higher power light micrographs of tissue showing the densely labeled nonpyramidal cells in layer IV of the young kitten (left) and of pyramidal cells in layers V and VI of the adult cat cortex (right). Scale bar for lower panels = 50 μm.

stellate cells. The binding clearly outlines the cell bodies with some dendritic involvement as well. The lower right panel of Fig. 10 is a high-power view of layer V binding in the adult animal. Here again the binding is concentrated on neuronal somata with some receptors clearly distributed along apical dendrites. In this case, however, it is the *pyramidal* cells of layer V that appear to be heavily labeled. Thus, in 28-day-old kittens, stellate cells of layer IV preferentially express muscarinic binding sites, whereas these neurons no longer express this binding site in adult animals. Instead pyramidal cells of layer V and other pyramidal cells of the superficial layers (not shown here in high power) seem to preferentially express this receptor. It thus appears that receptors are transiently expressed by some neuronal populations during the critical period. They are then lost and instead are expressed by other neurons at later ages.

SUSPICIOUS COINCIDENCES AND CORTICAL PLASTICITY MECHANISMS

Ocular dominance plasticity has been the most heavily investigated form of selective rearing. It is clear that the major effects occur in cortical layer IV and that a sharply defined critical period, peaking at approximately 4 weeks of age, exists during which only a few hours of unequal visual exposure can shift cortical ocular dominance. This effect depends on: (a) unequal input from the eyes, (b) the ability of the cortical cell to respond to the unequal visual inputs and the pre- and postsynaptic activity correlation, and (c) the presence of some sort of enabling or gating signal that may be neuromodulatory in origin. Paralleling this physiologically defined critical period we observe alterations in the number and distribution of neurotransmitter-neuromodulator receptors in the visual cortex. For several different receptors that we have studied (see Fig. 6), there is evidence of transient expression within layer IV of the cortex early in life, with a loss of these binding sites from layer IV as the age-related plasticity wanes. The evidence from monoclonal antibodies indicates that this loss of binding sites represents the transient expression of these binding sites by neurons in layer IV and subsequent expression of similar receptors by different neurons in other cortical layers. The nature of extracortical input can influence both the duration of the critical period and the timing and extent of receptor redistributions.

How might the alteration of receptors that we have observed contribute to the mechanisms of critical period plasticity? The short answer is that we still do not know. However, one can imagine several distinct but nonexclusive mechanisms based on *coincidences* in the distribution of neurotransmitter receptors in animals of different ages. For instance, if one recalls the developmental distribution of muscarinic and nicotinic receptors (Fig. 5) in the kitten visual cortex, it is clear that muscarinic receptors are vacating layer IV at the same time that nicotinic binding sites are becoming more numerous in this layer. There is, however, a brief window of time, from approximately 20 to 35 days of postnatal age during which both these binding sites are concentrated within layer IV. It is established that the nicotinic binding sites are located presynaptically, on LGN terminals, and that the muscarinic sites are postsynaptic (38,41). The coincidence of pre- and postsynaptic sites in layer IV during the height of the critical period provides a mechanism by which the same transmitter, acetylcholine, could simultaneously modulate both pre- and postsynaptic function with these two receptor populations in this layer. It could hence force correlations by coincident activation of pre- and postsynaptic targets. It may be that this forced correlation, when combined with an asymmetry in the inputs from the two eyes, is a necessary substrate of the mechanism by which ocular dominance modification occurs during the critical period. Similar effects may also occur with other classes of receptor such as $GABA_A$ and $GABA_B$ receptors.

A second, possibly interrelated mechanism refers to the striking concentration of several putative postsynaptic receptor binding sites within layer IV during the critical period. Thus, β-adrenergic, muscarinic, cholecystokinergic, opiatergic, and other binding sites are all found concentrated in layer IV near the height of the critical period. In general when neurotransmitter receptors are stimulated they produce intracellular effects via activation of second messenger systems. There is evidence that simultaneous activation of the *same* second messenger system via two *different* receptors can cause much more intense activation than input via either receptor alone (47). Strong activation of a given second messenger system might then result in phosphorylation of intracellular substrates, leading to long-term alterations of membrane proteins and/or ion channels. One can readily make the argument that plasticity should not occur in response to every ongoing stimulus. Rather only specific situations, which meet certain stringent requirements, should enable long-term neuronal modifications to take place. These requirements might include unequal input from the two eyes, and activity in two or more of the neuromodulatory receptor systems (27). The simultaneous presence of two or more of the receptor populations previously listed on the same postsynaptic cells in cortical layer IV would be crucial to the function of such a mechanism, and it may not function after the critical period because these receptor populations have vacated layer IV.

Another form of coincidence that may be required for cortical ocular dominance to shift with unequal visual exposure in the two eyes is the coincidence of neurotransmitter receptors and the second messenger system with which they may be associated. Figure 7, illustrating the distribution of PKC in the developing kitten visual cortex, shows that this marker for the inositol lipid second messenger system changes its distribution during postnatal development. Using antibodies against this binding site (W.-G. Jia and M. Cynader, *unpublished data*), we have shown that it too appears to be transiently expressed within a population of cortical neurons during development and then expressed in different populations of neurons in adulthood. The simultaneous redistributions of neurotransmitters and second messengers may result in unique coincidences. Certain receptors may be associated with a particular second messenger system in given cell types only at particular times during postnatal development. One would expect that the presence or absence of a particular second messenger system within a given cell population would determine the long-term consequences of activation of a particular receptor system.

CONCLUSION

The cortex normally develops according to rules that lead to an effective information processing system, appropriate to the visual world in which the organism was reared early in life. Unfortunately, with peripheral anomalies such as refractive errors, cataracts and astigmatism, that visual world may not always be the same as that experienced by a normally sighted individual. Since cortical function can normally be altered only during the critical period, a major goal of current research has been to understand the mechanisms by which this occurs and to discover ways in which the critical period can be reinstated later in life. We are still far from achieving this goal but our emerging understanding of the neurochemistry of the cortex and its transmitter systems during the critical period surely constrain any theory that can be constructed to account for the ways in which visual inputs shape visual processing mechanisms.

ACKNOWLEDGMENT

This work is supported by the Medical Research Council of Canada (PG-29).

REFERENCES

1. Hubel DH, Wiesel TN. Receptive fields of cells in striate cortex of very young, visually inexperienced kittens. *J Neurophysiol* 1963;26:994–1002.
2. Buisseret D, Imbert M. Visual cortical cells: their developmental properties in normal and dark-reared kittens. *J Physiol (Lond)* 1976;255:511–525.
3. Cynader M, Berman N, Hein A. Recovery of function in cat visual cortex following prolonged deprivation. *Exp Brain Res* 1976;25:139–156.
4. Imbert M, Buisseret P. Receptive field characteristics and plastic properties of visual cortical cells in kittens reared with or without visual experience. *Exp Brain Res* 1975;22:25–36.
5. Sherk H, Stryker MP. Quantitative study of cortical orientation selectivity in visually inexperienced kitten. *J Neurophysiol* 1976;39:63–70.
6. Pettigrew JD. The effect of visual experience on the development of stimulus specificity by kitten cortical neurones. *J Physiol (Lond)* 1974;237:49–74.
7. Cynader M, Chernenko G. Abolition of directional selectivity in the visual cortex of the cat. *Science* 1976;193:504–505.
8. Pasternak T, Schumer R, Gizzi MS, Movshon JA. Abolition of cortical direction selectivity affects visual behaviour in cats. *Exp Brain Res* 1985;61:214–217.
9. Hirsch HVB, Spinelli DN. Visual experience modifies distribution of horizontally and vertically oriented receptive fields in cats. *Science* 1970;168:869–871.
10. Blakemore C, Cooper GF. Development of the brain depends on the visual environment. *Nature* 1970;228:477–478.
11. Stryker MP, Sherk H. Modification of cortical orientation selectivity in the cat by restricted visual experience: a reexamination. *Science* 1975;190:904–906.
12. Stryker MP, Sherk H, Leventhal AG, Hirsch HVB. Physiological consequences for the cat's visual cortex of effectively restricting early visual experience with oriented contours. *J Neurophysiol* 1978;41:896–909.
13. Cynader M, Berman N, Hein A. Cats raised in a one-directional world: effects on receptive fields in visual cortex and superior colliculus. *Exp Brain Res* 1975;22:267–280.
14. Tretter F, Cynader M, Singer W. Modification of direction selectivity of neurons in the visual cortex of kittens. *Brain Res* 1975;84:143–149.
15. Wiesel TN, Hubel DH. Single-cell responses in striate cortex of kittens deprived of vision in one eye. *J Neurophysiol* 1963;26:1003–1017.
16. Wiesel TN, Hubel DH. Comparison of the effects of unilateral and bilateral eye closure on cortical unit responses in kittens. *J Neurophysiol* 1965;28:1029–1040.
17. Wiesel TN, Hubel DH. Effects of visual deprivation on morphology and physiology of cells in the cat's lateral geniculate body. *J Neurophysiol* 1963;26:978–993.
18. Levay S, Stryker MP, Shatz C. Ocular dominance columns and their development in layer IV of the cat's visual cortex: a quantitative study. *J Comp Neurol* 1978;179:223–244.
19. Hubel DH, Wiesel TN. Receptive fields, binocular interaction and functional architecture in the cat's visual cortex. *J Physiol (Lond)* 1962;160:106–154.
20. Cynader M, Chernenko G. Some factors influencing the development of ocular dominance in

the cat striate cortex. Presented at the Association for Research in Vision and Ophthalmology, Sarasota, FL, April 1976.
21. Hubel DH, Wiesel TN, Levay S. Plasticity of ocular dominance columns in monkey striate cortex. *Philos Trans R Soc Lond [Biol]* 1977;278:377–409.
22. Mitchell DE. Effect of early visual experience on the development of certain visual capacities in animals and man. In: Walk RD, Pick HL, eds. *Perception and experience.* New York: Plenum Press, 1978;37–75.
23. Duke-Elder SS, Wybar K. *System of ophthalmology. Ocular motility and strabismus,* vol VI. London: Kimpton, 1973.
24. Guillery RW. Binocular competition in the control of geniculate cell growth. *J Comp Neurol* 1972;144:117–130.
25. Cynader M, Mitchell DE. Monocular astigmatism effects on kitten visual cortex development. *Nature* 1977;270:177–178.
26. Kasamatsu T, Pettigrew JD. Preservation of binocularity after monocular deprivation in the striate cortex of kittens treated with 6-hydroxydopamine. *J Comp Neurol* 1979;185:139–162.
27. Bear M, Singer W. Modulation of visual cortex plasticity by acetylcholine and noradrenaline. *Nature* 1986;320:172–176.
28. Daw NW, Robertson TW, Rader RK, Vedeen TO, Cosica CJ. Substantial reduction of noradrenaline by lesions of adrenergic pathways does not prevent effects of monocular deprivation. *J Neurosci* 1984;4:1354–1360.
29. Shaw C, Cynader M. Disruption of cortical activity prevents alterations of ocular dominance in monocularly-deprived kittens. *Nature* 1984;308:731–734.
30. Reiter HO, Stryker MP. Neural plasticity without postsynaptic action potentials: less active inputs become dominant when kitten visual cortex cells are pharmacologically inhibited. *PNAS* 1988;85:3623–3627.
31. Hubel DH, Wiesel TN. The period of susceptibility to the physiological effects of unilateral eyelid closure in kittens. *J Physiol (Lond)* 1970;206:419–436.
32. Cynader M, Timney BN, Mitchell DE. Period of susceptibility of kitten visual cortex to the effects of monocular deprivation extends beyond six months of age. *Brain Res* 1980;191:515–550.
33. Cynader M, Mitchell DE. Prolonged sensitivity to monocular deprivation in dark-reared cats. *J Neurophysiol* 1980;43:1026–1040.
34. Cynader M. Prolonged sensitivity to monocular deprivation in dark-reared cats: effects of age and visual exposure. *Dev Brain Res* 1983;8:155–164.
35. Mower GD, Berry D, Burchfiel JL, Duffy FH. Comparison of the effects of dark-rearing and binocular suture on development and plasticity of cat visual cortex. *Brain Res* 1981;220:255–267.
36. Needler MC, Shaw C, Cynader M. Characteristics and distribution of muscimol binding sites in cat visual cortex. *Brain Res* 1984;308:347–353.
37. Shaw C, Needler MC, Cynader M. Ontogenesis of muscarinic acetylcholine binding sites in cat visual cortex: reversal of specific laminar distribution during the critical period. *Dev Brain Res* 1984;14:295–300.
38. Prusky G, Shaw C, Cynader MS. Nicotine receptors are located on lateral geniculate nucleus terminals in cat visual cortex. *Brain Res* 1987;412:131–138.
39. Shaw C, Cynader M. Unilateral eyelid suture increases $GABA_A$ receptors in cat visual cortex. *Dev Brain Res* 1988;40:148–153
40. Prusky GT, Cynader MS. [^{3}H]Nicotine binding sites are associated with mammalian optic nerve terminals. *Visual Neurosci* 1988;1:245–248.
41. Shaw C, Prusky G, van Huizen F, Cynader M. Cellular localization of receptor populations in cat visual cortex using quinolinic acid lesions. Presented at the Society for Neuroscience, New Orleans, 1987.
42. Cynader M, Shaw C. Mechanisms underlying binocular competition in cat visual cortex. In: Kellar E, Zee D, eds. *Adaptive processes in visual and oculomotor systems.* New York: Pergamon Press, 1986;53–61.
43. Shaw C, Wilkinson MW, Cynader M, Needler MC, Aoki C, Hall SE. The laminar distributions and postnatal development of neurotransmitter and neuromodulator receptors in cat visual cortex. *Brain Res Bull* 1986;16:661–671.
44. Needler MC, Wilkinson M, Prusky G, Shaw C, Cynader M. Development of phorbol ester (protein kinase C) binding sites in cat visual cortex. *Dev Brain Res* 1988;42:217–227.

45. Shaw C, Needler MC, Wilkinson M, Aoki C, Cynader M. Modification of neurotransmitter receptor sensitivity in cat visual cortex during the critical period. *Dev Brain Res* 1985;22: 67–73.
46. Van Huizen F, Strosberg AD, Cynader M. Cellular and subcellular localisation of muscarinic acetylcholine receptors during postnatal development of cat visual cortex using immunocytochemical procedures. *Dev Brain Res* 1988;44:296–301.
47. Morrison JH, Magistretti PJ, Benoit R, Bloom FE. The distribution and morphological characteristics of the intracortical VIP-positive cell: an immunohistochemical analysis. *Brain Res* 1984;292:269–282.
48. Wong-Riley M. Changes in the visual system of monocularly sutured or enucleated cats demonstrable with cytochrome oxidase histochemistry. *Brain Res* 1979;171:11–28.

The Development of Visual Function in Infants

Davida Y. Teller

Departments of Psychology and Physiology/Biophysics, University of Washington, Seattle, Washington 98195

There are at least two motivations for studying the development of visual capacities during human infancy. The first is that adult-like visual function requires adult-like neural information processing, and different immaturities of neural functioning at a variety of critical loci can be expected to limit particular visual functions in infants. Insofar as we understand which neural elements are necessary for particular visual functions, functional development may challenge hypotheses concerning neural development, and vice versa. The second is that assessment of visual functions such as acuity and stereopsis could potentially play an important role in clinical diagnosis and in monitoring the effects of clinical treatments.

This chapter provides a brief summary of current knowledge concerning the development of visual acuity, contrast sensitivity, flicker fusion, stereopsis, and color vision during the first postnatal year. For a more comprehensive review of the development of vision and the visual system in human and nonhuman primates, and extensive citations of the basic and clinical literature, the reader is referred to (1). For a recent review of infant perceptual development, see (2).

MEASUREMENT TECHNIQUES

In the past 15 years, a variety of behavioral and electrophysiological techniques have been developed and refined for estimating the visual capacities of infants.

Preferential Looking

The most common behavioral techniques used in infant vision testing are variants of *preferential looking* techniques (3). Preferential looking techniques depend on the fact that infants will preferentially fixate and track patterned stimuli. In acuity testing, for example, the infant is confronted with a stimulus display containing a black and white acuity grating on one side and a blank field of matched space-average luminance on the other. The spatial frequency of the grating varies from trial to trial. An adult observer who is blind to the stimulus location watches the infant through a peephole and judges the direction of preferential fixation. A consistent preference for the grating over the blank field indicates that the infant can resolve the grating. In *forced-choice preferential looking,* the observer is required to judge the location of the grating on each trial; above-chance performance over a series of trials indicates that the infant can resolve the grating (4).

Operant Testing

Infants over 6 months of age rapidly become bored with preferential looking techniques. Operant reinforcers, such as animated toys and pieces of cereal, can be used to help sustain the necessary behavior (5,6).

Visual Evoked Potentials

Averaged visually evoked cortical potentials resulting from the presentation of flashed or phase-alternated visual patterns can be recorded from scalp electrodes. Recent advances in visual evoked potential (VEP) techniques include presentation of the stimuli in a rapid "sweep" rather than sequentially, and the use of sophisticated signal-to-noise analyses and scoring techniques (7).

Clinical Testing

All of these techniques have been used to test infants who are at risk for visual disorders, but, as yet, few are efficient enough or have high enough success rates for routine clinical use. A more efficient variant of preferential looking has been developed recently for clinical use (8,9).

DEVELOPMENT OF VISUAL FUNCTIONS

Grating Acuity

Typical behavioral data describing the development of grating acuity are shown in Fig. 1. One-month-old infants resolve approximately 1 cycle/deg (20/600 Snellen equivalent). Grating acuity improves over a long, slow time course, reaching 30 cycle/deg (20/20 Snellen equivalent) at about age 3. Forced-choice preferential looking and operant data together indicate a continuous slow emergence of visual resolution, both in group data and in individual infants tested longitudinally (10).

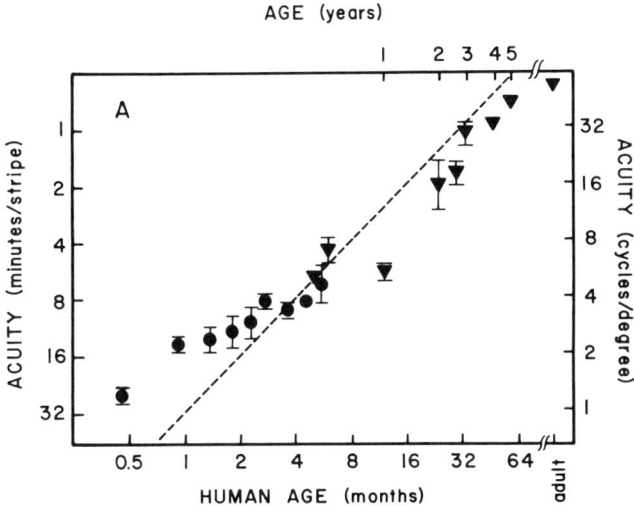

FIG. 1. The development of visual acuity as measured by forced-choice preferential looking (●) and operant preferential looking (▲). (From ref. 30.)

VEP measures of acuity in infants show a similar gradual emergence of visual resolution but uniformly give acuity estimates 1 to 2 octaves higher than those found with behavioral measures. VEP acuities as high as 20 cycle/deg can be found at 6 to 12 months (Fig. 2). Discrepancies between behavioral and VEP measures are partially attributable to differences in signal averaging and data scoring strategies for the two techniques and partially to a presumed loss of information between the sites of generation of the VEP and the sites of initiation of the behavioral responses.

Contrast Sensitivity Functions

The behaviorally measured contrast sensitivity functions (CSFs) of infants are extremely immature at birth, both in overall sensitivity and in shape. The CSFs of very young infants may lack a low-frequency falloff (11) but become bandpass by 2 to 3 months post-natally. Sensitivity to low frequencies matures earlier than sensitivity to high frequencies in infant monkeys (12) and presumably in human infants. Similar results are obtained with VEPs, except that sensitivity is higher at all ages; the most recent VEP results show sensitivity to low spatial frequencies approaching that of adults at 10 weeks post-natally (13).

Many factors converge to limit the spatial resolution capacities of adults, and the slow and smooth development of spatial resolution likewise suggests the involvement of many factors in infants. Since the optics of the eye are clear and well developed in early infancy, the limited acuity of infants is

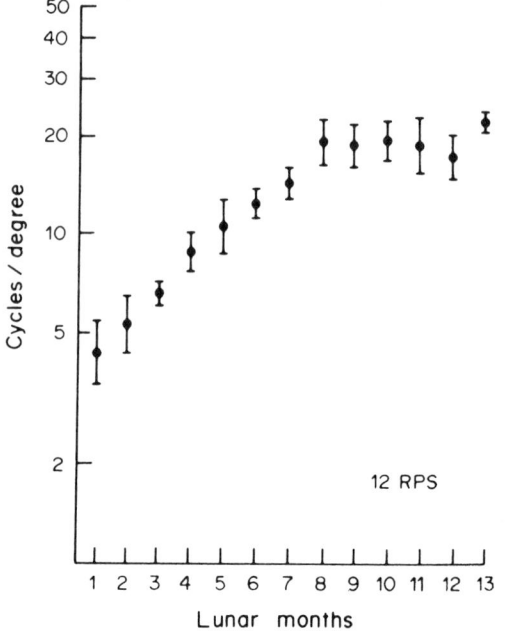

FIG. 2. Development of visual acuity as measured by the "sweep" VEP. (From ref. 7.)

usually attributed to neural immaturities. Current theorizing (14–16) emphasizes the immaturity of the fovea (17), particularly the limited quantum-catching efficacy of the immature cone outer segments and the coarser grain of foveal receptive fields caused by the immature packing density of foveal cones. It is suggested (18) that the relatively high sensitivity of the infant to low spatial frequencies is caused by the relative maturity of extrafoveal as opposed to foveal structures.

Flicker Fusion

In contrast to the major spatial resolution deficits seen in young infants, temporal resolution is apparently remarkably good (19). Behaviorally measured critical flicker fusion frequencies (CFFs) for 1-, 2-, and 3-month-old infants have been reported at approximately 40, 50, and 52 Hz, respectively, as shown in Fig. 3. No specific theoretical account of the development of CFF has been presented, but the general fit with several broad theoretical structures is good.

Rods, Cones, and Color Vision

The dark-adapted spectral sensitivity curves of young infants conform closely to the standard adult scotopic curve and to the absorption spectrum of

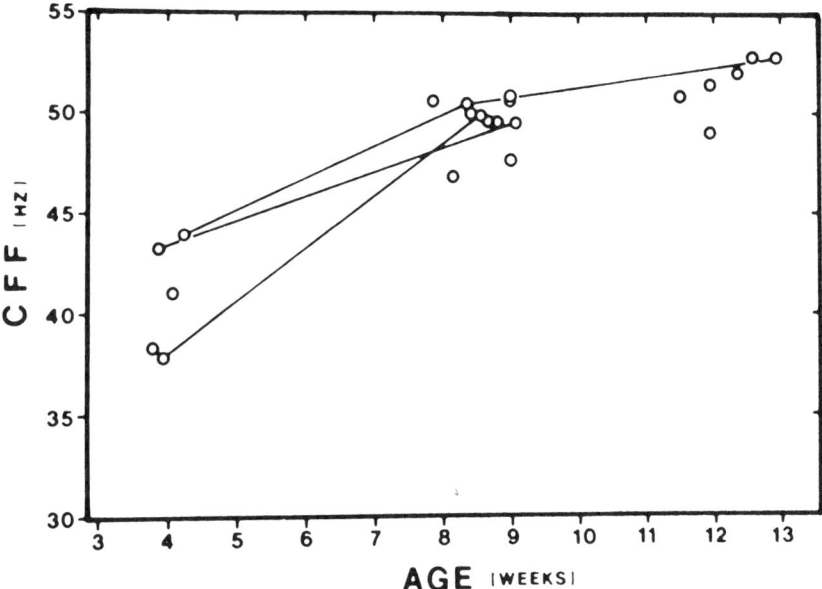

FIG. 3. Development of critical flicker frequency (CFF). (From ref. 19.)

rhodopsin; thus, rods are clearly functional in young infants. Light-adapted spectral sensitivity curves are broader, indicating the presence of additional receptor types.

Recently, the presence of "blue" cones has been confirmed in 4- to 6-week-old infants by means of VEP techniques (20). In addition, the presence of "red" and "green" cones and a chromatically opponent red/green channel have been confirmed by demonstration of a Sloan notch in 3-month-olds (21) (Figs. 4 and 5).

Behavioral paradigms have been worked out that allow testing of the capacity to make wavelength discriminations in the absence of brightness artifacts. To date, infants have been tested only with a few, widely spaced wavelength differences, usually intended to be diagnostic of the presence of individual cone types. So far, it has been difficult to demonstrate wavelength discrimination in 1-month-old infants. Two-month-olds do better, and 3-month-olds have succeeded in the cases in which they have been tested. (For a review, see [22].)

Overall the data suggest improvements in chromatic discrimination capacities during the first few postnatal months. However, behavioral testing is a laborious process, and only a few of the many aspects of color vision have yet been investigated. It is too soon to characterize the overall time course of development of color vision or to make any important guesses concerning the time periods of onset of major aspects of color vision other than minimal wavelength discrimination capabilities.

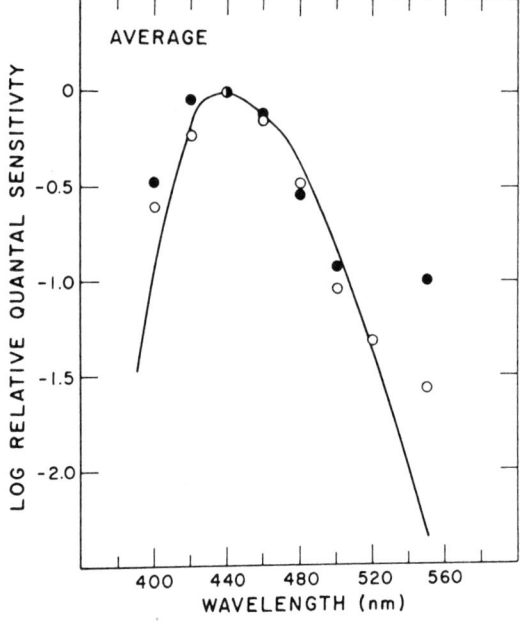

FIG. 4. "Blue" cones in 4- to 6-week-old infants, as revealed by use of visual evoked potentials. (○) adult; (●) infant. (From ref. 20.)

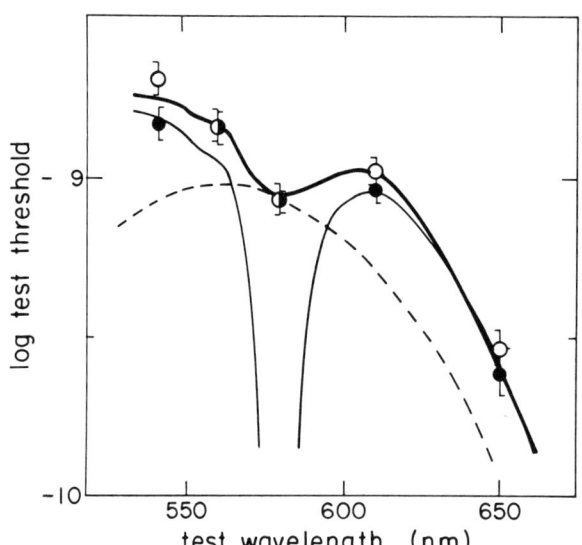

FIG. 5. Spectral sensitivity of 3-month-olds measured against a 580 nm adapting field, as tested by behavioral techniques. The minimum in sensitivity at 580 nm reveals a classical "Sloan notch" and indicates the presence of "red" and "green" cones. (From ref. 21.)

Stereopsis

The onset of response to binocular disparity, or to variations in binocular correlation, has been studied with both VEP and behavioral paradigms and with the use of both line and random-dot stereograms. All techniques so far are in remarkable agreement. By all techniques, few infants show a response to disparity cues prior to 3 to 4 months post-natally; virtually all show such responses by 6 to 7 months post-natally. In addition, and unlike the case of visual acuity, the onset of responses to binocular disparity and of stereoacuity has been reported to be extremely rapid within individual infants (Figs. 6 and 7) (23).

The rapid onset of response to binocular disparity coincides at least roughly with the time at which cortical ocular-dominance columns are presumed to be forming in the infant cortex. This temporal coincidence leads to the speculation that absence of a single neural process (such as the preservation of eye-of-origin information or the disparity tuning of cortical cells) prohibits the response to binocular disparity and that the abrupt onset of such a process allows the onset of response to stereo cues (24).

THEORETICAL CONSIDERATIONS

In summary, 1-month-old infants can certainly see, in the sense that they stare at bold patterns, detect light in both scotopic and photopic ranges, and

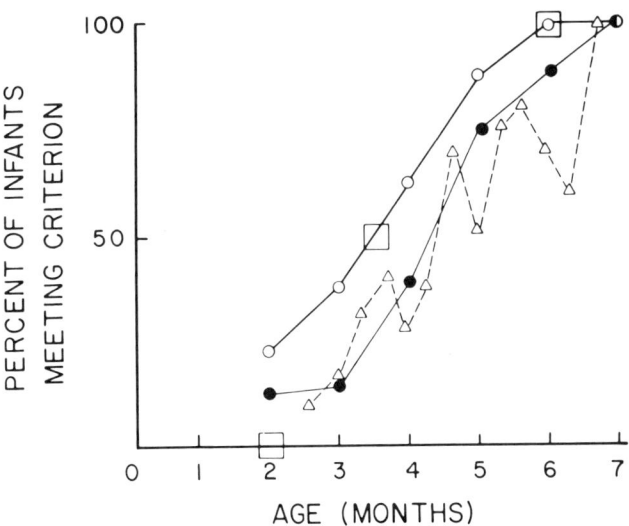

FIG. 6. Development of stereopsis, as measured by various authors using random-dot stereograms and VEPs (□), random-dot stereograms and preferential looking (△), and line stereograms and preferential looking (○,●). (From ref. 31.)

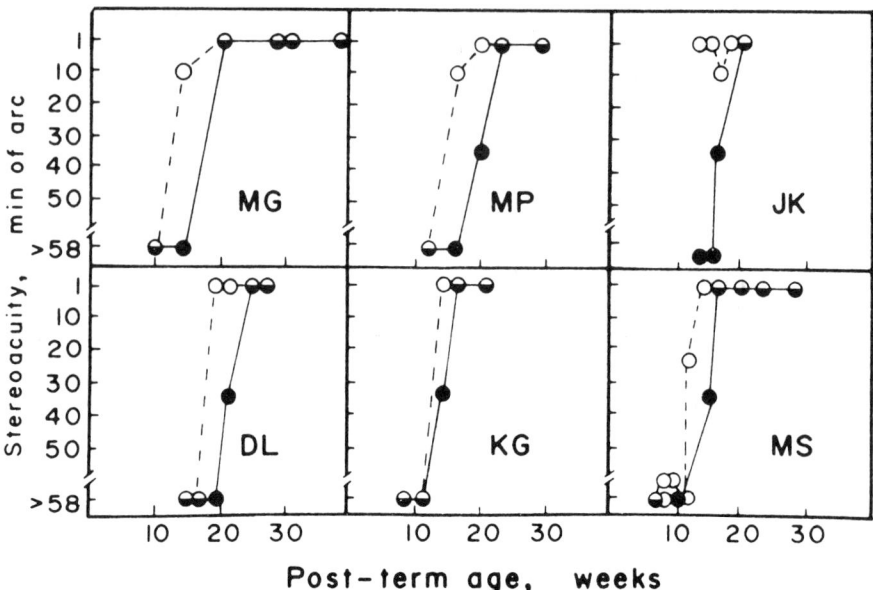

FIG. 7. Rapid development of stereoacuity in individual infants. (From ref. 23.)

show measurable VEPs, and their flicker resolution is remarkably good. However, to date they have not demonstrated responsiveness to stereo disparities, their acuity is very limited, and their color vision is apparently poor to nonexistent. Stereovision and related functions show a rapid onset during the fourth through sixth postnatal month, whereas visual resolution develops with a stately time course during at least the first postnatal year.

The fact that different aspects of visual function emerge with different time courses and in different postnatal epochs suggests that the emergence of different aspects of vision is limited by the maturation of different neural elements and combinations of elements. The differences in developmental time course also open the possibility that different visual functions may have different critical or sensitive periods, during which visual deprivation may irreversibly perturb the emergence of normal vision.

In addition to specialized theoretical accounts of the neural basis of development of specific visual functions previously mentioned, several authors have proposed more general schemes concerning the overall limits imposed on visual function by neural development. For example, it has sometimes been argued that infant visual development may be governed by shifts from subcortical to cortical functioning (25) or by the development of cortical/subcortical connections (26). The immaturity of the infant fovea tempts comparisons of infant vision to adult peripheral vision (27,28). Alternatively, it has been suggested that differences in the development of X and Y pathways may govern the broad course of human visual development (29). Although all of these theories are worthy of consideration, the suggested schemes are overlapping and in the main not mutually exclusive, and the quality of the visual development data to date is insufficient to allow a clear choice among alternatives.

In the context of this volume, it is natural to suggest that different time courses of development of the different visual information processing "streams" could be a useful overall theoretical framework for understanding the development of visual functions. Earlier development of the magno system could account qualitatively for the early emergence of good flicker resolution, and later development of the parvo system could provide a qualitative rationale for the long slow emergence of grating acuity. It is tempting to speculate that more detailed and quantitative developmental data of the future could assist us in choosing among different models of the numbers, functions, and interactions among parallel processing "streams" in the human visual system.

ACKNOWLEDGMENTS

Preparation of this chapter was supported by grants EY 02920 and EY 04470 from the National Eye Institute.

REFERENCES

1. Boothe RG, Dobson V, Teller DY. Postnatal development of vision in human and nonhuman primates. *Ann Res Neurosci* 1985;8:495–545.
2. Salapatek P, Cohen LB, eds. *Handbook of infant perception: from sensation to cognition, vol 1.* New York: Academic Press, 1987.
3. Fantz RL, Ordy JM, Udelf MS. Maturation of pattern vision in infants during the first six months. *J Comp Physiol Psychol* 1962;55:907–917.
4. Teller DY. The forced-choice preferential looking procedure: a psychophysical technique for use with human infants. *Inf Behav Dev* 1979;2:135–153.
5. Mayer DL, Dobson V. Visual acuity development in infants and young children, as assessed by operant preferential looking. *Vision Res* 1982;22:1141–1151.
6. Birch EE, Gwiazda JA, Bauer J, Naegele J, Held R. Visual acuity and its meridonial variations in children aged 7–60 months. *Vision Res* 1983;23:1019–1024.
7. Norcia AM, Tyler CW. Spatial frequency sweep VEP: visual acuity during the first year of life. *Vision Res* 1985;25:1399–1411.
8. Teller DY, McDonald M, Preston K, Sebris SL, Dobson V. Assessment of visual acuity in infants and children: the acuity card procedure. *Dev Med Child Neurol* 1986;28:779–789.
9. Sebris SL, Dobson V, McDonald MA, Teller DY. Acuity cards for visual acuity assessment of infants and children in clinical settings. *Clin Vis Sci* 1987;2:45–58.
10. Allen J. The development of visual acuity in human infants during the early postnatal weeks. PhD thesis, University of Washington, 1979.
11. Banks MS, Salapatek P. Contrast sensitivity function of the infant visual system. *Vision Res* 1976;16:867–869.
12. Boothe RG, Kiorpes L, Williams RA, Teller DY. Operant measurements of contrast sensitivity in infant macaque monkeys during normal development. *Vision Res* 1988;28:387–396.

13. Norcia AM, Tyler CW, Hamer RD. High visual contrast sensitivity in the young human infant. *Invest Ophthalmol Vis Sci* 1988;29:44–49.
14. Brown AM, Dobson V, Maier J. Visual acuity of human infants at scotopic, mesopic and photopic luminances. *Vision Res* 1987;27:1845–1858.
15. Wilson HR. Development of spatiotemporal channels in infant vision. Paper presented at the Annual Meeting of the Optical Society of America, Seattle, 1986.
16. Banks MS, Bennett PJ, Schefrin B. Foveal cones and spatial vision in human neonates. *Invest Ophthalmol Vis Sci* 1987;28(suppl):4.
17. Yuodelis C, Hendrickson A. A qualitative and quantitative analysis of the human fovea during development. *Vision Res* 1986;26:847–855.
18. Norcia AM, Tyler CW, Hamer RD. High visual contrast sensitivity in the young human infant. *Vision Res* 1988;29:44–49.
19. Regal DM. Development of critical flicker frequency in human infants. *Vision Res* 1981;21:549–555.
20. Volbrecht V, Werner JS. Isolation of short wavelength-sensitive cone photoreceptors in 4–6-week-old human infants. *Vision Res* 1987;27:469–478.
21. Brown AM, Teller DY. Chromatic opponency in 3-month-old human infants. *Vis Res* 1989;29:37–45.
22. Teller DY, Bornstein MH. Infant color vision. In: Salapatek P, Cohen LB, eds. *Handbook of infant perception*. New York: Academic Press, 1987;185–236.
23. Birch EE, Gwiazda J, Held R. Stereoacuity development for crossed and uncrossed disparities in human infants. *Vision Res* 1982;22:507–513.
24. Held R. Binocular vision—behavioral and neural development. In: Mehler J, Fox R, eds. *Neonate cognition: beyond the blooming, buzzing confusion*. Hillsdale, NJ: Erlbaum, 1984;37–44.
25. Bronson GW. The postnatal growth of visual capacity. *Child Dev* 1974;45:873–890.
26. Atkinson J. Human visual development over the first 6 months of life: a review and a hypothesis. *Hum Neurobiol* 1984;3:61–74.
27. Hamer RD, Alexander KR, Teller DY. Rayleigh discriminations in young human infants. *Vision Res* 1982;22:575–587.
28. Norcia AM, Tyler CW, Hamer RD. High visual contrast sensitivity in the young human infant. *Invest Ophthalmol Vis Sci* 1988;29:44–49.
29. Maurer D, Lewis TL. A physiological explanation of infants' early visual development. *Can J Psychol* 1979;33:232–252.
30. Teller DY. The development of visual acuity in human and monkey infants. *Trends in Neurosci* 1981;4:21–24.
31. Teller DY. Scotopic vision, color vision, and stereopsis in infants. *Curr Eye Res* 1983;2:199–210.

Vision and the Brain,
edited by B. Cohen and I. Bodis-Wollner.
Raven Press, Ltd., New York © 1990.

Segregation of Form, Color, Movement, and Depth Processing in the Visual System: Anatomy, Physiology, Art, and Illusion

Margaret Livingstone

Department of Neurobiology, Harvard Medical School, Boston, Massachusetts 02115

It would be interesting if some real authority investigated carefully the part which memory plays in painting. We look at the object with an intent regard, then at the palette, and thirdly at the canvas. The canvas receives a message dispatched . . . from the natural object. But it has come through a post office *en route*. It has been transmitted in code. It has been turned from light into paint. It reaches the canvas a cryptogram. Not until it has been placed in its correct relation to everything else that is on the canvas can it be deciphered, is its meaning apparent, is it translated once again from mere pigment into light. And the light this time is not of Nature but of Art.

Winston S. Churchill, *Painting as a Pastime*

The process of seeing is much more complicated than most people think. In an age when accurate representations of the visual world can be made, stored, and transmitted using a variety of photographic and electronic methods, we are tempted to think of the visual system as just another kind of camera. But it is not: no matter how sophisticated a representation of the world you have, you still need to look at it to know what it shows, and that is what the visual system does. As Churchill surmised, your visual system analyzes light patterns and converts the information into code, a code powerful enough and flexible enough to furnish you with an enormous amount of information about your environment, from an almost infinite variety of images. That is something no video system or computerized camera has come close to being able to do. The strategies that the visual system uses to extract information from light patterns are often surprisingly simple and sensible, but they are not obvious—indeed none of them was predicted before they were actually discovered.

As I will describe, not all light information from an image is equally important to the visual system, and, furthermore, the same light pattern is analyzed in several ways to encode different aspects of the scene. Even though the underlying neurobiological explanations for many of the phenomena I will describe have only recently been worked out, many artists and designers seem to have been empirically aware of some of the principles. Nevertheless it may be easier to maximize particular desired visual effects if you have some understanding of how the brain processes visual information.

Recent findings about the anatomy, physiology, and psychology of the visual system allow us to make some predictions about the influence of pattern and color on our ability to organize and relate the visual information in a single scene. Most people know that borders, contours, and lines can do more than just indicate the outlines of objects: they can also determine how we perceive their three-dimensional shape and position. What may not be so obvious is that a contour formed by the abutment of two bright, vivid colors may be very noticeable, even strident, but nevertheless be surprisingly ineffective in telling us about position, depth, or movement. Moreover, that same edge formed instead by two different shades of the same hue, or even two shades of gray, although less noticeable, may nevertheless have a much stronger effect. For example, converging lines in a flat drawing usually give a strong illusion of depth; the apparent shape of a torso can be altered by lines in a garment that draw the eye along one direction; a few well-placed contour lines or stippling can transform a flat outline into an image that produces an impression of a vividly three-dimensional object. But the contour can be more or less effective in generating a sense of depth or organization depending on the colors that generate it.

It can be hard to pick out in an image the color borders or contours that are the most important in determining the relative positions of elements in the picture and in generating a sensation of depth. But a simple black and white photograph of that color picture can reveal the organizing strengths of different contours and indicate how to make a given border more or less powerful. As I will describe, the part of your visual system responsible for generating a sense of depth and for perceiving spatial relationships is independent of other parts of the visual system, and unlike the other parts, it sees colors as shades, like black and white photography. The simple strategy of taking a black and white photograph of a colored image, to distinguish strong from weak color combinations, should be interesting and perhaps useful to people involved in the visual arts, fashion, and advertising; we, in turn, would be interested to find out how well our laboratory findings apply to other fields.

THE PROCESSING OF DIFFERENT KINDS OF VISUAL INFORMATION IN ANATOMICALLY SEGREGATED PATHWAYS

The brain extracts biologically relevant information from patterns of light by analyzing the information in a series of stages, starting in the eye and extending through dozens of processing steps in the brain. At each stage the input from the previous stage is analyzed in a more complicated way. In the first step, the light receptors in the eye, the only information you have is the light intensity at millions of tiny points in a two-dimensional array. The light receptors turn this light into electrical signals. In the next processing stages, still within the eye, these signals are transformed into a code that gives information about the difference in light intensity between each point in the scene and the average light intensity surrounding that point. When you get to the brain the information is processed to encode the location and orientation of borders or edges. At still higher brain levels, the information is correlated with information from memory, and you have such sophisticated functions as the recognition of familiar faces and the ability to read.

But the brain does not process visual information in only one such hierarchical system. Rather it feeds the same raw data into at least three separate computational systems that act independently and in parallel (Fig. 1). Each of these separate subsystems seems to have specific visual functions: one deals with the perception of shape, another with color, and the third with position, movement, and depth. Each subsystem processes visual information in a different way, in order to extract the type of information needed for its particular visual function.

It may seem strange to think of vision as multipartite rather than a single process; strange to think that your perception of the shape of an object, its color, its position in space, and its movement are each handled by separate parts of your brain—but anatomical, physiological, and psychological studies strongly support this idea. We are not intuitively aware that our visual perception is fragmented, so presumably the three systems respond simultaneously and independently to different aspects of the same visual scene and the summed information is interpreted by the brain as a unified perception—just as when you experience a person speaking, you are not really aware that hearing his or her words and seeing his or her mouth move are processed independently. It is only with unusual types of visual stimuli that one system can be active and the others quiet, and then things can look quite peculiar.

The first split in the visual system occurs at a stage within the eye, before the information even reaches the brain; here there are already major differences between the two subsystems in the type of information transmitted, especially in the handling of information about color. I will concentrate first on how you see color, especially on how the three subsystems differ in their processing of color information. The predictions arising from these differences are of general interest and somewhat surprising.

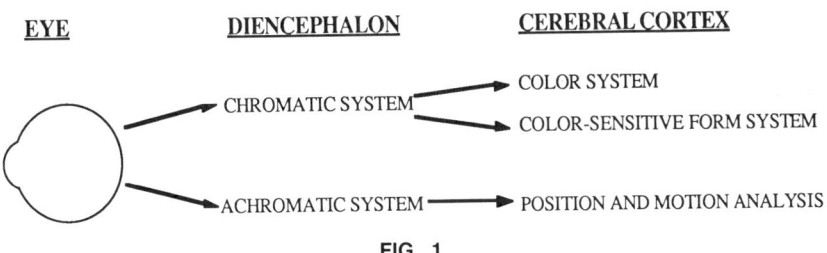

FIG. 1.

HOW DO WE SEE COLOR?

We are constantly bombarded by electromagnetic radiation of a wide range of wavelengths, and light, the type of energy we can see, is only a small subset of these energies. We cannot see the other wavelengths because the light-sensitive pigments in our eyes respond to only a particular range of wavelengths. As Isaac Newton discovered, ordinary white light from the sun contains a mixture of wavelengths, which can be separated by a prism to produce a spectrum or by water droplets to produce a rainbow.

We can distinguish different wavelengths of light as different colors because we have three visual pigments that each absorb (and can therefore emit a signal in response to) a different range of wavelengths. The cells containing these light-absorbing pigments are called cones. Each cone contains only one of the three types of pigments; thus we have three types of cones that respond best to different ranges of wavelength: one type responds best to longer wavelengths (red and orange light); the second to intermediate wavelengths (green light); and the third to still shorter wavelengths (blue and violet).

Each cone type responds to a relatively broad range of wavelengths, and, because the ranges overlap, it is only by *comparing* or *subtracting* the responses of the three cone types that we can discriminate colors. A red cone responds optimally to a bright red spot. It will give a weaker response to either a dim red spot or a bright yellow or green spot. It is only when the red-cone response is *compared* with the green- and blue-cone responses that the nature of the stimulus can be determined unambiguously.

We have a fourth type of photoreceptor, the rods, which are much more light sensitive than the cones and are used in very dim light. In light that is too dim to be visible to the cones but bright enough for the rods, such as moonlight, we cannot see colors even when we can distinguish shapes and see shades of gray. (The next time the moon is full and you wake up in the middle of the night, check this out for yourself.) This is because the rod system has only a single kind of pigment, so it cannot produce a differential response to different wavelengths. For the rest of this discussion I will be concerned only with daylight vision and will not need to consider the rod system.

THE THREE SUBDIVISIONS OF THE VISUAL SYSTEM

The idea that different types of information from common sensory receptors can be processed along separate pathways is far from new. Evidence that the mammalian visual system consists of at least two separate subpathways originates with the observation that the retinas project both to the lateral geniculate bodies, and from there to the cortex and to the superior colliculi. I will not discuss the pathway to the superior colliculus or any other subcortical pathways, which are concerned with eye movements; in this chapter I will be concerned only with the geniculocortical part of the visual system, which is responsible for what we think of as vision or conscious visual perception.

The geniculocortical pathway is itself subdivided: the first anatomically obvious division is in the lateral geniculate body (one of several knee-shaped structures deep in the brain) and a second division occurs in the visual cortex; from there these three pathways then seem to remain separate. The fact that the visual system consists of several subdivisions was discovered with anatomical techniques, and we are beginning to understand the functional significance of dividing up the processing of visual information in this way by recording from neurons at different stages in each of the pathways and finding out what aspects of visual information are encoded by each neuron.

After the eyes, the next stage in the visual system is the lateral geniculate bodies, a pair of peanut-sized structures, one on each side of the brain. The geniculates have two distinct subdivisions, *magnocellular* and *parvocellular*, so named because of a conspicuous difference in cell sizes. Each eye sends projections to both subdivisions; the two sets of geniculate layers then project to separate sublayers in the primary visual cortex. Subdivisions in the primary and secondary visual cortical areas can be seen by staining for the mitochondrial enzyme cytochrome oxidase; the differences in staining among the subdivisions probably reflect differences in activity levels. In Visual Area 1 we see small round, dark-staining areas, called "blobs" because of their shape, surrounded by lighter-staining interblob regions; Visual Area 2 has three types of subdivisions, also distinguishable by cytochrome-oxidase staining, arranged in stripes: two types of dark-staining stripes, thin and thick, interdigitating with lighter-staining interstripes. The magno-recipient parts of Visual Area 1 project to the thick stripes of Visual Area 2 and to the higher cortical area MT. The parvo-recipient upper layers of Visual Area 1 are themselves further subdivided, into blob and interblob regions. The interblobs project to the pale interstripes of Visual Area 2. The input to the blobs is not entirely clear: they may receive input from the magno as well as from the parvo system. The blobs project to the thin stripes in Visual Area 2. These pathways seem to remain independent in their projections to still higher cortical areas: the thick stripes project to area MT; the thin stripes to area V4; and the projections of the interstripes are unclear. A diagram of these independent pathways is shown in Fig. 2.

FUNCTIONAL DIFFERENCES BETWEEN THE SUBDIVISIONS

As mentioned earlier, the first step in all the subdivisions of the visual system is to compare the amount of light at each point on the retina with the amount of light in the immediately surrounding area. This comparison, which amounts to a subtraction, is essential for our ability to extract useful informa-

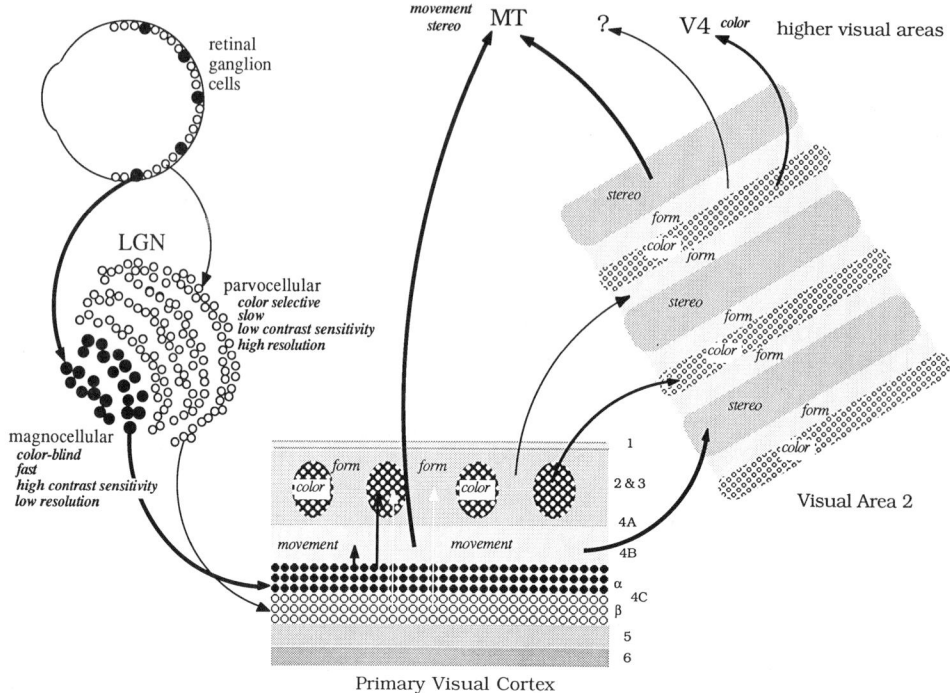

FIG. 2. Functional segregation in the primate visual system.

tion from patterns of light without having to know what the illumination intensity is. For example, if you look at a newspaper in ordinary lamplight, the headline looks black and the paper white; if you take the same newspaper outside on a sunny day, the amount of light coming to your eye from the headline is 100 times greater than the amount of light that had previously been coming from the white paper under lamplight; nevertheless, the print still looks black and the paper white. The reason for this constancy is that center/surround antagonism converts the visual input of absolute amounts of light into information about the relative brightness at any point compared with its immediate surround.

Although in both the parvo and the magno pathways the first step in information processing is a center/surround comparison, in the parvo pathway the subtraction also involves a comparison of different colors or cone types, and in the magno pathway it does not. As shown in Fig. 3, in the parvo pathway, the center/surround antagonism involves the *subtraction* of the inputs of the three types of cones (in different combinations for different cells). This subtractive analysis of color inputs is essential for our ability to see colors, but physiological and psychophysical experiments indicate that it is also important

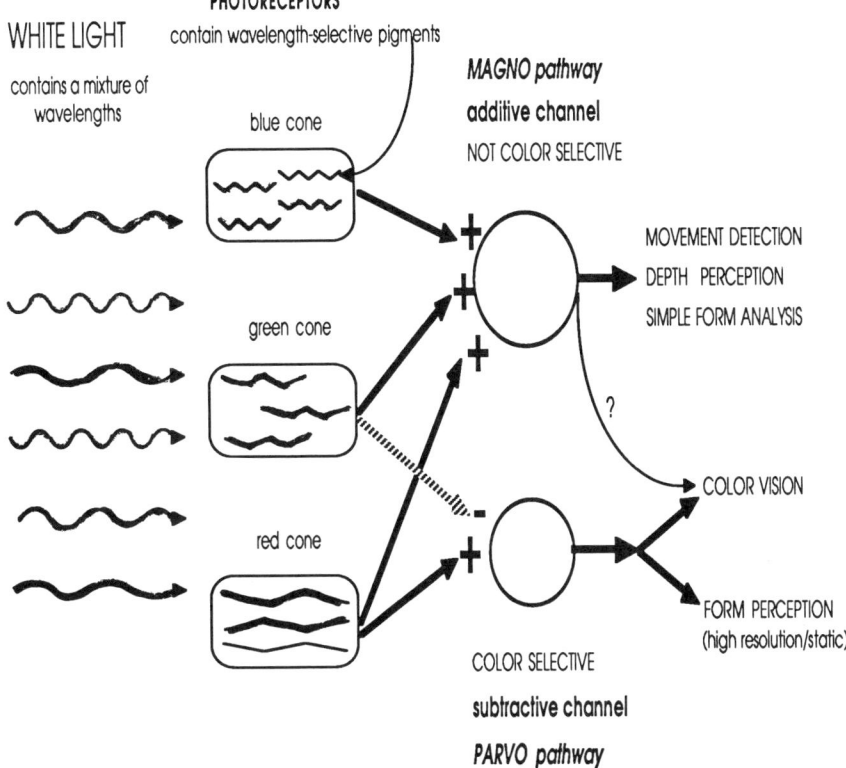

FIG. 3.

for our ability to use color differences to see borders for shape perception. In the further subdivisions of the parvo pathway, the blob system carries information about the color (including shades of gray) of objects, and the interblob system carries information about the shape or outline of objects using both brightness and color differences to detect edges.

The first step in the magno system is to *sum* the inputs from the three cone types. Because of this initial summing of cone inputs, this system, like night vision, cannot discriminate differences in color but can distinguish brightness differences.

The differences in the physiological properties of cells in these three anatomically defined pathways indicate that they handle different kinds of visual information. Some of the most important differences probably originate in the retina, but they have been studied most extensively in the geniculate. Parvocellular and magnocellular neurons differ markedly in three other ways besides their color properties: contrast sensitivity, temporal resolution, and acuity. The magno system, compared with the parvo system, has a higher sensitivity to brightness contrast, faster response times, and lower acuity.

The striking differences in the physiological properties between the magno and parvo geniculate divisions suggest that they serve very different visual functions, but what these functions are is not evident from the properties of cells at these early stages. There are, nevertheless, some hints from the response properties of cells at higher levels. For example, physiological studies in Semir Zeki's (1) laboratory suggest that the higher visual cortical area MT is especially important in motion perception, because cells in this area are very sensitive to moving stimuli and are often selective for the direction of motion. Zeki (2) has also reported that another higher cortical area, V4, seems to contain a high proportion of cells conveying information about color. Until recently, however, it was not known what the relationship was between these higher cortical visual areas and the subdivisions of the geniculate. Recent work that David Hubel and I (3,4) have done on the connections and physiological properties of the different subdivisions at intermediate levels, visual areas 1 and 2, has allowed us, in a sense, to complete the puzzle. Because we now know which of the lower level pathways provide input to these higher visual areas, we can begin to assign functions to the different pathways and then to predict how differences in the geniculate properties should be reflected in different types of visual tasks.

Taken together, the physiology and anatomy suggest that we can assign the following functions to the three subdivisions of the geniculocortical visual system:

1. The *magnocellular* ➡ *thick-stripe* ➡ *MT* pathway is characterized by cells that are selective for movement and stereoscopic depth.

2. The *parvocellular* ➡ *interblob* ➡ *pale-stripe* system seems to be responsible for high resolution static form perception. Cells in this system respond to both luminance- and color-contrast borders, but they are probably not concerned with the perception of color as such since most of them are not wavelength or contrast-sign selective. This system is probably responsible for our being able to see form and shape using either color-contrast or brightness-contrast edges and for our ability to see in detail the stationary elements of a scene. It can use color differences to detect borders that might be invisible or camouflaged to the achromatic magno system, but it nevertheless does not carry the information about what the colors are that form the border. It can detect a red spot on an equiluminant green background, but it probably does not carry information about the color of the spot or the background.

3. The *blob* ➡ *thin stripe* ➡ *V4* system is concerned with color but not with movement, shape discrimination, or stereopsis. This system has a lower acuity than the interblob system by a factor of approximately three or four.

The physiological properties of these functional divisions should have some obvious psychophysical consequences, and David Hubel and I tested such predictions by reviewing the psychophysical literature, repeating some experiments, and doing some of our own. We asked if human depth and movement perception, as compared with shape and color perception, are consistent with the physiological differences between the magno and parvo systems. For example, are movement and depth perception, compared with high-resolution form perception, less sensitive to color, more sensitive to luminance contrast, and do they have lower spatial and higher temporal resolution? Many psychophysical experiments suggest that these predictions are indeed largely true, and I will describe some of the evidence that motion perception and stereoscopic depth perception are color-blind and have low acuity, a very high sensitivity to luminance contrast, and fast temporal resolution.

THE DISTINCTION BETWEEN COLOR CONTRAST AND LUMINANCE CONTRAST

A border formed between a red object and a green one (or between a red object and a green background) is a strong stimulus for the color-sensitive parvo system, because it produces a maximum response in cells that compares green and red inputs. The parvo system can distinguish between red and green at all relative brightnesses of the two. The achromatic magno system is like black and white photography, in that it carries information about the brightness of surfaces but not about their colors, so reds and greens simply appear as different shades of gray, as in a black and white photograph. For any pair of colors, say red and green, there is a narrow range of relative red-to-green brightnesses for which they will appear as the same shade of gray in a black and white photograph, and hence any border or edge between them will vanish. Similarly, for the magno system, over a narrow range of relative red-to-green brightnesses the red and green will be equally effective. The two colors are then called *equiluminant.* A border between two equiluminant colors has color contrast but no luminance contrast. The exact brightness ratio between two colors at which a border between them becomes invisible to the achromatic part of the visual system may be different for different people, just as different black and white films may be relatively more sensitive to particular colors. Kodak Panatomic films have approximately the same relative red/green sensitivity as many people, but Kodak Orthochromatic films are much less sensitive to red relative to green. Panatomic film will therefore more closely represent what your achromatic magno system sees, but Orthochromatic film will exaggerate some contours and miss others.

I have used the term color-blind to describe the magno system, but this system is really much more color-blind than a person with ordinary color blindness. Someone with red/green color blindness, the most common kind, is missing only one of the three types of cones. He or she can therefore still use the other two cone types subtractively to discriminate wavelengths. Although he or she will not be able to distinguish between some colors that appear different to a normal observer, he or she will nevertheless still be able to distinguish most pairs of colors from each other no matter what their relative brightness. This is much less color-blind than everyone's magno system or night vision.

We therefore asked what visual functions are lost at equiluminance, to try to find out the functions of the magno system. Physiological studies had suggested that both movement and stereopsis are carried by the magno system, and there was already some human psychophysical evidence that both are insensitive to color.

Patrick Cavanagh, Christopher Tyler, and Olga Favreau (5) at Université de Montréal put moving red and green sinewave gratings (alternating red and green stripes) on a TV screen; they found that when the red and green were equiluminant, the perceived speed of movement was greatly reduced, or the stripes even appeared to stop moving completely. Other studies have confirmed that at least some aspects of motion perception are color-blind and moreover are sensitive on low luminance contrasts, consistent with the idea that motion perception is mainly a function of the magno system but not the parvo system.

Stereopsis is the ability to judge depth using differences between the images in the two eyes. In a three-dimensional scene, the images on the two retinas are different because the two eyes view the same scene from slightly different angles, and the visual system can interpret these differences as distance. You use stereoscopic depth perception when you look in a stereoscope or see a 3-D movie. Cary Lu and Derek Fender (6) from California Institute of Technology found that the ability to see stereoscopic depth is lost when images contain only equiluminant colors. There had been some controversy about the validity of their finding, probably due to technical difficulties in achieving exact equiluminance, so we tested it for ourselves. Our results, in agreement with the original report of Lu and Fender, are that stereopsis is indeed lost at equiluminance. Figure 4 is a graph of a subject's ability to use stereopsis to judge the distance of a uniform green object against a uniform red background for a range of relative red-to-green brightnesses. When the object was nonequiluminant with the background, the subject could guess correctly 100% of the time whether it was nearer or farther than a reference point. When the object was equiluminant with the background (when the relative brightness was 1), he could not guess correctly more often than chance (you get 50% correct just by chance).

Probably because it can easily be quantified, stereopsis is the depth cue studied most often by visual physiologists, but it is not the only one and is not essential for depth perception. Looking at photographs or paintings, you ignore or override the stereoscopic information that the picture is actually flat in order to experience any illusion of depth from the picture. This is why, as Leonardo da Vinci pointed out, you can increase the depth illusion from a picture by closing one eye.

When we found that depth from stereopsis was color-blind and likely to be

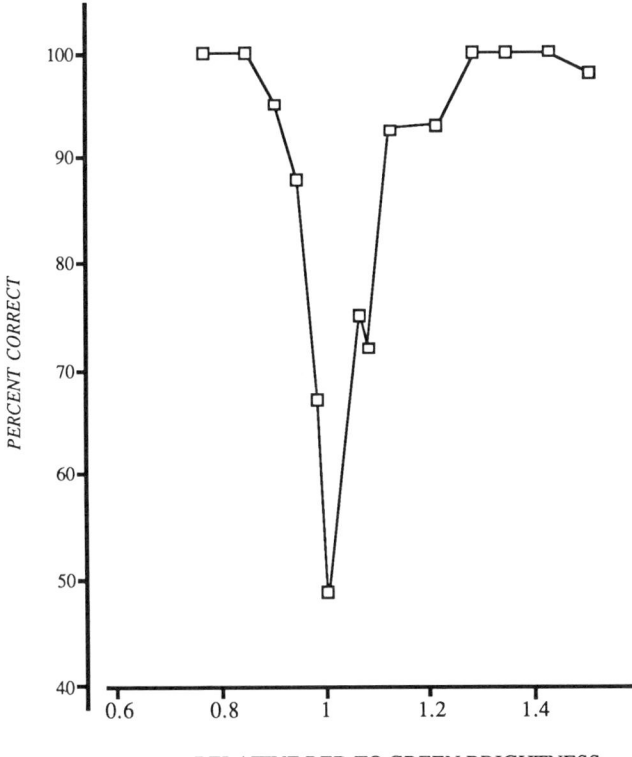

FIG. 4. Graph of a subject's ability to judge stereoscopic depth of a green target on a red background as a function of the red to green brightness.

carried by the magno system, knowing that other kinds of visual information can be used to perceive depth, we immediately asked whether other nonstereoscopic depth cues might also be color-blind. The other cues used by the visual system to see depth include (a) perspective and relative size of objects, (b) relative movement of objects (move your head sideways—near objects will move more than far objects), (c) shading and shadows, and (4) gradations in texture. We had expected that depth from movement might be color-blind simply because movement perception in general is, but to our surprise we found that all of these different types of information fail to produce a perception of depth when they are made equiluminant. This suggests that all aspects of depth and distance perception are carried by the achromatic magno system, with little or no contribution from the parvo system. The temporal properties, contrast sensitivity, and acuity of these functions further support this idea. I will describe ways many different types of depth and positional cues can be made ineffective or misleading by manipulating their luminance contrast and color contrast independently.

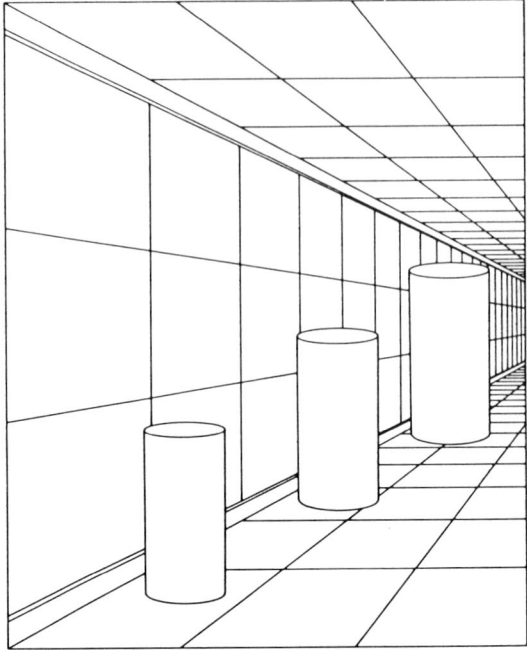

FIG. 5. James Gibson's corridor illusion.

The three cylinders in James Gibson's corridor illusion shown in Fig. 5 may not appear to be the same size, but you can convince yourself they are by measuring them. The one on the right appears larger because the perspective cues provided by the converging lines suggest that it is farther away. Perspective is the principle that the image of an object gets smaller the farther away it is.

A reduction in image size with increasing distance from an observer occurs when light passes through a focusing lens, as in an eye or a camera. You can see from the diagram in Fig. 6 that an object of a given size will produce a smaller image on the back of the eye or a camera film the farther away it is. The diagram also shows how a flat projection or drawing can mimic this size distortion and thus convey the same depth effect.

The information that the visual system starts with is a two-dimensional image on the retina, but it uses information about perspective and other depth cues to deduce the real size and position of objects in three-dimensional space. These seemingly sophisticated calculations happen automatically, probably because the visual system incorporates rules about the geometry of space into the way it handles information about contours and converging lines. You do not have to remember your geometry to see depth and the influence of apparent depth on perceived object size in the corridor illusion shown above; indeed, the calculation is so automatic that it is difficult not to see a receding hallway or to

FORM, COLOR, MOVEMENT, DEPTH PROCESSING 131

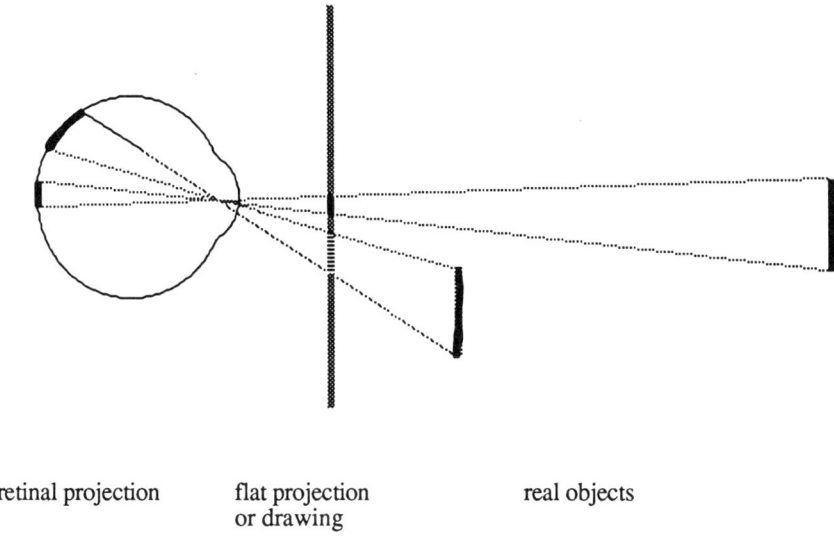

retinal projection flat projection real objects
or drawing

FIG. 6.

see the cylinders as all being the same size. The fact that we automatically and unconsciously perceive the visual world as a three-dimensional space rather than as the two-dimensional image that actually forms on our retina makes it difficult for most untrained people to make a drawing that looks like what they see.

We found that if we drew the corridor illusion with red lines on an equiluminant green background, it stopped looking like a hall receding into the distance and appeared to be a flat surface with a pattern that gets finer toward the right, and, furthermore, the cylinders then appeared to be the same size (as they actually are). Thus for converging lines or textures to generate a sensation of depth and to influence the apparent position and size of other objects they must have some luminance contrast with the background. This is consistent with our hypothesis that perspective is carried by the magno system. The geometrical basis for perspective was understood by the time of the Renaissance, but the fact that only luminance contrast and not color contrast information can generate depth from perspective is new.

The relative movement of objects provides very strong depth information; it is primarily this depth cue that makes ordinary movies seem so three dimensional. This depth cue has the same geometrical basis as perspective in that the retinal distance traversed in a given time is smaller the farther away the object is. For example, as you drive along a road, the trees at the edge of the road seem to zip past the car much more rapidly than the more distant fields; the fields seem to move faster than the still more distant mountains, and the sun seems to move along with you. You can get a very accurate estimate of the distance of objects simply by moving your head sideways and seeing how things move in your visual field relative to each other. We found that, like other depth cues, the ability to use relative movement to see depth is color-blind and depends solely on luminance contrast.

Shading is the variation in the amount of light reflected from different parts of an object because of its three-dimensional shape or because another object lies between it and the light source; not surprisingly, it is an important cue for the perception of depth and shape. For a single source of light, shading will consist mainly of differences in brightness but not color. In nature, even with more than one source of light, such as direct and reflected sunlight, the wavelength composition of the different sources is usually very similar. The depth information conveyed by shading and shadowing is thus almost always purely luminance-contrast information, so the part of the visual system coding shape-from-shading might as well not bother to carry any color-contrast information. This does not mean that it necessarily has to be color-blind, only that it has no need to carry color information.

Studies of human depth perception by Cavanagh and Leclerc (7) suggest that shape-from-shading is indeed color-blind: a shadow can be any hue, it only needs to be darker than the rest of the surface to convey a sense of depth. The fact that the color of a shadow is unimportant for conveying depth information seems to have been known by many artists. For example in Matisse's *Portrait de l'artiste en Maillot,* the green color of the shadows is peculiar, but the perceived three-dimensional shape nevertheless seems normal. It would take very unusual illumination to produce such colored shadows, but the strange color of the shadows does not interfere with their ability to generate a perception of shape: the only important criterion is that they be darker than the rest of his skin—their hue is irrelevant, at least for indicating shape. A black and white photograph shows that the green shadows are in fact darker.

Besides color sensitivity, another difference between the magno and parvo systems is that the magno system has approximately two- to threefold lower acuity. You can see the effect of this difference in resolution in Bridget Riley's painting (Fig. 7) by looking at it at different distances: close up the depth sensation should be very vivid, but as you move farther away, the impression of depth should be lost before you lose the ability to see the lines clearly. There should be a range of distances where the line spacing is too fine for your magno system but is still resolvable by the high-resolution form system. Thus, at the farthest distances at which you can still see the wavy lines, the surface they indicate will look much flatter than it does up close.

FIGURE-GROUND DISCRIMINATION

A particular border in a visual scene can be generated by the edge of an object against a background, by an edge of one object in front of another object, or by a shadow or bend, and so on. The gestalt psychologists analyzed

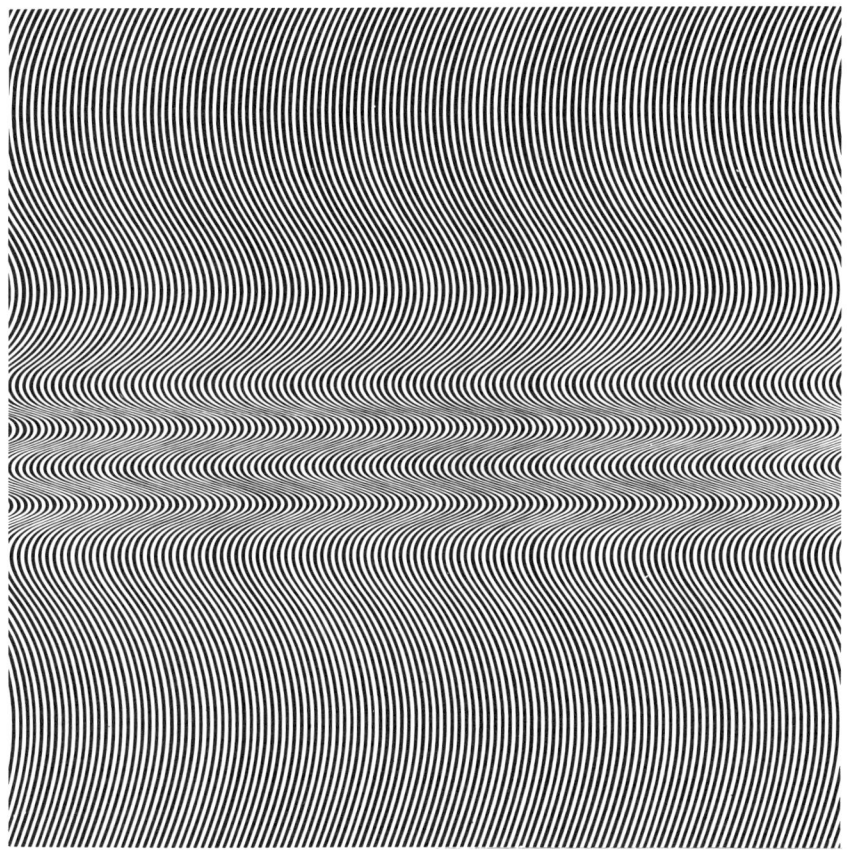

FIG. 7. Reprinted with permission. RILEY, Bridget. *Current.* 1964. Synthetic polymer paint on composition board, 58 ⅜" × 58 ⅞". Collection, The Museum of Modern Art, New York. Philip Johnson Fund.

the cues that are used to determine which contours belong to the same object and to segregate objects from the background. The differentiation of objects from each other and from the background seems to depend on many of the cues that break down at equiluminance, such as occlusion, stereopsis, and relative movement. Suzanne Liebmann (8) in 1926 described the difficulty in distinguishing figure from background at equiluminance, and K. Koffka (9) pointed out in 1935 that luminance differences are strikingly more important than color differences: "Thus two greys which look very similar will give a perfectly stable organization if one is used for the figure and the other for the ground, whereas a deeply saturated blue and a grey of the same luminosity which look very different indeed will produce practically no such organization." Edgar Rubin's popular illustration of the problem of deciding between figure and ground is the vase/face shown in Fig. 8. At nonequiluminance the

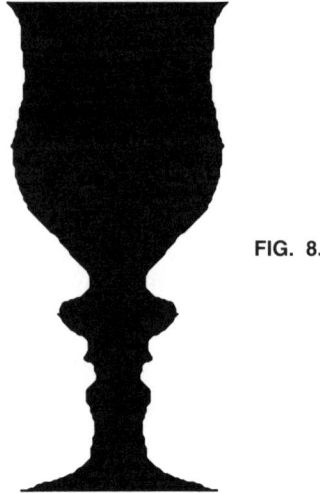

FIG. 8.

percept is bistable, so that one sees either the face or the goblet, but usually not both at the same time. At equiluminance the two percepts reverse rapidly, and one can occasionally see both the goblet and the faces simultaneously; that is, the distinction between figure and ground gets weaker or even disappears entirely.

A SUBSYSTEM FOR SPATIAL ORGANIZATION: LINKING

It was the loss of stereopsis at equiluminance that prompted us to examine perspective, size constancy, parallax, relative motion, shading, and occlusion because we wondered whether all kinds of information about depth might be carried by a color-blind system. Although we have not exhausted the list of possible depth cues or exhaustively examined any one of them, our overall impression is that they all deteriorate dramatically at equiluminance. Since it is clear that not all visual abilities are lost at equiluminance—shape recognition, for example, including high-resolution shape discrimination, is hardly impaired at all—we wondered whether all the abilities that are lost at equiluminance are functionally related as part of a single visual subsystem, a subsystem whose functions include the perception of motion, depth from various different types of information, and perhaps other functions involved in analyzing three-dimensional spatial organization.

Why should such a wide assortment of functions be carried by the magno system and not by the parvo system? What they may all have in common is the ability to help distinguish objects one from another and from the background, to correlate parts of the visual field that belong to the same objects, and to assign relative positions to objects in space. The gestalt psychologists suggested that certain visual properties of objects are used to group together parts of an image, to integrate figures, and to separate objects from each other and from the background; properties Horace Barlow (10) of Cambridge University called "linking features." These include direction and velocity of motion, depth (e.g., stereopsis, occlusion), collinearity, lightness, and texture. The fact that these are all functions that fail at equiluminance suggested to us that the ability to link together related parts of the visual scene, to discriminate figure from ground, and to perceive the correct spatial relationships of objects might all be carried by the magno system. This hypothesis would explain why cells selective for movement and stereopsis are found in the same brain region: movement-selective cells may be carrying information not about motion as such, but rather about spatial relationships conveyed by relative movement. You do not want to know the exact velocity of each dark spot moving in your visual field, you only need to know that a cluster of spots moving together means that a leopard is moving towards you. Barlow and the gestalt psychologists included color as a linking feature, but our results suggest that it is the brightness difference between two colors rather than wavelength difference that is used for linking.

An example of the use of colinearity as a linking feature is shown in Fig. 9 (10). Here you immediately know which lines belong to the same object even when they are discontinuous because they are occluded by other objects. You can tell the three-dimensional shape of each of the objects and how they are arranged in space. We found that at equiluminance this order broke down and we saw only a jumble of lines, instead of a pile of blocks. Like many other phenomena that break down at equiluminance, our ability to see the spatial organization in this figure was still possible with very low brightness-contrast images, consistent with the idea that linking by colinearity is carried by the magno system.

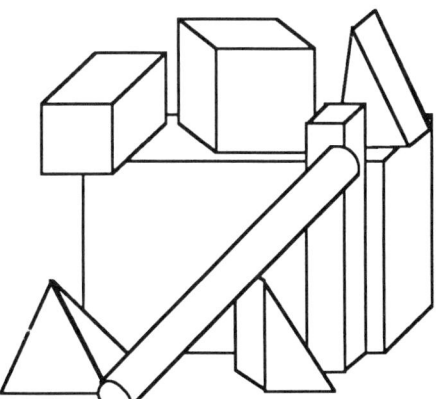

FIG. 9. Example of the use of colinearity as a linking feature.

WHERE VERSUS WHAT IN HIGHER VISUAL AREAS

Since shape discrimination is possible at both low luminance contrasts and equiluminance we have to conclude that both the magno and parvo systems have some ability to discriminate form. But the highest resolution form discrimination and the ability to use color-contrast information to determine shape both seem to be carried only by the parvo system. We have suggested that the magno system is responsible for the ability to determine depth and spatial relationships. The idea that even higher visual functions may also be so subdivided, with the subdivisions carried by anatomically separate pathways, receives some support from studies in Mortimer Mishkin's (11) laboratory at NIH. These studies suggest that visual areas higher than Visual Area 2, MT, and V4 can also be divided into two separate pathways, one that seems to be important for recognition of objects and the other for determining their spatial relationships. Spatial discrimination learning (remembering the location of objects) requires the posterior parietal cortex but not the temporal cortex, whereas the reverse is true for object discrimination tasks, a distinction described by Mishkin as where versus what. From anatomical connections, we suspect that the object recognition pathway probably represents a further continuation of the parvocellular pathway, and the localization pathway may correspond to the continuation of the magnocellular pathway. The clinical observation that people with strokes can lose specific visual abilities, such as the loss of color perception with loss of form perception or the loss of the ability to recognize faces, for half or even all of the visual field provides strong evidence that in humans as well different visual functions are carried out in separate brain regions.

SOME CONSEQUENCES OF THE SEGREGATION OF VISUAL FUNCTIONS

Some of the peculiar effects of op art probably arise from using color combinations that are strong activators of the parvo system but weak stimuli for the achromatic magno system. Objects that are equiluminant with their background look vibrant and seem somehow unstable in position. Equiluminant figures have been described in the psychophysical literature as "jazzy," "jelly-like," or "disorganized." Since the chromatic parvo system tells you the shape and color of an object, you can tell its shape quite well, but the magno system tells you where it is so its position in space is less definite. In paintings and prints, a figure that is equiluminant with the background will seem to float in an ambiguous depth plane, neither clearly in nor out of the plane of the picture. And since your magno system is responsible for motion analysis, your ability to tell whether it is moving is also impaired; thus without any information from the magno system, it can seem to jump around, drift, or vibrate.

MISREPRESENTATION OF VALUES USING COLORS

Mapmakers, engineers, and computer scientists often use colors to represent a third dimension, in order to display gradations of values (such as elevation, temperature, or speed) on a two-dimensional surface. The use of colors rather than gray levels makes it easier for the viewer to assign a unique value to a given point, because different colors are easier to name than different grays. But in choosing particular colors to represent the gradation of values, the artist often loses the benefit that gray levels have of conveying the overall pattern. The overall pattern, especially one of relative depth or height, is seen best by the achromatic system, so you need to provide the correct luminance-contrast information in order to see it.

These same principles can be applied to fashion. The overall impression of the shape of a garment can be influenced by lines in the material or trim, but the lines must have luminance contrast to be effective; the higher the luminance contrast, the greater the effect. Moreover, you can have patterns that do not interfere with the line of a garment if they are formed by colors that are close to equiluminant. If you want to wear horizontal stripes, but do not want to appear shorter and broader, then make sure that the stripes are close to equiluminant or very narrow. Wearing a kelly green shirt with bright royal blue pants is a combination that gives you a vibrant border, and the horizontal border will not contribute much to the overall impression of shape or draw the eye. So the combination will probably make you look taller than the same pants worn with a shirt of the same hue but a different shade, such as sky blue or navy.

The evidence is strong that the visual system is divided into several subsystems operating independently and in parallel, sharing some properties but differing significantly in others. Although we can see evidence of this subdivision in our own visual perception, we nevertheless do not understand the functional significance of this organization; we do not know whether it is a salutary design principle or an accident of evolution. Subdividing a single system might facilitate interactions, such as center-surround opponency, among cells carrying the same type of information. Moreover, segregation of different functions could allow each subdivision to acquire properties that might be particularly suited to its specialization. For example, the fast temporal properties of the magno system should be particularly useful in movement analysis. The slower temporal properties of the parvo system might make it capable of discriminating stationary objects, which the magno system might be blind to. The benefits of other differences, such as having the magno system insensitive to color or the parvo system less sensitive to luminance contrast, are less obvious.

From considerations of both development and evolution, there are hints that the magno system is older and more primitive than the parvo system, which is well developed only in primates. The magno system may be homologous to the entire visual system of lower mammals like cats and dogs. Thus, it may be that we should not ask what the magno system is specialized for but rather what is added on by the parvo system. An animal whose parvo system, or its homologue, is not well developed may be perfectly well able to carry out what we have been considering as the essential functions of vision, such as detecting, identifying, and following objects, especially moving ones, and determining their positions in space so the animal can navigate through its environment. But such an animal might nevertheless see the world very differently from the way we see it: it should see only the outlines of objects, with all homogeneous surfaces appearing the same, not differing in color or lightness, and it should be able to distinguish well only moving objects.

I have shown a few examples of how knowledge about the segregation of functions in the visual system could be useful to artists, advertisers, and designers; this knowledge might also be useful in designing surveillance systems, in devising ways to see blurry, low-contrast, or camouflaged images, and in designing video systems for robotics or automatic navigation. Because of the high-contrast sensitivity and movement selectivity of the magno system, we would predict that hard-to-see objects would become much easier to see if one could produce relative movement of the image—by moving the object or moving the observer relative to the object, by introducing stereoscopic depth, or by having two images of the scene taken from different positions. This sort of approach could make fuzzy images such as clinical X-ray photographs much easier to interpret and would be less expensive than CAT scans. Similarly, what we know about strategies used by the magno system for distinguishing objects from the background might be useful in designing automatic navigating systems. For example, such a machine could calculate the relative positions of objects that need to be avoided or followed with a very low resolution system simply by using parallax, without ever needing to identify the shape of the object.

REFERENCES

1. Zeki SM. *Proc R Soc Lond* 1980;207:239–248.
2. Zeki S. *Nature* 1980;284:412–418.
3. Livingstone MS, Hubel D. *Science* 1988;240:740–749.
4. Livingstone MS, Hubel DH. *J Neurosci* 1987;7:3416–3468.
5. Cavanaugh P, Tyler C, Ravreau O. *J Opt Soc Am [A]* 1984;1:893–899.
6. Lu C, Fender D. *Invest Ophthalmol* 1972;11:482–490.
7. Cavanaugh P, Leclerc Y. *Invest Ophthalmol* 1985;26:282.
8. Liebmann S. *Psychol Forsch* 1926;9:300–353.
9. Koffka K. *Principles of gestalt psychology.* New York: Harcourt, Brace, 1935;126–127.
10. Barlow H. *Proc R Soc Lond* 1981;212:1–34.
11. Mishkin M, Ungerleider LG. Macko KA. *Trends in Neurosci* 1983;6:414–417.

> Vision and the Brain,
> edited by B. Cohen and I. Bodis-Wollner.
> Raven Press, Ltd., New York © 1990.

The Neural Computation of the Velocity Field

Ellen C. Hildreth

Massachusetts Institute of Technology Artificial Intelligence Laboratory and Center for Biological Information Processing, Cambridge, Massachusetts 02139

The measurement and use of visual motion is a fundamental ability of biological vision systems, serving many essential functions. For example, a sudden movement in the scene might indicate an approaching predator or a desirable prey. The rapid expansion of features in the visual field can signal an object about to collide with the observer. Discontinuities in motion often occur at the locations of object boundaries and can be used to carve up the scene into distinct objects. Motion signals provide input to centers controlling eye movements, allowing objects of interest to be tracked through the scene. Relative movement can be used to infer the three-dimensional (3-D) structure and motion of object surfaces, and the movement of the observer relative to the scene, allowing biological systems to navigate quickly and efficiently through the environment.

The pattern of movement in the changing image is not given to the visual system directly but must be inferred from the changing intensities that reach the eye. The 3-D shape of object surfaces, the locations of object boundaries, and the movement of the observer relative to the scene can in turn be inferred from the pattern of image motion. Typically, the overall analysis of motion is divided into these two stages: first, the measurement of movement in the changing two-dimensional (2-D) image, and second, the use of motion measurements, for example to recover the 3-D layout of the environment. It is not yet clear whether motion analysis in biological systems is necessarily performed in two distinct stages, but this division has served to facilitate theoretical studies of motion analysis and to focus empirical questions for perceptual and physiological studies.

This chapter examines one aspect of the computation of an instantaneous 2-D velocity field, which captures the direction and speed of movement of image features. Early motion detection mechanisms in biological systems generally provide only partial information about image motion, due to a problem often referred to as the *aperture problem*. To compute a full velocity field, it is necessary to integrate motion information over an extended area of the image. An issue that arises in both computational and perceptual studies is whether this integration occurs along oriented features in the image, such as edge contours, or over 2-D areas. This chapter reviews both theoretical and experimental work that addresses this issue and presents a hypothetical neural model that combines both strategies for integrating motion information.

THE APERTURE PROBLEM

The goal of the velocity field computation is illustrated in Fig. 1. Figure 1a shows two frames from a sequence of images taken from an airplane flying over terrain. Figure 1b shows, superimposed on one of the two images, the instantaneous 2-D velocity field. The orientation and length of the line segments indicate the direction and speed of movement of features in the image, as the plane flies along. Figure 1c shows three views of a 3-D wireframe object undergoing rotation about a central axis in space. Figure 1d shows the projected velocities of individual points on the object as it rotates. In this chapter, we formulate the goal of the velocity field computation as the derivation of these descriptions of the local direction and speed of movement, from the changing retinal image. We assume implicitly that the human visual system also derives at least some approximation to this velocity field. Such a computation, for example, might underlie the short-range motion measurement process (1,2).

The earliest mechanisms for detecting image movement, both in computer and biological vision systems, examine only a limited part of the visual field. As a consequence, they often can provide only partial information about the 2-D pattern of movement in the changing image, due to the aperture problem (3-8). Consider the computation of the projected 2-D velocity field for the rotating wireframe object illustrated in Fig. 1. Suppose that the movement of features on the object were first detected using operations that examine only a limited area of the image, such as those performed by neural mechanisms with spatially limited receptive fields. The information provided by such mechanisms is illustrated in Fig. 2a. The extended edge E moves across the image and its movement is observed through a window defined by the circular aperture A. Through this window, it is possible to observe the movement of the edge only in the direction perpendicular to its orientation. The component of motion along the edge is invisible through this limited aperture. Thus, it is not possible to distinguish between motions in the directions b, c, and d. This is

FIG. 1. The velocity field. **a:** A natural image sequence, taken from a camera mounted on an airplane. **b:** At evenly spaced points in the image, the velocity field is represented by black line segments superimposed on one of the two images. The orientation and length of the line segments represent the direction and speed of motion. **c:** Three views of a 3-D wireframe object that is rotating about a central vertical axis. **d:** The projected 2-D image and motion of the object. *Arrows* represent the projected 2-D velocity of individual points on the object.

NEURAL VELOCITY FIELD COMPUTATION

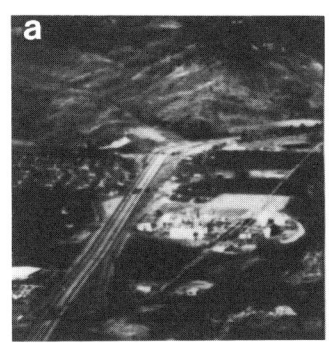
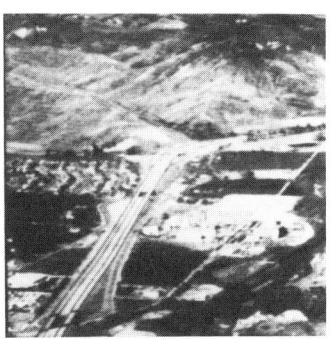

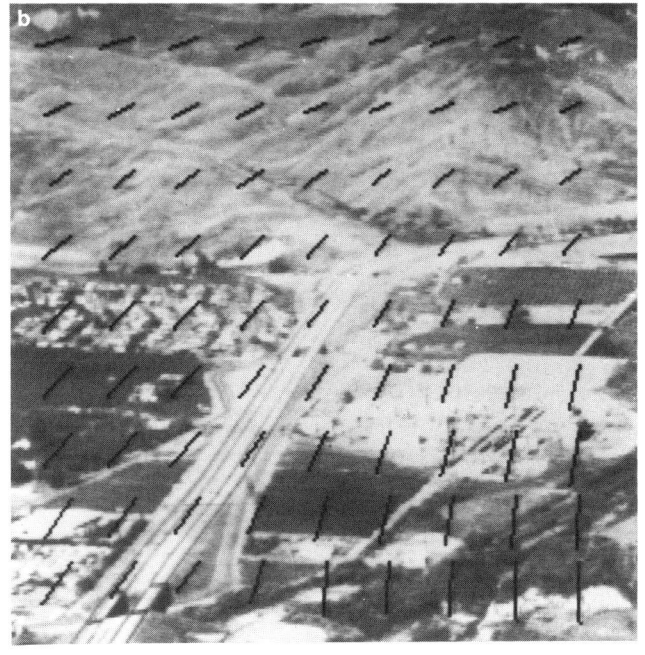

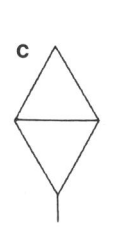
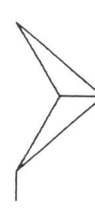
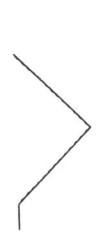
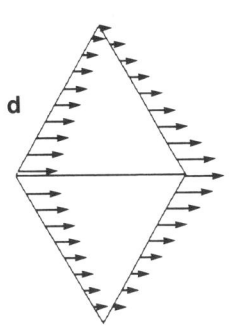

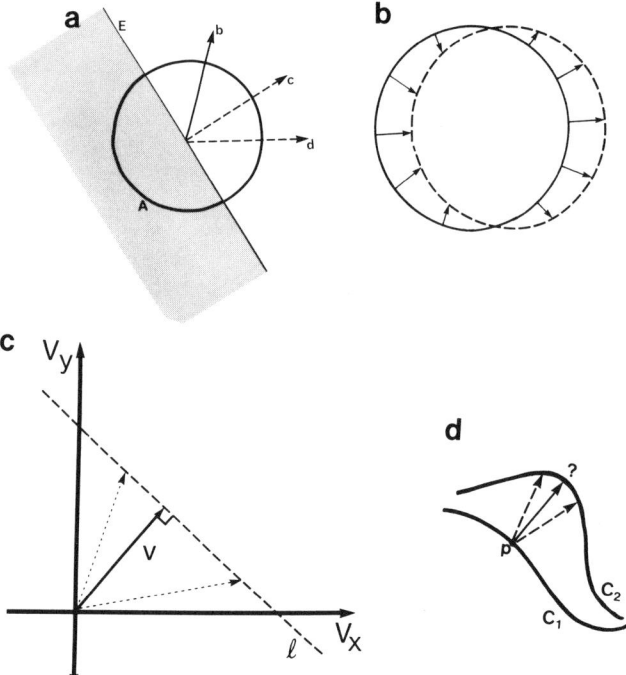

FIG. 2. The aperture problem in motion measurement. **a:** An operation that views the moving edge E through the local aperture A can compute only the component of motion c in the direction perpendicular to the orientation of the edge. The true motion of the edge is ambiguous. **b:** The circle undergoes pure translation to the right; the *arrows* represent the perpendicular components of velocity that can be measured from the changing image. **c:** The vector V represents the perpendicular component of velocity at some location in the image. The true velocity at that location must project to the line *l* perpendicular to V; examples are shown with *dotted arrows*. **d:** The curve C_1 rotates, translates, and deforms over time to yield the curve C_2. The velocity of the point p is ambiguous.

the aperture problem and is inherent in any motion detection operation that examines only a limited area of the image.

As a consequence of the aperture problem, the measurement of motion in the changing image requires two stages of analysis: the first stage measures components of motion in the direction perpendicular to image features; the second combines these components of motion to compute the full 2-D pattern of movement in the image. In Fig. 2b, a circle undergoes pure translation to the right. The arrows along the contour represent the perpendicular components of velocity that can be measured directly from the changing image. These component measurements each provide some constraint on the possible motion of the circle, as illustrated in Fig. 2c. The bold vector V represents the local perpendicular component of motion at a particular location in the image. The possible true motions at that location are given by the set of velocity vectors whose endpoint lies along the line *l* oriented perpendicular to the vector V. Examples of possible true velocities are indicated by the dotted vectors.

The movement of image features such as corners or small spots can be measured directly. In general, however, the first measurements of movement provide only partial information about the true movement of features in the image and must be combined to compute the full pattern of 2-D motion. In this chapter, we address only the second stage of combining the initial motion components; mechanisms for measuring the components themselves are reviewed in Hildreth and Koch (9).

The measurement of movement is made even more difficult by the fact that in theory, there are infinitely many patterns of motion that are consistent with a given changing image. For example, in Fig. 2d, the contour C_1 rotates, translates, and deforms to yield the contour C_2 at some later time. The true motion of the point p is ambiguous. Additional constraint is required to identify a unique solution. In general, it may not be possible to recover the 2-D projection of the true 3-D field of motions of points in space from the changing image intensities (10). Factors such as changing illumination, specularities, and shadows can generate patterns of optical flow in the image that do not correspond to the real movement of surface features. The additional constraint used to measure image motion can yield at best a solution that is most plausible from a physical standpoint.

Another issue that arises regarding the solution to the aperture problem is the question of whether the early motion measurements are integrated over 2-D areas of the image or along oriented features such as edge contours. Figure 3 illustrates the distinction between these two strategies. The original image shown in Fig. 3a consists of a single extended contour surrounded by a background texture of smaller contours. Suppose that the extended contour undergoes a vertical translation and the background texture moves to the right. Consider the early detection of movement of a segment of the contour, as shown in Fig. 3b. This measurement identifies the component of motion in the direction perpendicular to the contour but does not specify the true 2-D direction and speed of movement of the contour. In order to derive the true direction and speed of movement, this local measurement of motion must be combined with other measures computed nearby. Two strategies for combining these measurements are shown in Fig. 3 c and d. In Fig. 3c, all measurements within a 2-D area of the image are combined to resolve the direction and speed of movement, whereas in Fig. 3d, only measurements along the connected contour are integrated. In this case, where the extended contour actually undergoes a different motion from the surround, it is more desirable to integrate motion measurements along the contour. In the next section, in which we explore possible computational solutions to the velocity field problem, we discuss in more detail the advantages and disadvantages of the two strategies illustrated in Fig. 3.

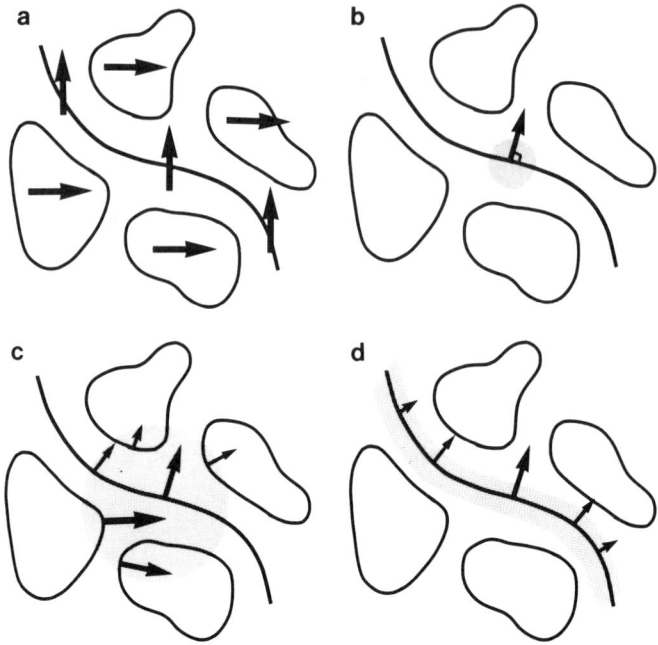

FIG. 3. Contour-based versus area-based integration of motion information. **a:** An image consisting of a single extended contour translating upward, surrounded by a background texture of smaller contours translating to the right. **b:** The detection of movement of a segment of the contour within a limited aperture. This measurement identifies the component of motion in the direction perpendicular to the contour, but does not specify the true 2-D direction and speed of movement of the contour. **c:** Measurements within a 2-D area of the image, highlighted with shading, are combined to resolve the direction and speed of movement. **d:** Only measurements along the connected contour are integrated, as suggested by the shaded region.

SOLVING THE APERTURE PROBLEM

We first consider possible additional assumptions that could be used to compute a unique 2-D velocity field from the initial components of motion at the locations of image features. Perhaps the simplest assumption that one could make is that objects in the scene just undergo pure translation or that the pattern of movement can at least be approximated locally by pure translation. This assumption has been used extensively, both in computer vision studies and in biological models of motion measurement (4,7,8,11–16). In theory, the use of this constraint is quite simple. Figure 4a shows a square translating to the right, with two perpendicular components of motion illustrated by the solid arrows on two sides of the square. The possible velocities of the overall figure that are consistent with the local measurements must extend from the points on the square to the solid lines drawn perpendicular

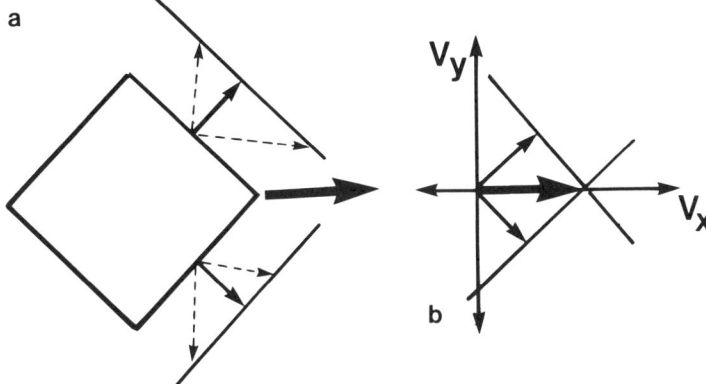

FIG. 4. Using the assumption of pure translation. **a:** A square translating to the right, with two perpendicular components of motion indicated by the *solid arrows* on two sides of the square. The possible velocities of the overall figure that are consistent with the local measurements must extend from the points on the square to the solid lines drawn perpendicular to the two components. Examples of possible velocity vectors consistent with each component are shown with *dashed arrows*. **b:** Constraint on the overall direction of motion imposed by the two components is illustrated in a *velocity space,* in which the X and Y axes represent the horizontal and vertical components of velocity. There is only one overall motion vector that is consistent with both of these components, given by the intersection of the two solid *constraint lines.*

to the two components. Examples of possible velocity vectors consistent with each component are shown with dashed arrows. To see how these two measurements interact, they are transferred to a common origin in a *velocity space,* in which the X and Y axes represent the horizontal and vertical components of velocity. As shown in Fig. 4b, there is only one overall motion vector that is consistent with both of these components, given by the intersection of the two solid *constraint lines.* This intersection point corresponds to translation to the right.

The assumption of pure translation may be useful for tasks such as tracking objects, detecting discontinuities in motion, or detecting sudden movements in the periphery, for which only a rough measurement of motion may be necessary. When a 3-D object undergoes rotation or translation through space, however, it typically generates a pattern of image motion that changes from one location to the next, as shown in Fig. 1. It is important to preserve this variation, because it provides a vital cue to the 3-D structure and motion of the object surface relative to the viewer. The analysis of these variations in motion requires the use of a more general physical assumption.

Other possible assumptions have been considered for the solution of the aperture problem. For example, one could assume that the pattern of image motion corresponds to the motion of a rigid object in the image plane (17), or to the projection of smooth objects moving rigidly in space (18–20). (For reviews of other work, see [9,21–26]). These other assumptions may still be inadequate for analyzing complex patterns of motion. First, there are situations in which we observe simple rigid motions but perceive them as distorting (27–29), and second, objects can be nonrigid themselves. It may therefore be overly restrictive to assume that the pattern of image motion will correspond to the projected movement of rigid objects.

A more general assumption that has been considered is one that is often referred to as the *smoothness assumption* (6,30–34). The assumption rests on the principle that physical surfaces are generally smooth; that is, variations in the structure of a surface are usually small compared with the distance of the surface from the viewer. When surfaces move, nearby points tend to move with similar velocities. There exist discontinuities in movement at object boundaries, but most of the image is the projection of relatively smooth surfaces. Thus, it is natural to assume that image velocities vary smoothly over most of the visual field. A unique pattern of movement can be obtained by computing a velocity field that is consistent with the changing image and has the least amount of variation possible. In other words, a pattern of movement is derived for which nearby points in the image move with velocities that are as similar as possible.

In order to compute a velocity field with the least amount of variation, we need some means for measuring variation in velocity. One such method is illustrated in Fig. 5. Hildreth (30) proposed a computational model in which the initial measurements of the components of motion are computed at the locations of significant intensity changes or edges. These measurements are then integrated along connected edge contours to derive the full 2-D velocity field. Figure 5a shows a piece of contour with two nearby velocity vectors V_1 and V_2. In Fig. 5b, these two velocities are shown with a common origin in velocity space. The difference between the two velocities is given by the dotted arrow shown between their endpoints. In continuous mathematical terms, if we let $V(s)$ denote the velocity field along the contour (the parameter s denotes distance along the contour), then this difference between nearby velocity vectors can be described as the derivative of the velocity field with respect to the curve, $\partial V/\partial s$. A scalar measure of this change can be obtained by taking the magnitude of the difference vector. To measure how much variation there is in the velocities along the entire contour, one can simply

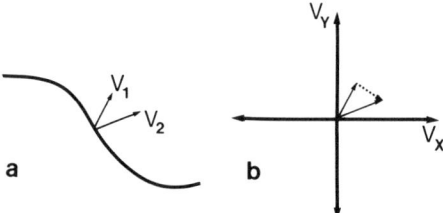

FIG. 5. Measuring variation in the velocity field. **a:** A segment of a contour with two nearby velocity vectors V_1 and V_2. **b:** The two velocities are shown with a common origin in velocity space. The difference between the two velocities is given by the *dotted arrow* shown between their endpoints and can be described in continuous mathematical terms as $\partial V/\partial s$.

sum the local changes everywhere along the contour. Formally, variation in the velocity field can be measured with the following function:

$$\int \left| \frac{\partial V}{\partial s} \right|^2 ds \qquad [1]$$

In the case of moving contours, the initial components of motion are first measured everywhere along the contour, and then a 2-D velocity field is computed that is consistent with these measurements and minimizes the above measure of variation. Another way to describe this model is to say that a velocity field is computed for which nearby velocity vectors are as similar as possible to one another, while being consistent with the initial components of motion. The above measure of variation simply provides a formal means of assessing the difference between adjacent velocity vectors. The velocity fields shown in Fig. 1 were computed using this model.

The use of the smoothness assumption for motion measurement has several important attributes from a computational perspective. First, it allows general motion to be analyzed. Surfaces can be rigid or nonrigid, undergoing any movement in space. It is always possible to compute a projected velocity field that preserves the variation in the local pattern of movement. Second, the smoothness assumption can be embodied in the motion measurement computation in a way that guarantees a unique solution (30). Third, it can be shown that the solution that is obtained is physically plausible (35); there are many situations, in fact, where this computation will yield the correct projected velocity field (30,36). The smoothness assumption incorporates the assumption of pure translation as a special case. Finally, the velocity field of least variation can be computed straightforwardly, using standard computer algorithms (6,30,32), as well as simple analog resistive networks that have properties believed to be similar to those of neural hardware (37,38).

As we noted above, a second issue that arises regarding the computation of the velocity field is the question of whether the early motion measurements are integrated over 2-D areas of the image or along oriented features such as edge contours. Some models integrate these measurements over areas (6,31–34), whereas others integrate motion measurements along connected contours (17,18,20,30,39).

From a computational perspective, there are advantages and disadvantages to the use of these two strategies. If the image is very textured within a local region, it may be advantageous to combine all of the motion information available within this region. If the region is small, then chances are that the direction and speed of movement does not vary significantly, so one could use a simple scheme to combine the motion components that assumes pure translation (i.e., that the direction and speed of movement are actually constant within this region). In this way, the true direction and speed of movement can be computed very quickly within textured image regions.

On the other hand, suppose that a region of the image is not very textured but consists of an extended, oriented pattern, such as an extended object boundary. Because of the aperture problem, it is not possible to resolve the true direction and speed of movement of the edge by combining the components of motion over small image areas, if the local image features all have similar orientations. In this case, motion information must be combined over longer distances in the image. One approach to achieving long-distance interactions is simply to combine the motion components over larger 2-D areas of the image. This strategy has a problem, however—there may be object boundaries within a larger 2-D area, across which the direction and speed of movement change, because the two surfaces on either side of the boundary are undergoing different motions. A better strategy in this case would be to combine motion information along connected edge features, which are more likely to be contained within a single object. Such connected edges might, for example, run along the boundary of an object or along some surface marking or texture. In natural scenes, connected edge contours rarely run across the surfaces of two different objects. Furthermore, if motion information is integrated over a longer distance, there is a greater likelihood that the direction and speed of movement varies over such a long distance, especially if the object rotates or deforms over time. To preserve these variations in motion, which may be important for recovering the 3-D shape of the object, it is necessary to use a strategy for combining the motion components that incorporates a more general assumption about the velocity field, such as the smoothness assumption.

We propose that one can achieve the best properties of both strategies by considering a hybrid model, which combines motion components over small 2-D areas of the image, using the simple assumption of pure translation, while also allowing motion components to be combined along extended edge features when necessary, using the more general smoothness assumption. In the next sections, we present perceptual evidence by Nakayama and Silverman (40,41) and others, which supports such a possibility, as well as a hypothetical neural implementation of this hybrid model.

THE PERCEPTUAL STUDY OF THE VELOCITY FIELD COMPUTATION

This section describes some perceptual studies that address three of the computational issues that arise regarding the velocity field computation. The first issue is whether the human visual system analyzes motion in two stages, where the first stage extracts the components of motion in the direction perpendicular to the orientation of image features and the second stage combines these components to derive the full pattern of 2-D image motion. The second issue is whether the human system integrates motion information along extended edge contours or over 2-D areas of the image. The third issue is the nature of the underlying physical assumptions that allow the human system to compute a unique pattern of image motion.

The issue of whether the motion measurement computation is performed in two stages was addressed in both perceptual and physiological studies by Movshon et al. (16). We describe here the perceptual experiments. These studies used visual patterns that consist of superimposed sinewave gratings of two different orientations, each moving perpendicular to their orientation. In the schematic drawing in Fig. 6, for example, two obliquely oriented gratings moving downward to the right and upward to the right, respectively, are shown superimposed. Typically, when the two components are shown together, observers perceive a single rigid checkerboard pattern moving in one direction that is consistent with the two components. In general, this direction is determined by the geometric construction illustrated in Fig. 4. In the case of the components of the pattern in Fig. 6, their combined motion corresponds to pure translation to the right.

Visual patterns of the type shown in Fig. 6 were used to test whether the human visual system analyzes the combined pattern in two distinct stages. In one experiment, oriented dynamic noise was added to the combined sinewave pattern. The noise appeared as a rapidly and randomly moving pattern of parallel stripes of varying widths. It was argued that if the human visual system first extracts the motions of the two individual sinewave components independently and then combines the two motions in a second stage of analysis, then only noise patterns whose orientation is aligned roughly with one of the two components should significantly disrupt the perception of coherent 2-D motion of the pattern. On the other hand, if the motion measurement computation consists of a single nonoriented analysis of image motion (for example, based on a tracking of the intersections of the two gratings), then masking noise at any orientation is expected to disrupt the perception of coherent motion. The experiments revealed that the masking noise disrupts the perceived motion of the pattern only when its orientation is roughly aligned with the orientation of one of the two component gratings, lending support to a two-stage motion measurement computation.

In a second experiment by Movshon et al. (16), the subjects were first

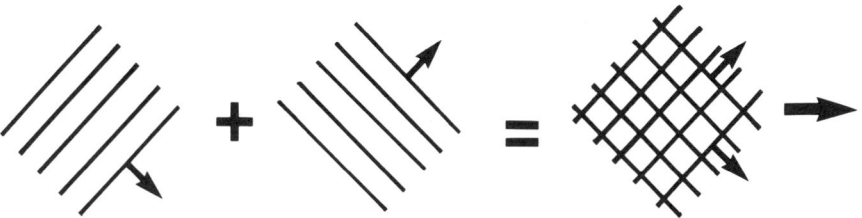

FIG. 6. The stimuli used by Movshon et al. (16). Two sinewave gratings, shown schematically, are superimposed to form a single rigid pattern moving to the right.

adapted either to single oriented and moving sinewave gratings, or to a combined pattern of two moving gratings. The effect of these two forms of adaptation on the perceived motion of both single and compound grating patterns was then tested. If was found, for example, that adaptation to a single oriented grating affected the perceived coherence of a combined pattern only when the orientation of the single grating was aligned roughly with that of one of the components of the combined pattern. Thus, adaptation to a single vertically oriented grating moving to the right had little effect on the perceived coherence of a rightward moving pattern that consisted of two oblique components (as shown in Fig. 6). These observations lend further support to the idea that in the human visual system, motion may be analyzed by first extracting the oriented components of motion and then combining these components to resolve the 2-D direction and speed of movement of image features.

The local perpendicular components of motion are not always combined by the human visual system. The conditions governing whether these measurements are combined were studied by Adelson and Movshon (8,16) and by Nakayama and Silverman (40). The Adelson and Movshon study (8) used superimposed grating patterns of the type shown in Fig. 6. Under some conditions, the gratings do not form a single coherent pattern perceptually; rather, the two components appear to split and move independently of one another. The coherence of the combined pattern was found to decrease with an increase in any of the following factors: (a) the difference in contrast between the two gratings, (b) the angle between the primary directions of the gratings, (c) the difference between the two spatial frequencies, and (d) the speed of movement of the overall pattern. In a later study by Adelson (42), it was shown that the two components of motion also appear to split if they were presented binocularly on different depth planes. This observation suggests that stereodisparity enters into the solution to the aperture problem in motion.

Nakayama and Silverman (40) used stimuli consisting of sinewave lines undergoing pure translation, as shown in Fig. 7. When the range of orientations spanned by the sinewave is greater than approximately 30°, as shown in Fig. 7a, the moving line is perceived as undergoing a rigid translation. If the span of orientations is less than approximately 30°, however, the perceived movement of the line is nonrigid, with each component of the sinewave appearing to move in the direction perpendicular to itself, as shown in Fig. 7b. Nakayama and Silverman argue that, in principle, the components of motion

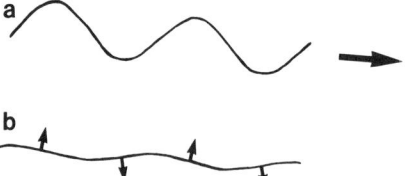

FIG. 7. The stimulus used by Nakayama and Silverman (40). **a:** A sinewave line undergoing pure translation to the right. The range of orientations spanned by the sinewave is greater than 30°. **b:** A sinewave line with a span of orientations less than 30°. *Arrows* indicate the perceived direction of motion of segments of the sinewave.

should not be combined in this case, because the noise inherent in these measurements would lead to an unstable solution to the velocity field computation (also see [30], Fig. 4.27).

A second issue that we raised concerning the computation of a velocity field regards whether motion information is integrated over 2-D areas of the image or along oriented features such as edge contours. This issue was addressed in another recent perceptual study by Nakayama and Silverman (41). This study used a simple distorted line, as shown in Fig. 8, which was oscillated up and down. When viewed alone, as shown in Fig. 8a, the central diagonal section of the line appears to move in an oblique direction, so that the entire figure appears nonrigid. The figure can be made to appear to move more rigidly up and down by the introduction of additional features to the pattern that are unambiguously moving up and down. Nakayama and Silverman introduced both breaks on the contour, as shown in Fig. 8b, and short segments off the contour, as shown in Fig. 8c. It was found that both the breaks on the line and the segments off the line could cause the central part of the line to appear to move up and down, but the features on the contour had a much stronger effect, in that their distance from the center could be much larger. The segments off the contour had to be very close to the line in order to exert any influence on the perception of its motion.

The observations of Nakayama and Silverman suggest that the integration of motion constraints along contours may play a strong role in the human visual system. This conclusion is also supported by a number of qualitative perceptual demonstrations presented by Wallach (3) and Hildreth (30). Wallach described a demonstration in which an obliquely oriented line was drawn on a textured wallpaper pattern, and the entire pattern was moved vertically downward behind a horizontally oriented rectangular aperture. Even with a clear vertical movement of the background, the line appeared to split from the background and move horizontally (its perceived direction of motion without the background). Wallach, Weisz, and Adams (27) observed that a circle drawn on the periphery of a rotating turntable, as shown in Fig. 9a, appears to remain upright as it rotates, even when the background rota-

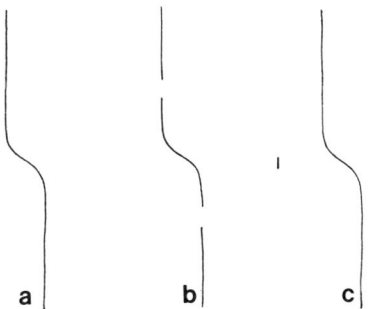

FIG. 8. The stimulus used by Nakayama and Silverman (41). **a:** This distorted line was translated up and down. **b:** Breaks on the contour also moved up and down. **c:** Segments off the contour moved up and down.

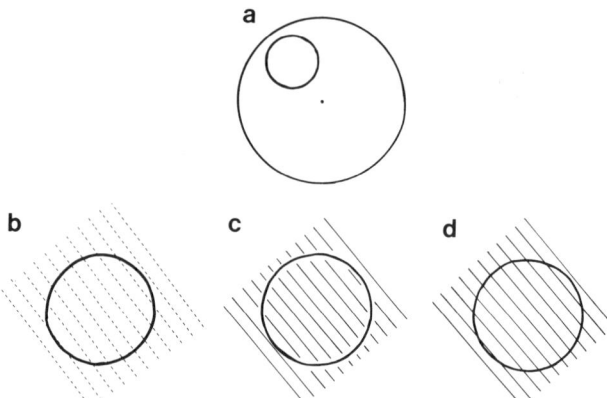

FIG. 9. Integrating motion information along contours. **a:** A circle is placed on the periphery of a turntable and rotated. **b:** Background lines of lower contrast than that of the circle, shown schematically with *dashed lines,* are added to the circle. **c:** Lines are added to the circle that do not intersect. **d:** The lines and circle intersect and appear with the same contrast.

tion of the turntable is clear. Hildreth (30) explored some variations on this experiment, shown in Fig. 9 b–d. The three patterns shown were drawn on white paper and mounted on the periphery of a rotating turntable. The figures were then viewed with fixation maintained at the center of the turntable. If the background lines in the pattern are either of very different contrast (indicated by the dotted lines in Fig. 9b) or are disconnected from the circle, as suggested in Fig. 9c, the circle appears to split from the background and remain roughly upright as the turntable rotates. If the background is of sufficient contrast and intersects the circle, as shown in Fig. 9d, then the circle appears to rotate as the turntable rotates. Thus the motion of the background appears to influence the perceived motion of the circle only when the background and circle are connected (or nearly connected) in the image.

With regard to the issue of what physical assumptions are used to compute a unique velocity field, one can ask, for example, whether the human visual system derives patterns of movement that are consistent with those predicted by a computation that uses the smoothness assumption. In particular, one can ask whether an incorrect pattern of motion is perceived in situations where a computer algorithm also fails. The method for computing the velocity field suggested by Hildreth is guaranteed to yield the correct solution for at least two classes of motion: (a) pure translation and (b) general motion (translation and rotation) of rigid 3-D objects whose edges are essentially straight. The moving object of Fig. 1c is an example of the second class of objects for which a correct velocity field is derived. For the case of smooth curves undergoing rotation, this computation sometimes yields a solution that differs from the correct projected velocity field. The human visual system also appears to derive an incorrect perception of motion in these situations (30). Three examples of this phenomenon are shown in Fig. 10. The short line segments along the smooth contours represent the directions and speeds of movement of individual points on the contours. The smoothest velocity fields that are consistent with the changing image are shown on the right in Fig. 10, while the true velocity fields are shown on the left. The first example is a logarithmic spiral whose image rotates about its center. Human observers perceive an expansion

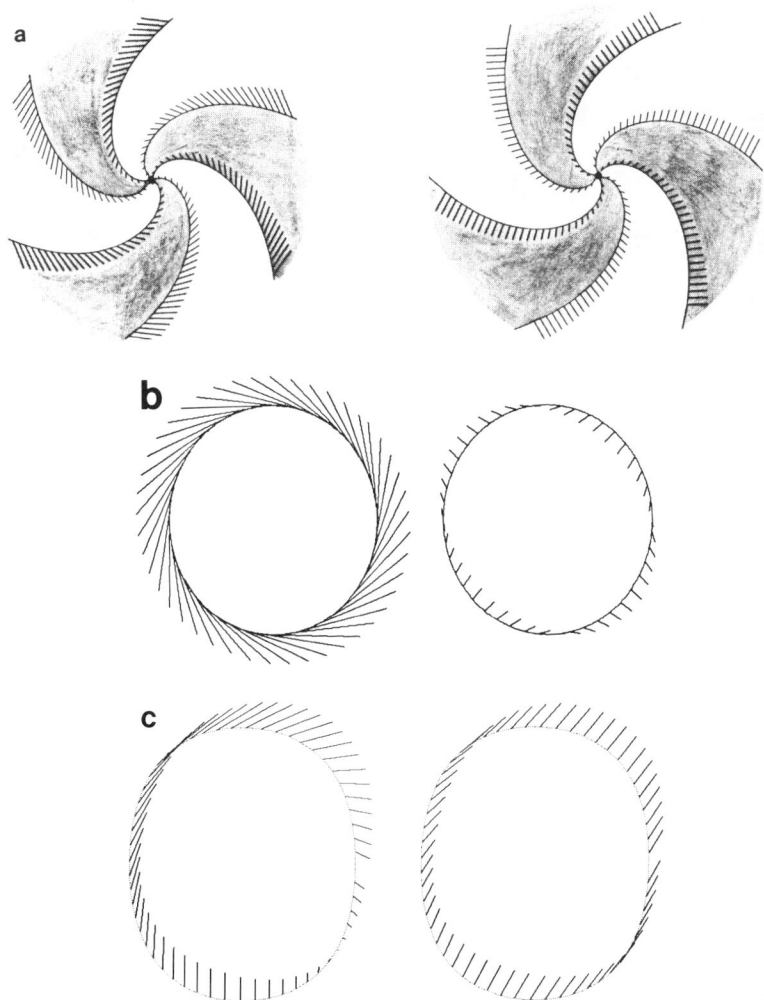

FIG. 10. Motion illusions. **a:** On the left is the true velocity field for a logarithmic spiral rotating around its center. The line segments along the contour represent the direction and speed of movement of individual points. On the right is the smoothest velocity field. **b:** The true velocity field (*left*) and smoothest velocity field (*right*) for an ellipse that is almost circular and rotating around its center. **c:** A contour formed by wrapping a circle around the surface of a cylinder is rotated in space around an oblique axis. The true projected velocity field is shown on the *left* and the smoothest velocity field on the *right*.

or contraction of a rotating spiral, depending on its direction of rotation (43). The true motion is pure rotation, but the perceived motion contains a large radial component. Consistent with this perception, there is a large radial component in the smoothest velocity field, particularly toward the center of the spiral. The second example is an ellipse that is almost circular and rotating about its center. Wallach et al. (27) showed that human observers do not perceive the rotation of the ellipse in this case; rather, they perceive the major and minor axes of the ellipse as pulsating inward and outward. This perception is also consistent with the smoothest velocity field shown on the right in Fig. 10b. Finally, the contour shown in Fig. 10c was formed by wrapping a circle onto the side of a cylinder. The contour was then rotated in space around an oblique axis, generating the projected velocity field shown on the left. At this moment in the trajectory of the contour, it is perceived as undergoing a rough translation up and to the right, consistent with the smoothest velocity field shown on the right.

The question of whether a smoothness assumption might be used in the measurement of motion in the human system was addressed in a more quantitative way in the study by Nakayama and Silverman (41). These experiments used variations of the pattern shown in Fig. 8b. If the human system integrates motion information along contours in a way that attempts to minimize the variation in direction and speed of movement along the contour, then one would expect to observe the following: (a) as the breaks on the line are moved closer to the center of the pattern, they should exert a stronger influence on the perceived motion of the center, causing the overall pattern to appear more rigid; (b) if the speed of motion of the breaks is decreased relative to the speed of motion of the central part of the figure, they should exert less influence, and hence the overall pattern should appear less rigid; and (c) if stationary breaks are placed between the remote, moving breaks and the center of the figure, then these stationary breaks should "block" the influence of the remote breaks, so that the central part of the figure should still appear nonrigid. Experimental observations by Nakayama and Silverman largely confirmed all three expectations, lending support to the use of a smoothness assumption. They argue, however, that there is a tendency for the visual system to perceive local segments of the contour as moving in a direction that is somewhat closer to their perpendicular direction than that expected from Hildreth's formulation of the velocity field computation. Nakayama and Silverman propose that the human visual system might instead try to minimize a measure of variation in velocity given by the following expression:

$$\int \int \left[\left| \frac{\partial V}{\partial s} \right|^2 + F(\psi, V_L) \right] ds \qquad [2]$$

where the first term is the same as that suggested by Hildreth (see Eq. 1), and the second is a monotonic function of the difference, ψ, between the computed direction of velocity and the direction perpendicular to the orientation of the contour, and V_L is the magnitude of the local velocity vector.

To summarize, the above perceptual studies suggest first that the measurement of motion in the human visual system may take place in two stages, corresponding to the extraction of the perpendicular components of motion and the subsequent combination of these components. Second, there are perceptual observations consistent with the idea that motion information is combined over 2-D areas within small regions of the image, whereas longer distance interactions may occur along extended features such as edge contours. Finally, demonstrations discussed by Hildreth (30), together with the Nakayama and Silverman (41) study, support the use of a general assumption such as smoothness in the computation of the velocity field.

These conclusions should perhaps not be taken too strictly, however. For example, strict connectivity of image features is not essential to the solution of the aperture problem. Consider the moving pattern shown in Fig. 11, where vertical and horizontal line segments moving perpendicular to themselves are shown in separate regions of the image. If one views this pattern for a short time, say 100 to 200 msec, the dominant perception is of the separate horizontal and vertical motions of the two components. Over longer viewing periods, however, it is possible to imagine that the disconnected segments are actually part of a connected square that is viewed through a set of windows. In this case, the two components combine to yield a perception of the connected square as moving rigidly in an oblique direction downward and to the right. The components are not physically connected in the image but can be grouped perceptually and give rise to an apparent motion corresponding to the combination of the disconnected components.

Finally, there are many phenomena that have been observed in the percep-

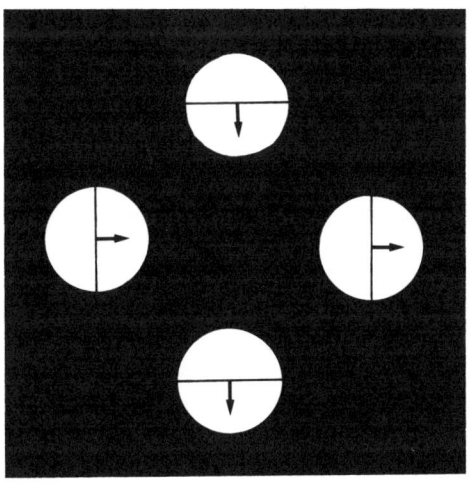

FIG. 11. Variation on the aperture problem. Vertical and horizontal line segments are moving perpendicular to themselves in separate regions of the image. The pattern is also consistent with a rigid square translating downward and to the right, viewed behind a set of apertures.

tion of continuous motion that are not yet considered in this hybrid model of the velocity field computation. Among them are the phenomenon of motion capture (44), the perception of coherent global motions from random local motion fields (45,46), and the potential interaction between short-range velocity-based motion measurement mechanisms and long-range motion correspondence (47–51).

THE PHYSIOLOGICAL STUDY OF THE VELOCITY FIELD COMPUTATION

The motion measurement problem can also be examined from a physiological perspective. Early movement detectors in biological systems have spatially limited receptive fields and therefore face the aperture problem. Stimulated by a theoretical analysis of the aperture problem, Movshon et al. (16) sought and found direct physiological evidence for a two-stage motion measurement computation in the primate visual system. This section reviews this evidence and describes a hypothetical neural implementation of a solution to the aperture problem that uses the hybrid model described earlier.

Two visual areas that include an abundance of motion-sensitive neurons are cortical areas V1 and MT. MT is the middle temporal area of extrastriate cortex, located in the posterior bank of the superior temporal sulcus (52–58). The explicit role of area MT in the cortical analysis of visual motion was confirmed recently by Newsome et al. (59), who showed that small restricted chemical lesions in area MT of the macaque monkey led to a behavioral deficit in monkeys' ability to match the velocity of smooth pursuit eye movements with the velocity of visual targets. Andersen and Siegel (60) showed that restricted lesions in area MT also lead to a deficit in monkeys' ability to recover 3-D structure from motion.

Movshon et al. (16) explored the type of motion analysis taking place in area MT of the macaque monkey, using the same visual patterns with superimposed sinewave gratings shown in Fig. 6. A simplification of the logic behind the physiological experiments is illustrated in Fig. 12. Figure 12a shows three patterns of gratings whose overall 2-D direction of motion differs. The patterns on the left and in the center are formed from horizontal and vertical components, and the pattern on the right has oblique components. Suppose that a given class of cells performs the function of extracting single oriented components of motion and that a particular cell within this class detects vertically oriented components moving to the right, as shown in Fig. 12b. One would expect this cell to respond to the leftmost and central patterns in Fig. 12a, because they each contain a vertically oriented component moving to the right. On the other hand, such a cell should not respond to the pattern on the far right, which does not contain a vertically oriented component. Suppose, on the other hand, that another class of cells combines the components of

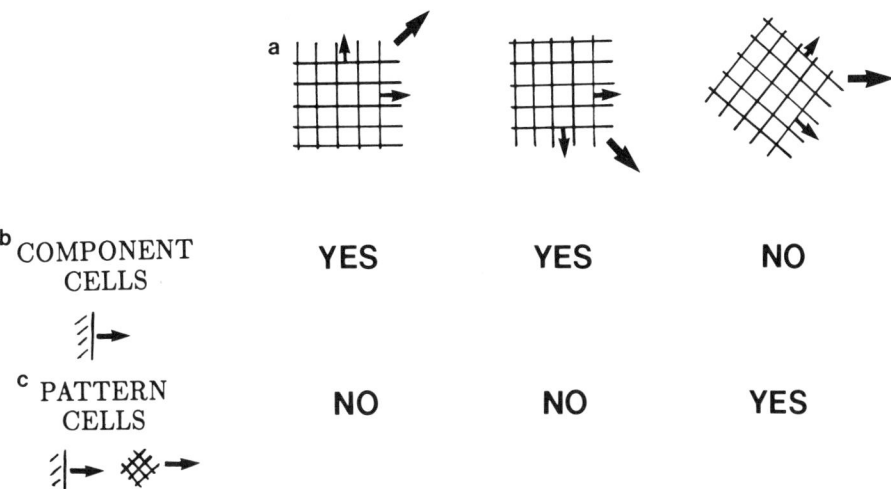

FIG. 12. The Movshon et al. (16) physiology experiments. **a:** Three patterns of gratings whose overall 2-D direction of motion differs. The patterns on the left and in the center are formed from horizontal and vertical components, whereas the pattern on the right has oblique components. **b:** The expected responses of a component cell that detects vertically oriented components moving to the right. **c:** The expected responses of a pattern cell that prefers overall motion of the pattern to the right.

motion to compute the overall 2-D direction of motion and that a particular cell within this second class detects motion to the right, as shown in Fig. 12c. This cell is not expected to respond to the leftmost or center patterns in Fig. 12a, because their overall motion is in oblique directions. The cell should respond, however, to the rightmost pattern whose overall motion is to the right. Thus, the two classes of cells are expected to have a very different signature in their response to the three combined grating patterns. This is the essence of the logic behind the experiments conducted by Movshon et al. (16).

The results of these experiments indicate that the selectivity of neurons in area V1 for direction of movement is such that they could provide only the component of motion in the direction perpendicular to the orientation of image features. These neurons essentially respond to only a single component of the combined grating pattern, independent of the presence of the second grating, and were referred to as *component cells* in the study. In area MT, roughly 40% of the cells analyzed behaved like component cells; this population was concentrated in layers 4 and 6. It was found, however, that area MT also contains a subpopulation of cells, referred to as *pattern* cells, that appear to respond to the 2-D direction of motion of the combined grating pattern, independent of the individual components. These cells formed roughly 25% of the MT cells studied and were concentrated in layers 2, 3, and 5. This latter population of neurons may serve to combine motion components to compute the real 2-D direction of velocity of a moving pattern.

Albright (54) examined the selectivity of MT neurons in the macaque both to the direction of movement of isolated spots and random dot patterns and to the orientation of a stationary flashed bar of light. Roughly 60% of the MT cells studied were selective for a direction of movement of the spot or random dot pattern that was perpendicular to the optimal orientation of the stationary bar. Another 30% were selective for a direction of movement of the spot or dot pattern that was parallel to the preferred bar orientation. Albright argued that the behavior of the first class corresponds to what one would expect from component cells, whereas the second is consistent with the behavior of pattern cells. Rodman and Albright (61) showed recently that the two classes identified by Albright (54) do, in fact, correspond to the component and pattern cell classes established by Movshon et al. (16).

With regard to the computation of the velocity field, Movshon et al. (16) proposed a simple model by which pattern cells in area MT could combine component measurements to determine the overall 2-D direction of movement of a pattern. This model assumes that the direction and speed of motion is roughly constant within the region of the image over which the component measurements are combined. The essence of the model is illustrated in Fig. 13. (A similar model is also described by Rodman and Albright [61].) In the example shown, the pattern cell prefers motion directed downward and re-

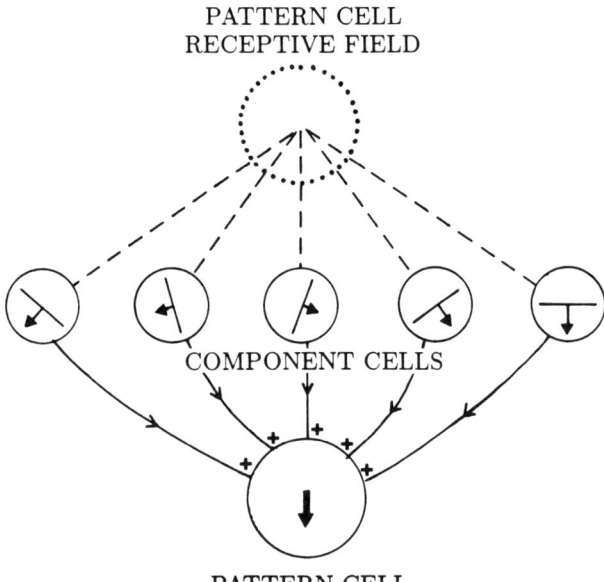

FIG. 13. A neural model that assumes pure translation. A pattern cell that prefers motion directed downward receives direct input from component cells whose responses would be consistent with an overall downward movement of a pattern. The particular model proposed by Movshon et al. (16) suggests a facilitative interaction between component and pattern cells.

ceives direct input from component cells whose responses would be consistent with an overall downward movement of a pattern. The particular model proposed by Movshon et al. suggests a facilitative interaction between component and pattern cells, although one could also consider a modification of the model in which the pattern cell receives inhibitory input from component cells whose responses would be inconsistent with the preferred direction of motion of the pattern cell.

In principle, the component cell inputs could come from V1 directly or from component cells within MT. Experiments by Movshon and Newsome (62) indicate that most of the input from V1 to MT does arise from directionally selective cells with component behavior. Movshon et al. (16) showed, however, that the pattern cells appear to be concentrated in layers 2, 3, and 5 of area MT, and the direct input from V1 converges onto cells in layer 4 (63). Thus, if the MT pattern cells do receive direct input from component cells, they are likely to be those within area MT.

As we noted earlier, models for the velocity field computation that assume pure translation may be useful for tasks such as tracking objects, detecting discontinuities in motion, or detecting sudden movements in the periphery, for which only a rough measurement of motion may be necessary. When 3-D objects undergo rotation or translation through space, however, they typically generate a pattern of image motion that changes from one location to the next. The analysis of these variations in motion requires the use of a more general physical assumption. At the end of the section on the aperture problem, we presented a hybrid model for the velocity field computation that combines motion components over small 2-D areas of the image, using the simple assumption of pure translation, while also allowing motion components to be combined along extended edge features when necessary, using the more general smoothness assumption.

Figure 14 illustrates a possible neural implementation of this hybrid model for the velocity field computation. The larger circles represent pattern cells. In order to implement the strategy of computing the smoothest velocity field, we need communication between neighboring pattern cells, because the computed direction and speed of motion at one location should be similar to motions computed nearby. In the particular example shown in Fig. 14, the network consists of pattern cells that are each selective for a similar direction and speed of movement (obliquely upward to the right), and the interactions between pattern cells are facilitatory. One can, of course, consider a model in which pattern cells selective for very different directions or speeds of motion also inhibit one another.

In the model shown in Fig. 14, each pattern cell also receives direct input from component cells within a smaller region of the image, whose activity would be consistent with the preferred direction of motion of the pattern cell (these inputs are illustrated only for the central pattern cell). This aspect of the model is similar to that of Movshon et al. (16). Over this small region, the

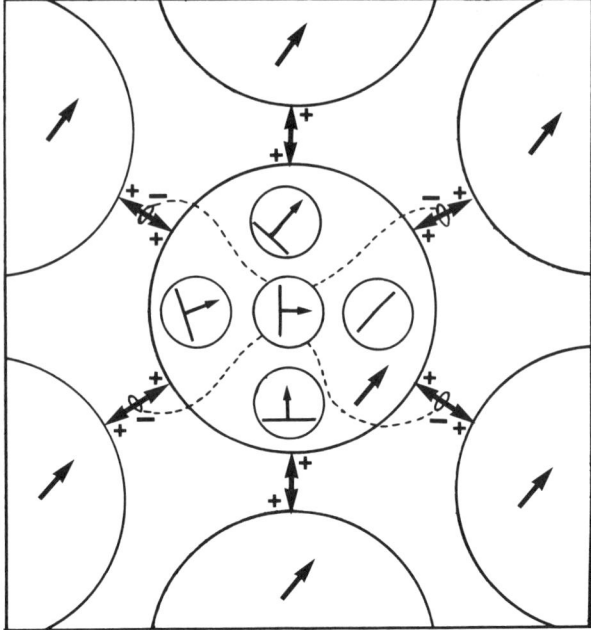

FIG. 14. A neural implementation of the hybrid velocity field computation. The *larger circles* represent pattern cells, which have facilitatory interactions between them. Each pattern cell also receives direct input from component cells (*smaller circles*) within a smaller region of the image, whose activity would be consistent with the preferred direction of motion of the pattern cell. Component cell inputs are shown only for the central pattern cell. Component cell inputs also inhibit the interactions between the pattern cell for which they form a direct input and neighboring pattern cells located in a direction roughly perpendicular to the preferred orientation of the component cell. This inhibition is illustrated by *dashed lines* for only one component cell.

components could be combined with the assumption that direction and speed of velocity are constant. We argued that it would be advantageous for longer distance interactions between pattern cells to take place along oriented features in the image, such as extended contours. One way to achieve this is for the component cell inputs to inhibit the interactions between the pattern cell for which they form a direct input and neighboring pattern cells located in a direction roughly perpendicular to the preferred orientation of the component cell. This inhibition is illustrated for one component cell in Fig. 14, by the dashed lines. The other component cell inputs could similarly inhibit interactions in the directions roughly perpendicular to their preferred orientations. This sort of inhibition would tend to promote interactions between pattern cells along connected edges, which are likely to maintain a similar orientation along a significant extent.

Consider the behavior of the model shown in Fig. 14 when presented with a textured image pattern, such as a random dot pattern, moving in the preferred direction for this network of pattern cells. In this case, many of the direct component cell inputs will be active, which has two consequences: first, they will lead to direct excitation of the central pattern cell, and second, they will inhibit any interaction between the central pattern cell and its neighbors. For textured patterns, however, direct communication with neighboring pattern cells is not essential, because there is sufficient motion information within the smaller image region to resolve the real 2-D direction and speed of movement of the pattern.

Now consider the behavior of the model when the smaller region of the image contains only an extended contour. In particular, suppose that the orientation of this contour is roughly vertical and that its perpendicular component of motion is directed to the right. For the model in Fig. 14, only the central component cell selective for vertically oriented features would be active. This response alone is not sufficient to resolve the real 2-D pattern of motion of the contour. This one component cell could provide some excitation of the pattern cell, and in addition, there will still be interactions with other pattern cells along the orientation of the active component, whose behavior could help to resolve the real direction of motion of the pattern. In the model illustrated in Fig. 14, the interactions between pattern cells are drawn only between pattern cells with identical preferred directions of motion, but there can also be interactions between pattern cells with nearby preferred directions.

Finally, we note that Poggio and Koch (37,38) presented a very different neural model of the smoothest velocity field computation. They began with the design of simple linear, electrical or chemical, analog networks that implement this computation. From these analog networks, a hypothetical neural circuit was then designed that behaves in a similar way.

The goal of the analysis here was to show that it is possible, in principle, to embed a more general model for the velocity field computation in neural circuitry, using simple local interactions. The use of longer distance interactions along oriented features such as edge contours and a more general assumption such as smoothness need not require a neural model that is vastly more complex than one could imagine exists in an early visual area such as MT. The physiological experiments conducted by Movshon et al. (16) and Albright (54) do not yet distinguish between the use of a simple model such as that shown in Fig. 13 and a more general scheme such as the hybrid model illustrated in Fig. 14. Stimulus patterns undergoing more complicated motions, together with an analysis of the time course of the pattern cell responses, are required to make such a distinction. There has been a recent excitement about interactions leading to responses of MT cells from stimuli well beyond the classical receptive field (55,56). Although we believe that even the simple computation of the velocity field can require extended spatial interactions, it remains a challenge to determine whether the particular interactions observed experimentally would be appropriate for this particular task.

ACKNOWLEDGMENTS

We thank M. Drumheller for valuable feedback on a draft of this manuscript. This chapter describes research done within the Artificial Intelligence Laboratory and the Center for Biological Information Processing (Whitaker College) at the Massachusetts Institute of Technology. Support for the A. I. Laboratory's artificial intelligence research is provided in part by the Advanced Research Projects Agency of the Department of Defense under Office of Naval Research contract N00014-85-K-0124. Support for this research is also provided by grants from the Office of Naval Research, Cognitive and Neural Sciences Division; the Sloan Foundation; the National Science Foundation, under contract IRI-8657824; and the McDonnell Foundation.

REFERENCES

1. Braddick OJ. A short-range process in apparent motion. *Vision Res* 1974;14:519–527.
2. Braddick OJ. Low-level and high-level processes in apparent motion. *Philos Trans R Soc Lond [Biol]* 1980;290:137–151.
3. Wallach H. On perceived identity: 1. The direction of motion of straight lines. In: Wallach H, ed. *On perception*. New York: Quadrangle, 1976.
4. Fennema CL, Thompson WB. Velocity determination in scenes containing several moving objects. *Comput Graph Image Proc* 1979;9:301–315.
5. Burt P, Sperling G. Time, distance, and feature trade-offs in visual apparent motion. *Psychol Rev* 1981;88:171–195.
6. Horn BKP, Schunck BG. Determining optical flow. *Artif Intell* 1981;17:185–203.
7. Marr D, Ullman S. Directional selectivity and its use in early visual processing. *Proc R Soc Lond [Biol]* 1981;211:151–180.
8. Adelson EH, Movshon JA. Phenomenal coherence of moving visual patterns. *Nature* 1982;300:523–525.
9. Hildreth EC, Koch C. The analysis of visual motion: from computational theory to neuronal mechanisms. *Annu Rev Neurosci* 1987;10:477–533.
10. Verri A, Poggio T. Motion field and optical flow: qualitative properties. *MIT Artif Intell Memo 917,* 1986.
11. Lappin JS, Bell HH. The detection of coherence in moving random dot patterns. *Vision Res* 1976;16:161–168.
12. Pantle AJ, Picciano L. A multistable display: evidence for two separate motion systems in human vision. *Science* 1976;193:500–502.
13. Anstis SM. The perception of apparent motion. *Philos Trans R Soc Lond [Biol]* 1980; 290:153–168.
14. Thompson WB, Barnard ST. Lower-level estimation and interpretation of visual motion. *IEEE Computer* August 1981;20–28.
15. Lawton DT. Processing translational motion sequences. *Comput Vis Graph Image Proc* 1983;22:116–144.
16. Movshon JA, Adelson EH, Gizzi MS, Newsome WT. The analysis of moving visual patterns. In: Chagas C, Gattas R, Gross CG, eds. *Pattern recognition mechanisms*. Rome: Vatican Press, 1985;117–151.
17. Davis L, Wu Z, Sun H. Contour-based motion estimation. *Comput Vis Graph Image Proc* 1983;23:313–326.
18. Wohn K. A contour-based approach to image flow. PhD thesis, Department of Computer Science, University of Maryland, September 1984.
19. Subbarao M. Interpretation of image motion fields: A spatio-temporal approach. *Proc IEEE Workshop on Motion: Representation and Analysis,* South Carolina, 1986;157–165.

20. Waxman AM. Image flow theory: A framework for 3-D inference from time-varying imagery. In: Brown C, ed. *Advances in computer vision*. Hillsdale, NJ: Erlbaum, 1988;165–224.
21. Ullman S. Analysis of visual motion by biological and computer systems. *IEEE Computer* August 1981;57–69.
22. Ballard DH, Brown CM. *Computer vision*. Englewood Cliffs, NJ: Prentice-Hall, 1982.
23. Barron J. A survey of approaches for determining optic flow, environmental layout and egomotion. *Univ Toronto Tech Rep Res Biol Comp Vis* RBCV-TR-84-5, 1984.
24. Jain R. Dynamic scene analysis. In: Kanal LN, Rosenfeld A, eds. *Progress in pattern recognition 2*. Amsterdam and New York: North-Holland, 1985;125–168.
25. Horn BKP. *Robot vision*. Cambridge, MA: MIT Press and McGraw-Hill, 1986.
26. Brown C, ed. *Advances in computer vision*. Hillsdale, NJ: Erlbaum, 1988.
27. Wallach H, Weisz A, Adams PA. Circles and derived figures in rotation. *Am J Psychol* 1956;69:48–59.
28. Braunstein ML, Andersen GJ. A counterexample to the rigidity assumption in the visual perception of structure from motion. *Perception* 1984;13:213–217.
29. Adelson EH. Rigid objects that appear highly non-rigid. *Invest Ophthalmol Vis Sci* 1985;26(suppl):56.
30. Hildreth EC. *The measurement of visual motion*. Cambridge, MA: MIT Press, 1984.
31. Nagel HH. Recent advances in image sequence analysis. *Proc Premier Colloque Image—Traitement, Synthese, Technologie et Applications*. Biarritz, France, May 1984;545–558.
32. Nagel HH, Enkelmann W. Towards the estimation of displacement vector fields by "oriented smoothness" constraints. *Proc 7th Int Conf on Pattern Recognition*, Montreal, Canada, July 1984;6–8.
33. Anandan P, Weiss R. Introducing a smoothness constraint in a matching approach for the computation of optical flow fields. *Proc IEEE Workshop on Computer Vision: Representation and Control*, Bellaire, MI, October 1985;186–194.
34. Anandan P. Measuring visual motion from image sequences. PhD thesis, Department of Computer and Information Science, University of Massachusetts, May 1987.
35. Ullman S, Yuille AL. Rigidity and smoothness of motion. *MIT Artif Intell Memo 989*, 1987.
36. Yuille AL. The smoothest velocity field and token matching schemes. *MIT Artif Intell Memo 724*, 1983.
37. Poggio T, Koch C. Ill-posed problems in early vision: from computational theory to analog networks. *Proc R Soc Lond [Biol]* 1985;226:303–323.
38. Poggio T, Torre V, Koch C. Computational vision and regularization theory. *Nature* 1985;317:314–319.
39. Waxman AM, Wohn K. Contour evolution, neighborhood deformation and global image flow: planar surfaces in motion. *Int J Robotics Res* 1985;4:95–108.
40. Nakayama K, Silverman GH. The aperture problem. I: Perception of non-rigidity and motion direction in translating sinusoidal lines. *Vision Res* 1988;28:739–746.
41. Nakayama K, Silverman GH. The aperture problem. II: Spatial integration of velocity information along contours. *Vision Res* 1988;28:747–753.
42. Adelson EH. Binocular disparity and the computation of two-dimensional motion. *J Opt Soc Am [A]* 1984;1:1266.
43. Holland HC. *The spiral aftereffect*. Oxford: Pergamon Press, 1965.
44. Ramachandran VS, Ginsburgh AP, Anstis SM. Low spatial frequencies dominate apparent motion. *Perception* 1983;12:457–461.
45. Williams DW, Sekuler R. Coherent global motion percepts from stochastic local motions. *Vision Res* 1984;24:55–62.
46. Williams DW, Phillips G, Sekuler R. Hysteresis in the perception of motion direction: evidence for neural cooperativity (*submitted*).
47. Clatworthy JL, Frisby JP. Real and apparent movement: evidence for unitary mechanism. *Perception* 1973;2:161–164.
48. Green M. Inhibition and facilitation of apparent motion by real motion. *Vision Res* 1983;23:861–865.
49. Green M, von Grünau M. Real and apparent motion: one mechanism or two? *Proc ACM Interdis Workshop on Motion: Representation and Perception*, Toronto, Canada, 1983;17–22.
50. Gregory RL. Movement nulling: for heterochromatic photometry and isolating channels for 'real' and 'apparent' motion. *Perception* 1985;14:193–196.

51. Mather G, Cavanagh P, Anstis SM. A moving display which opposes short-range and long-range signals. *Perception* 1985;14:163–166.
52. Maunsell JHR, Van Essen DC. Functional properties of neurons in middle temporal visual area of the macaque monkey. I. Selectivity for stimulus direction, speed and orientation. *J Neurophysiol* 1983;49:1127–1147.
53. Van Essen DC, Maunsell JHR. Hierarchical organization and functional streams in the visual cortex. *Trends Neurosci* 1983;6:370–375.
54. Albright TD. Direction and orientation selectivity of neurons in visual area MT of the macaque. *J Neurophysiol* 1984;52:1106–1130.
55. Allman J, Miezin F, McGuinness E. Direction- and velocity-specific responses from beyond the classical receptive field in the middle temporal area (MT). *Perception* 1985;14:105–126.
56. Allman J, Miezin F, McGuinness E. Stimulus specific responses from beyond the classical receptive field: neurophysiological mechanisms for local-global comparisons in visual neurons. *Annu Rev Neurosci* 1985;8:407–429.
57. Saito HA, Yukie M, Tanaka K, Hikosaka K, Fukuda Y, Iwai E. Interaction of direction signals of image motion in the superior temporal sulcus of the macaque monkey. *J Neurosci* 1986;6:145–157.
58. Maunsell JHR, Newsome WT. Visual processing in monkey extrastriate cortex. *Annu Rev Neurosci* 1987;10:363–401.
59. Newsome WT, Wurtz RH, Dursteler MR, Mikami A. Deficits in visual motion processing following ibotenic acid lesions of the middle temporal visual area of the macaque monkey. *J Neurosci* 1985;5:825–840.
60. Andersen RA, Siegel RM. Motion processing in primate cortex (*submitted*).
61. Rodman HR, Albright TD. Single-unit analysis of pattern-motion selective properties in the middle temporal visual area (MT) (*submitted*).
62. Movshon JA, Newsome WT. Functional characteristics of striate cortical neurons projecting to MT in the macaque. *Neurosci Abst* 1984;10:93.
63. Ungerleider LG, Desimone R. Cortical connections of visual area MT in the macaque. *J Comp Neurol* 1986;248:190–222.

Vision and the Brain,
edited by B. Cohen and I. Bodis-Wollner.
Raven Press, Ltd., New York © 1990.

Brain Mechanisms for Recognition of Faces, Facial Expression, and Gestures: Neuropsychological and Electroencephalographic Studies in Normals, Brain-Lesioned Patients, and Schizophrenics

Otto-Joachim Grüsser, Nina Kirchhoff, and Alexander Naumann

Department of Physiology, Freie Universität Berlin, 1 Berlin 33, West Germany

In everyday life, besides spoken and written language, nonverbal signals like facial expression and gestures are used for social communication. The knowledge and execution of some of these signals are acquired by daily experience and depend on the sociocultural background. The generation of some basic nonverbal social signals, however, is also determined by inborn neuronal mechanisms. On the perceptory and cognitive side, as a rule, such signals are "automatically" recognized by means of corresponding inborn neuronal networks. Therefore, some of the facial expressions and gestures are universally used and recognized. To our knowledge, this opinion was first expressed in Western philosophy by Nicolaus Cusanus (1401–1464 A.D.) in his last philosophical work *Compendium* (1).

The face is not only the source of expressive signals but also the most important and obvious characteristic structure of a human's individuality. Furthermore, the ability to recognize and differentiate between thousands of different faces during a lifetime constitutes an important factor in today's social life. The assumption that special structures of the brain control the execution and understanding of countenance and gestures is based on several findings:

1. *Prosopagnosia,* i.e., the inability to recognize previously known persons solely by their faces, is observed when circumscribed lesions have occurred on both sides, as a rule, of the basal and mesial occipitotemporal region in the cortical hemispheres of a human (2–7). Recently Landis et al. (8,9) and Bliestle et al. (10) provided evidence that extended unilateral lesions of this region in the right hemisphere might also lead to a serious impairment of face recognition and eventually to an at least transitory prosopagnosia.

2. These observations agree with other findings indicating that the right hemisphere is more important for some elementary mechanisms of face recognition than the left. A simple illustration of the left/right asymmetry in face perception is demonstrated by Fig. 1. For most observers, the left lower face has a greater similarity to the upper face. The results of such a comparison of photographs composed of double-left or double-right halves with the normal face deviate significantly from a 50% average (11–14). Right-handed subjects perceive double-right faces as being similar to the original photograph more frequently than double-left faces (Fig. 2).

3. When recording the *center of gaze position* of right-handed subjects inspecting human faces or photographs of the same (projected slides), one observes that the right side of the face is preferred approximately 60% to 70%

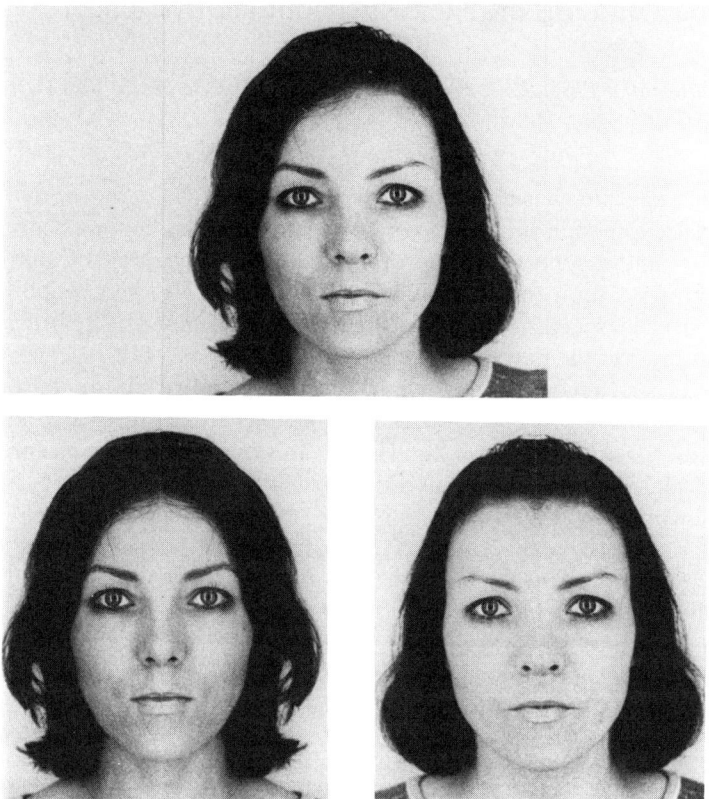

FIG. 1. Photograph of a test slide with a normal face (**upper**) and two artifical faces composed of double-right halves (**lower left**) and double-left halves (**lower right**). The observers had to judge which of the two lower faces best resembles the upper face. For this particular combination more than 90% of 162 medical students who had viewed this slide decided that the double-right face looks more similar to the normal face than the double-left face. (From ref. 48.)

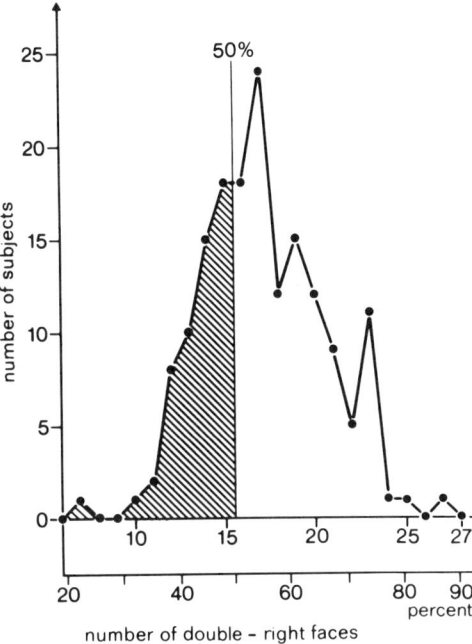

FIG. 2. Statistical results obtained in a lecture hall experiment (1978) with 31 slides of the type shown in Fig. 1 and 162 subjects. The slides were projected for 6 sec each, with a pause of 6 sec in between. The subjects had to decide whether the double-right or double-left face looked more similar to the normal face. They were not informed how the faces were constructed; positions of double-right and double-left faces were varied at random. The figure shows the frequency distribution of the preference for double-right faces for the 162 subjects. The two nonzero data points at the left end of the distribution were from left-handed subjects. The data of six further left-handed subjects are intermingled at random with those of the other right-handed subjects. The distribution differs significantly from symmetry around the 50% chance level. (From ref. 48.)

of the time in face recognition tasks and in tasks involving emotional decisions (cf. Fig. 4 in [48]). This side preference, however, is only partly face specific, since a tendency exists to scan objects placed in front of us by eye movements shifted more frequently toward the left field of gaze, i.e., the right side of the object (Jeannerod, 1980, *personal communication*). The tendency to asymmetric scanning of the face has its correlate in an asymmetric emotional expression: The left half of the human face is believed to express slight emotional changes more readily than the right half, which is considered the more "official" part of our face, akin to our "public mask" (15,16).

4. Several studies applying tachistoscopic presentation of faces to the right or left visual hemifield combined with recognition tasks evaluated by the measurement of reaction times also indicated a slight right-hemisphere preference for the processing of face stimuli (17–19). Face signals are also processed in the left hemisphere, of course (20, 21), and the importance of the left hemisphere in face recognition tasks presumably increases when linguistic competence and naming is required for face categorization (e.g. public faces/unknown faces).

5. During the past 6 years impressive results from microelectrode studies performed in awake monkeys (rhesus macaques) indicate that "face-specific" neuronal networks exist in the primate brain, located in the cortical area bordering on the deep central region of the superior temporal sulcus (22–26). The face-specific neurons of the temporal lobe most likely have connections with

part of the nucleus amygdalae, where neurons responding selectively to face stimuli have also been found (27,28). Creutzfeldt (29) described responses of neurons in the rostral area 19 of rhesus macaques sensitive to a threatening expression but not to friendly or neutral human faces. Recently, face-specific neurons were also demonstrated in the temporal lobe of sheep (30).

6. In all our studies we found a remarkably better performance in face recognition by female than by male subjects in both short- and long-term memory tests (31). Unresolved is whether this ability is genetically determined or essentially dependent on the different social attitudes and education of male and female subjects in our society. In a developmental study, we found that this female advantage in face recognition is first attained during adolescence and is not present in children below the age of 12 (31).

7. Observations in brain-lesioned patients, however, also indicate that correct face recognition and understanding of facial expressions may be impaired despite the absence of symptoms of prosopagnosia.

8. Every experienced psychiatrist knows from the reports of schizophrenic patients that impairment of face recognition and facial expression may develop during the course of this disease and can include mistaken identity, perception of offensive expressions in neutral or friendly faces, and the development of fear or even terror due to perceived changes in the faces and the expressions of other persons. Altered face perception seems to be especially frequent in schizophrenic children and adolescents: normal-appearing human faces are seen as monsters with large canines, huge threatening eyes, bushy eyebrows, and menacing changes in the appearance of the hair. We call this symptom, which was first described by Capgras, *paraprosopia* (32–35).

Considering the observations mentioned in these introductory remarks, it seems worthwhile to continue with systematic explorations of the face-specific mechanisms in the visual signal processing of the primate brain and search for methods to gain more insight into these mechanisms in the human brain, whereby a multidisciplinary approach would seem appropriate. During the past 8 years we have performed systematic studies on the ability to recognize faces and facial expressions in normal subjects, brain-lesioned patients, and schizophrenics, applying different types of neuropsychological tests, and in several additional studies we have tried to answer the question whether face-specific evoked potentials (EP) can be recorded in the human electroencephalogram (EEG).

TWO NEUROPSYCHOLOGICAL TESTS TO MEASURE THE ABILITY TO RECOGNIZE FACES, FACIAL EXPRESSION, AND GESTURES

Two different neuropsychological tests were applied in the studies described in the following sections.

Recognition of Black and White Photographs of Faces or Vases

During an inspection series the subjects looked at 60 slides (21 male and 23 female faces, 16 vases of the *art nouveau* style) for 6 sec each and were asked to put them in one of three categories: sympathetic, nonsympathetic, neutral. Six of the faces and four of the vases were presented upside-down (denoted as K). One hour after the inspection series, 18 slides were presented for 6 sec with a partner (6 male and 6 female faces, 6 vases), and the subjects had to decide which of the two items had been viewed an hour before (test 1, performed only with normal upright items [N]).

One week later 66 slides were shown (29 male and 27 female faces, 10 vases) that had been seen in the inspection series and/or test 1, together with an unknown item. In some of the slides the position of the items was changed from N to K or from K to N, compared with the inspection series or test 1. The distribution of the different items is shown in Table 1.

Subjects were 49 schizophrenic patients in two psychiatric state hospitals (Bezirkskrankenhaus Kaufbeuren, Landesnervenklinik Alzey) and 53 patients with a circumscribed brain lesion in the left hemisphere (LH) (35 patients) or right hemisphere (RH) (18 patients), excluding the occipital lobe. The latter group of 53 were either volunteer inpatients at the Department of Neurology, Landesnervenklinik Spandau (Dr. M. Larsen) or participated at our institute. A normal age- and social-status-matched control group (N1) was tested. All of the subjects were right-handed. The data were also compared with those obtained in a large group of 126 normal medical students (N2) including a few left-handed subjects. A detailed description of the test is given in (31).

TABLE 1. *Structure of the face recognition test: slides of black and white photographs with 6-sec presentation time*

	Faces		Vases	
Inspection series	38 N	6 K	12 N	4 K
Test 1 (1-hr delay)	12 NN		6 NN	
Test 2 (1-week delay)	11 NNN	12 NN		
	23 N-N	3 N-K	2 N-N	4 N-K
	4 K-N	2 K-K	2 K-N	2 K-K
	1 NN K			

N, normal position; K, upside-down.

A Movie Test for the Evaluation of Perception and Recognition of Faces, Facial Expression, and Gestures

In a second set of experiments, the elementary abilities to perceive and recognize faces, expressions, and gestures were studied by applying test movies. The test consisted of 13 different silent movie scenes, each 10 sec in duration. Seven female and seven male volunteers (21–28 years of age), all dressed in black, portrayed nausea, silence, fear, farewell, physical effort, offensive smell, noise, ignorance and perplexity, quiet grief, pain, fatigue, anger, and laughter in the movies spots. The 13 scenes were shown twice (parts 1 and 2), the second time with a delay of approximately 30 to 40 min in reverse order. Following each scene, the subjects had to solve five nonverbal multiple-choice tasks in part 1 of the test and five verbal or nonverbal multiple-choice tasks in part 2: T1, recognition of the person (1); T2, identification of facial expression and gestures; T3, recognition of expression in another person; T4, recognition of person and expression; T5, recognition of the person (2); T6, verbal description; T7, association of expression and fitting situation (selection of sketched scene); T8, verbal response 1 (reading); T9, verbal response 2 (listening); T10, same as T3.

In addition to 108 schizophrenic patients, a control group of 78 unpaid volunteers served as control subjects (34). Furthermore, 65 patients with LH (31 patients), RH (30 patients), and bilateral (4 patients) lesions were investigated with this test at our institute or at the Department of Neurology, University Hospital Zürich (Prof. G. Baumgartner) (Grüsser, Kiefer, and Landis, 1985, *unpublished data*).

IMPAIRMENT OF RECOGNITION OF FACES, FACIAL EXPRESSION, AND GESTURES IN PATIENTS SUFFERING FROM CIRCUMSCRIBED BRAIN LESIONS

Results with the Slide Test

All 35 patients suffering from a LH cortical lesion were afflicted with signs of aphasia: 15 suffered from Wernicke's sensory (fluent) aphasia (FL), 15 from Broca's motor (nonfluent) aphasia (NF), and 5 from amnesic aphasia (A). All of the patients and the age- and social-status-matched control group (N1) were right-handed. As Figs. 3 and 4 reveal, RH or LH lesions led to a significant impairment in face recognition, whereby recognition of faces was relatively more impaired than that of vases. It is interesting to note that significantly higher relative error scores were obtained in patients for the tasks in which the faces were presented during the inspection series, tests 1 and 2 in the N position (Fig. 5). The results of the study, described in detail by Grüsser and Kirchhoff (36), indicated that outside of the face-specific temporo-occipital

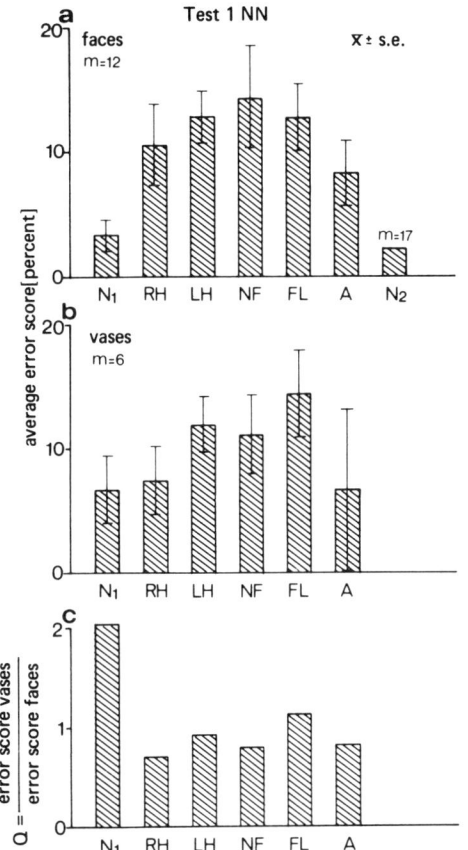

FIG. 3. Distribution of the error scores for recognition of upright faces (**a**) or vases (**b**) 1 hr after the inspection series for 15 normal subjects (N1) and 126 normal subjects (N2), 18 patients with right-hemispheric lesions (RH) and 35 patients with left-hemispheric lesions (LH). All LH patients were aphasics. Three columns in each graph represent the error scores in the LH patients belonging to the three different groups of aphasia. NF, 15 nonfluent Broca aphasics; FL, 15 fluent Wernicke aphasics; A, 5 amnesic aphasics. The relationship of error scores for recognition of vases and faces is given in (**c**). In normals, faces were better recognized than vases, whereas in brain-lesioned patients the opposite was true. (From Grüsser and Kirchhoff, 1985, *unpublished data.*)

cortical region, many other parts of the human brain contribute to the performance of simple face-recognition tasks.

Comparing the location of the different lesions (using computer tomograms [CT] as criteria), we could not find any specific site in the left or the right hemisphere (excluding occipital lobe lesions) that would affect face recognition in particular. It turned out, however, that the *size of the lesion* estimated by planimetry in three CT planes showed a positive correlation ($r = 0.67$) with the error score in the test (36).

Results with the Movie Test

Sixty-one patients with LH (30), RH (31), and bilateral (4) lesions were investigated with the movie test. In this series of experiments, we also included patients suffering from occipital lobe lesions (Grüsser, Kiefer, and Landis, 1985, *unpublished data*). As one can recognize from Fig. 6, the error scores in recognition of faces, facial expression, and gestures (averbal subtest

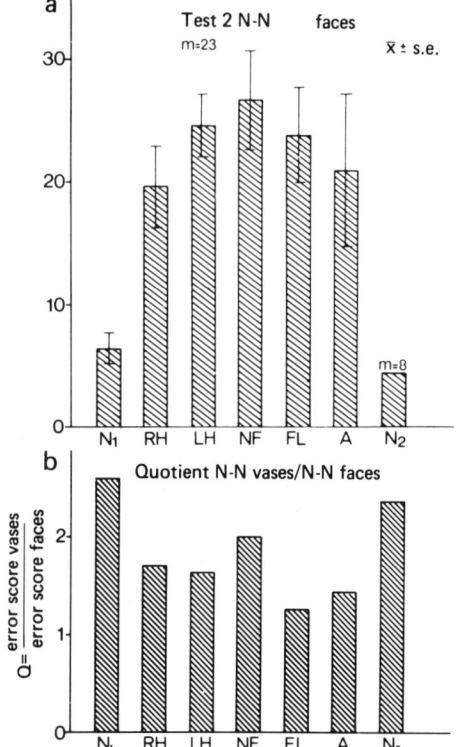

FIG. 4. Face recognition test after a delay of 1 week. Same subjects as in Fig. 3. **a:** Error score in percentages for the different groups of subjects for face recognition (upright position). **b:** Quotient between error scores for vase recognition and face recognition. (From Grüsser and Kirchhoff, 1985, *unpublished data.*)

1–5) were in all 65 patients higher on the average than in the verbal test (6, 8, 9) and the subtest 7, relating the expression to an adequate situation. The overall error score was higher in right-temporal and right-occipital lesioned patients than in patients suffering from a right-sided lesion in the frontal or parietal lobe or the insular region. The response pattern was quite different in LH-lesioned patients in which frontal lesions also led to considerable error scores in all three classes of subtests. LH patients had higher error scores in the verbal tests 5, 6, and 8 than RH patients (Fig. 7). For all tests and all movie scenes, error scores were significantly higher in LH and RH brain-lesioned patients than in the normal control group (Grüsser, Landis, and Kiefer 1985, *unpublished data*).

Conclusions

From the preceding studies we arrive at the following conclusions:

1. Lesions in any part of the cerebral cortex located outside the prosopagnosia region and outside the occipital lobe may lead to a considerable impairment in recognition of faces, facial expression, and gestures.

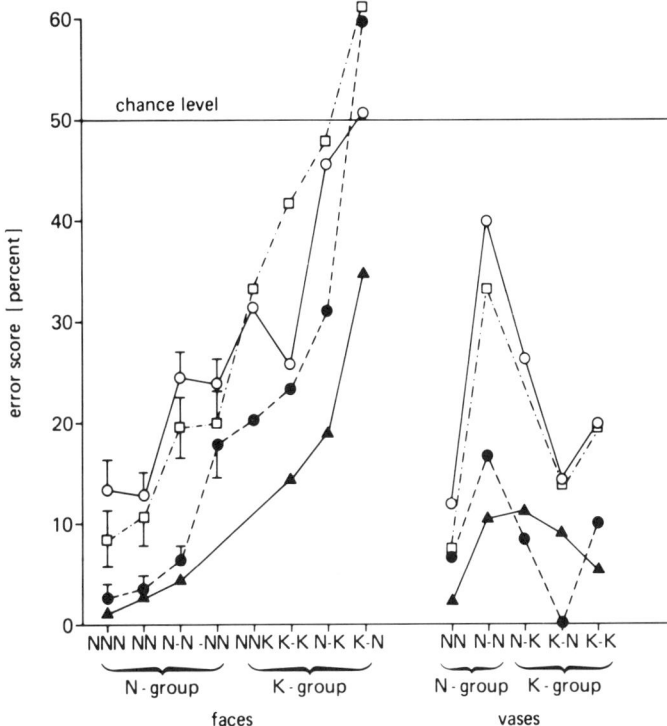

FIG. 5. Summary of data obtained in the recognition tests of faces and vases in normals (15 N1, ●; 126 N2, ▲) and brain-lesioned patients (35 LH, ○; 18 RH, □) under different stimulus conditions as indicated. NN, recognition of items in normal position after 1-hr delay. N-N, same after 1 week delay. NNN, items in normal position but seen in the inspection series, in test 1 after 1 hr and in test 2 after 1 week delay, error score for this test. K, items upside-down. For further explanation, see text. (From Grüsser and Kirchhoff, 1985, *unpublished data*.)

2. The size and extent of these lesions seem to be more important for test performance than the location.
3. A slight tendency to higher error scores in patients suffering from right temporal and occipital lesions was found in the movie tests compared with right frontal or parietal lesions.
4. Not surprisingly, the error scores obtained in the verbal tasks of the movie test were higher in LH than in RH patients, but the difference was surprisingly small, despite the aphasia present in most of the LH patients.
5. The static face-recognition test and the movie test were both very easy for normal subjects, and the differences between error scores obtained in brain-lesioned patients and in normal subjects were remarkable. Since only the static test with black and white photographs was time limited (6 sec projection and another 6 sec decision making), one can conclude from the data obtained in the time-unlimited movie test that it was not general

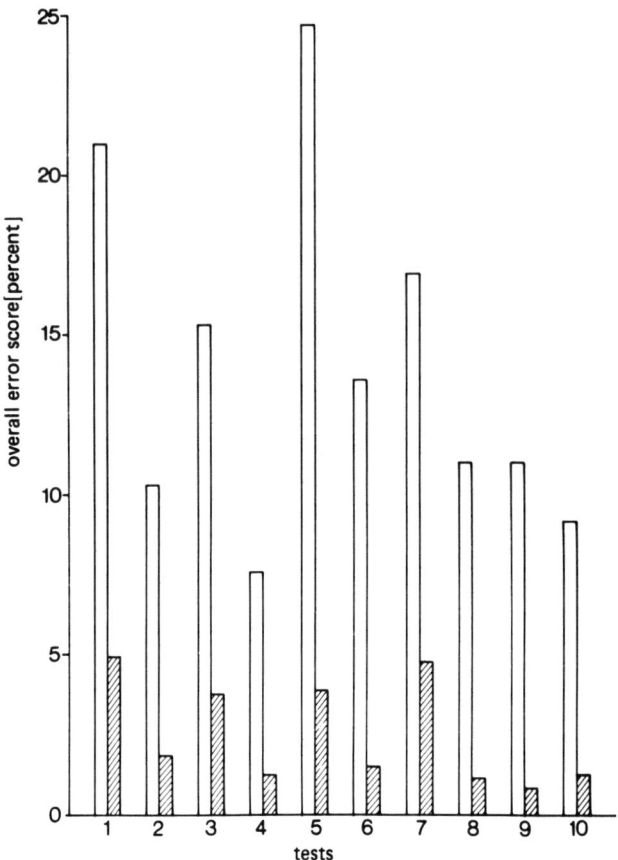

FIG. 6. Mimic, gesture, and person recognition. Average error scores of all 65 brain-lesioned (□) patients (31 RH, 30 LH, 4 bilateral) in the 10 different subtests of the movie test are compared with the average error scores of the 78 normal (▨) subjects. Tests 1–5 were averbal, tests 6, 8 and 9 verbal. See text for details. (From Grüsser, Kiefer, and Landis, 1986, *unpublished data.*)

slowing-down of perceptive and/or cognitive functions in brain-lesioned patients that led to these results.

IMPAIRMENT OF PERCEPTION AND RECOGNITION OF FACES, FACIAL EXPRESSION, AND GESTURES IN SCHIZOPHRENIC PATIENTS

The same two tests as described in the preceding sections were also applied in schizophrenic patients.

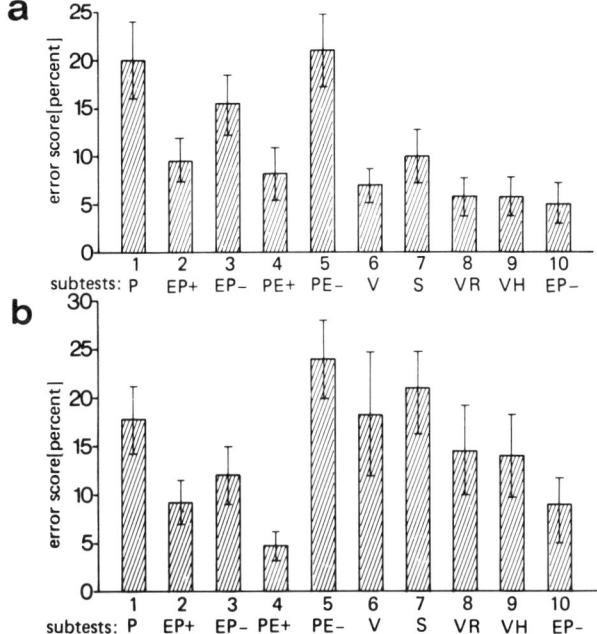

FIG. 7. Distribution of the error scores (±mean) in the 10 different subtests of the movie test for face, person, mimic, and gesture recognition obtained in RH ($n = 31$) and LH ($n = 30$) patients. Note the higher error scores in the verbal tasks (6, 8, 9) in LH patients (**b**) compared with the error scores in RH patients (**a**). (From Grüsser, Kiefer, and Landis, 1986, *unpublished data*.)

Face Recognition with a Static Slide Projection Test

The 49 patients participated on a voluntary basis and were informed that a scientific study was being carried out. Of these patients, 27 suffered from paranoic-hallucinatory schizophrenia (PH), 18 from hebephrenia (H), and four from a schizoaffective psychosis (SA). All patients fulfilled the diagnostic criteria of schizophrenia according to the DSM-III. A fairly extensive psychiatric exploration, based in part on the AMDP Manual 1981, was performed to classify and evaluate the psychopathological signs. A summary of the test results is shown in Fig. 8. It became evident that error scores in schizophrenic patients were as much as five times higher than in normals for the 1-hr and 1-week delayed recognition tests, when the items were presented in the N position. When rotation (K) was involved once or twice in the test tasks, however, the error scores of the schizophrenic patients no longer deviated significantly from those of the normal group matched in age and social conditions to the patients. Thus, the easier tasks led to relatively higher error scores

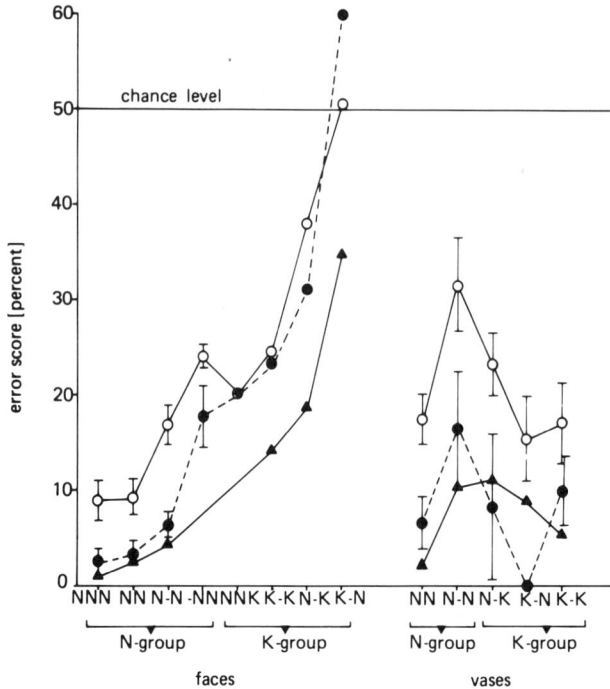

FIG. 8. Summary of error scores in the face and vase recognition test (as in Fig. 5) performed in normals (●, N1; ▲, N2) and 49 adult schizophrenic patients (○) See Fig. 5 for abbreviations. For explanation, see text. (From Grüsser and Kremer, 1986, *unpublished data*.)

in schizophrenic patients rather than the more difficult ones involving rotation of the faces. Since faces not only lose part of their emotional quality with rotation, but also part of their "faceness," it seems to be these components that are impaired by the pathological process underlying the clinical symptoms of schizophrenia (Grüsser and Kremer, 1986, *unpublished data*).

Results with the Movie Test

The movie test described in a previous section was applied in different groups of hospitalized schizophrenic patients. In the first study 81 patients (45 PH, 25 H, 8 SA, and three suffering from catatonic schizophrenia) were studied (33). In a second study a group of 28 adolescent schizophrenic patients (19 male and 9 female) with an average age of 19.0 ± 0.4 (S.E.) years were investigated and their performance in the test was compared with a middle-aged group of schizophrenic patients (40.0 ± 0.9 years) and two corresponding groups of normal subjects (18.2 ± 0.9 and 39.4 ± 1.1 years). The following data were obtained:

FACE, FACIAL EXPRESSION, GESTURE RECOGNITION 177

1. The overall error scores in schizophrenic patients increased as much as sevenfold than those of normals.
2. The error score for the averbal tests was higher on the average in paranoic patients than in the two other groups of schizophrenic patients, whereas the opposite was true for the error scores observed in the verbal tests (Fig. 9).
3. Age and sex had some impact on the test results. Whereas normal female subjects were slightly better in this test than male subjects, in schizophrenic patients the reverse was true. The relative impairment of adolescent schizophrenic patients (compared with adolescent normals) was, however, somewhat stronger than that of adult schizophrenics (Fig. 10). This supports the hypothesis that the defect found in this test was caused by the disease per se and not by other factors such as duration of illness or hospitalization.
4. In all patients the correlation between duration of disease and error score was low; less than 10% of the error scores could be attributed to factors related to length of illness or hospitalization.
5. Evaluation of psychopathological symptoms indicated that the stronger the schizophrenic defect, the higher the error score, but the impact of this psychopathological component was not more than 10% on the overall error scores (32–35).

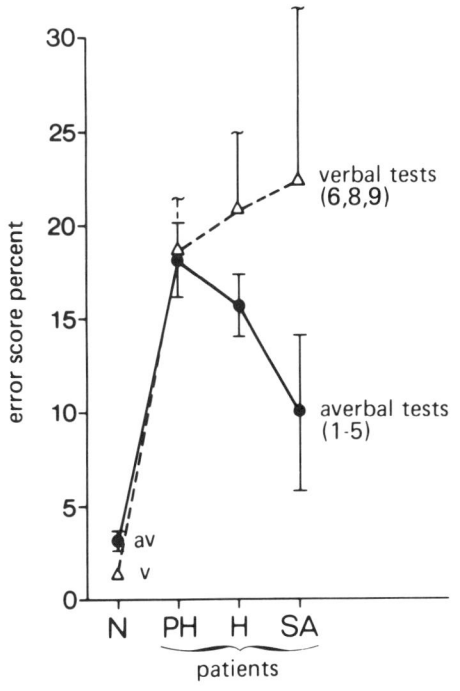

FIG. 9. Comparison of the average error scores for all verbal subtests of the movie test (T6, T8, T9) and all averbal subtests (T1–T5) for normals (●) and the three groups of schizophrenics (△). (From ref. 34.)

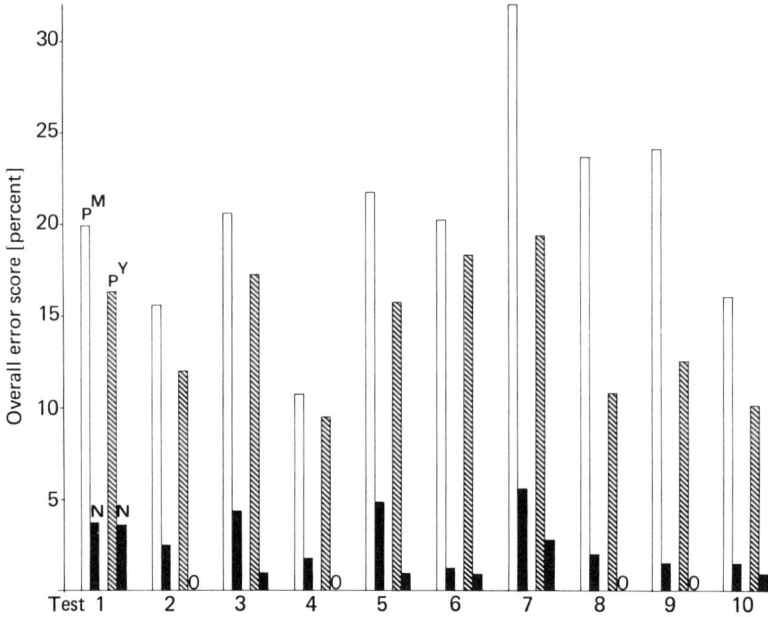

FIG. 10. Error score in the movie test obtained in normals (N) and schizophrenic patients (P) from adolescent (15–22 years) subjects (Y) and middle-aged (30–50 years) subjects (M). The errors are given in percentages (ordinate). In several subtests the group of young adolescent normals had no errors; this is marked with 0. Data from the 10 different subtests as described in text. (From ref. 35.)

Conclusions

The analysis of performance and test data in schizophrenic patients indicated that impairment in recognition of faces, facial expression, and gestures is most likely not only due to a general nonspecific impairment of cognitive functions but to a selective defect as well in the elementary cognitive visual functions necessary for averbal social communication. Since the recognition of facial and gestural expression is determined in part by genetic factors, i.e., the operation of inborn neuronal networks modified by experience and learning, one has to consider which part of the brain could be affected in schizophrenia leading to the defects found in the present study.

1. One could argue that due to the relatively general susceptibility of face-expression and gesture-recognition tasks to any lesion of the cerebral cortex, described in previous sections, the impairment of this function is primarily due to a nonlocalized change in brain function in schizophrenia.

2. Considering the idea supported by the EP responses to be discussed below, however, limbic structures are presumably essential in the tasks of face recognition. The data presented in this paragraph suggest a selective cognitive

impairment due to schizophrenia for tasks linked to "emotional components" of the communicative stimulus, for which limbic structures are of importance.

3. The data obtained in the movie test indicate that a disturbance in the "correct" perception of facial and gestural expression seems to be an elementary property of schizophrenia, perhaps one of the "core" symptoms of this disease. Should this be the case, many of the paranoic responses of schizophrenic patients related to their social field could be considerably secondary to the impairment in perception and cognition of highly relevant, social, averbal, communicative signals, and their misinterpretation.

ELECTRICAL BRAIN POTENTIALS EVOKED BY PICTURES OF FACES AND NONFACES: A SEARCH FOR "FACE-RESPONSIVE" COMPONENTS IN THE EVOKED POTENTIALS

Several laboratories have investigated changes in the EEG of human subjects when photographs (or slides) of faces were presented or other face-specific tasks had to be performed. Dumas and Morgan (37) found a suppression of EEG alpha activity that was more pronounced over the right cerebral hemisphere when their subjects called various faces to mind. Small (38) compared EEG potentials evoked by pictures of known and unknown faces and by geometric figures. She reported a high amplitude of the P-300 wave recorded over the right hemisphere with face stimuli as opposed to geometric figures and no differences in the EPs when responses to known and unknown faces were compared. Sobotka et al. (39) also reported some hemispheric differences in EEG potentials evoked by face stimuli. In contrast to these findings, Neville et al. (40) reported a higher P-300 amplitude in the EEG responses evoked by pictures of persons, paintings, or places known to the subjects as compared with the responses evoked by unknown items. Srebro (41,42) tried to localize the electrical brain activity related to face perception in human temporal lobe by applying a vector analysis technique. He used EEG potentials evoked by geometric figures and faces, computed the spatial Laplacian vector response and evaluated the differences between these responses to stimulus patterns recognized as "faces" and as "no face" (noise-masked patterns). These difference curves had a maximum at 206 msec. Srebro found similar differences, however, for faces and simple geometric figures. In his study only slight discrepancies existed in the EEG responses evoked by face and nonface stimuli with respect to shape and topographic location. More recently, Jeffreys and Musselwhite (43) reported on face-responsive EPs and described a midline positive response maximum at the electrodes Cz and Pz (international 10/20 recording scheme) peaking at 140 to 160 msec latency. Inversion or rotation through 90° increased this latency by 20 to 25 msec. Evidently these authors obtained potentials similar to those now to be described.

During the past 4 years in various experimental series we have systematically explored EPs in the EEG of normal human subjects, whereby face stimuli and similarly complex nonface stimuli were applied in the search for possible face-responsive or even face-specific EP components. In contrast to the EP studies mentioned, however, a new stimulation technique was employed by which face stimuli alternated in random sequence with nonface stimuli. Care was taken that only the structure of consecutive visual stimuli changed and not the overall average luminance (detailed description of the method in Häussler [44] and Bötzel and Grüsser [45]). Thus the recordings consisted of EEG responses to a sudden change in a complex visual stimulus pattern seen with the foveal and perifoveal retina (4×6° stimulus field). Altogether more than 70 subjects (unpaid male and female medical students, 19 to 32 years of age) served in these experiments. Their right-handedness had been confirmed by the Edinburgh inventory (46). The test persons were volunteers and were not informed in some of the tests that faces were the crucial stimuli until completion of the series. All subjects had normal binocular vision and no neurological, visual, or oculomotor impairment. They sat in a moderately comfortable chair, resting the head against the back, and were instructed to relax and fixate a small red light (0.05° diameter) 2 m away at eye level on a vertical reflecting white screen. The stimuli consisted of a sequence of slides projected onto this field for 2.5 to 4 sec. The stimulus duration was varied at random within these limits; the average luminance of the stimulus pattern was 12.5 cd/m^2 for the set of positive stimuli (black line drawings on a white background) or 0.5 cd/m^2 for the negative stimuli (white line drawings on a black background) and approximately 5 cd/m^2 for the black and white photographs. The background luminance of the experimental room was approximately 0.1 cd/m^2. Any acoustic signals were masked by continuous white noise transmitted through ear phones (approximately 70 dB SPL). The slides were projected alternately from one of two carousel slide projectors (Fig. 11). A shutter driven by a pneumatic system and controlled by means of an electromagnetic valve opened and closed the beams of the two projectors. The moment one beam was turned off, the other was turned on. The change required less than 6 msec. The shutter movement and slide change in the two carousel projectors were computer controlled.

The DC electronystagmogram and the EEG were recorded by standard EEG techniques with reference electrodes of "linked earlobes" or "linked mastoids." Responses from electrodes F_Z, C_Z, P_Z, T5 (left), and T6 (right) were used for recordings (international 10/20 system [47], bandpass 0.1–100 Hz, rejection of eye movement artifacts, standard averaging of 40–50 responses to items of the same class). The results described in the following indicate that with this technique some face-responsive components in the EPs can be detected, surprisingly not in the region of the temporal or temporo-occipital lobe but at the midline electrodes, especially C_Z and P_Z.

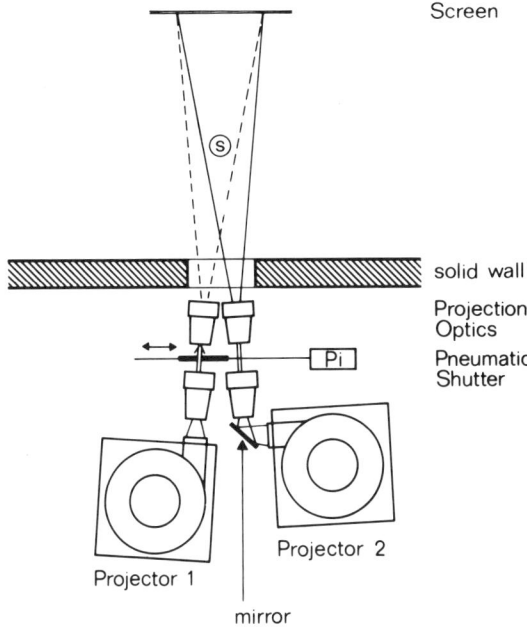

FIG. 11. Schematic drawing of the computer-controlled slide projection system. Two carousel projectors were used to project the stimuli alternately for 2.5–4-sec duration onto a reflecting screen. By means of a pneumatically driven, computer-controlled shutter one projector was turned off and simultaneously the other turned on within less than 6 msec. Size of the stimulus field 4 × 6°. (S) subject; (Pi) piston. (From ref. 45.)

Responses to Sketches of a Face, a Tree, and a Chair as Alternating Stimuli

The stimuli shown in Fig. 12 were presented in a semirandom order, whereby no slide of the 160 presented was followed by one of the same category. Especially at electrodes C_z and P_z, characteristic responses for schematic faces were found with three prominent peaks, absent with chair or tree stimuli (Fig. 12). The subtraction curves (face–chair, face–tree, chair–tree) and the auto- and cross-correlation functions between them supported the hypothesis of face-responsive EP components (45) (Fig. 13). The maxima of the cross-correlation functions between the difference curves (face–tree) and (face–chair) were significantly higher than the corresponding cross-correlation functions between the difference curves (face–chair/chair–tree) and (face–tree/chair–tree). All these observations were valid for P and N stimuli. It is interesting that the cross-correlation functions between the difference curves obtained for P and N stimuli reached higher values when face responses were involved (45).

182 FACE, FACIAL EXPRESSION, GESTURE RECOGNITION

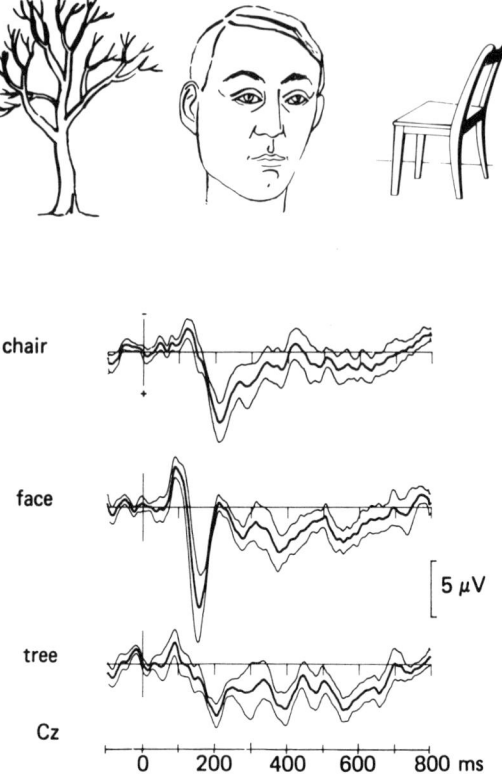

FIG. 12. Upper: Set of stimuli in the first experimental paradigm. Stimuli were black line drawings of a chair, face, or tree (P stimuli) or the same drawings with white lines on a black background (N stimuli). **Lower:** Grand averages (±standard error) of EPs recorded through electrode C_z in five female subjects; P stimuli. (From ref. 45.)

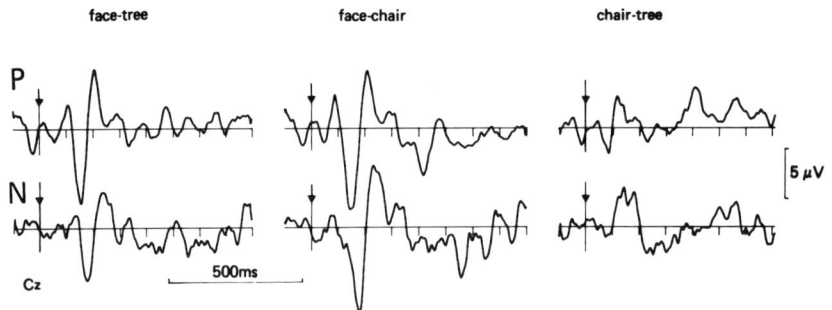

FIG. 13. Subtraction curves of the grand averages of EPs recorded in five female subjects with electrode C_z (paradigm 1: face–tree, face–chair, chair–tree). Note the considerably larger differences when face stimuli were involved for the responses obtained between 100 and 300 msec after stimulus change (*arrow*). Data obtained with P stimuli (P) in the upper row, with N stimuli (N) in the lower row. (From ref. 45.)

Responses Evoked by Black and White Photographs of Face and Nonface Stimuli

In a second series of experiments the set of stimuli consisted of 54 black and white photographs (slides) of different human faces of both sexes (frontal view) unknown to the subjects, 53 photographs of different vases, mostly ornamented and of the *art nouveau* style, and 53 photographs of different pairs of worn shoes, photographed from above. The grand averages of EPs obtained from 11 adult subjects showed an early negative peak occurring approximately 140 to 160 msec after the change in stimulus. This peak had the shortest latency and the highest amplitude at C_Z when the stimulus was a face. Amplitude and latency differences of different peaks were significant for face/vase and face/shoe stimuli at the 99% level for the electrodes C_Z and T6 (Wilcoxon test for matched pairs). The latencies of a large positive peak occurring between 210 and 240 msec were approximately the same for men and women (214 msec for faces, 230 msec for vases, and 234 msec for shoes). In most subjects a negative peak appeared at approximately 300 msec with face stimuli. In the responses to nonface stimuli, this peak was absent or small. In men it was considerably less pronounced than in women, and the negative peak at 300 msec did not reach the base line in the average EP of male subjects (45).

EPs During a Recognition Task: Learned and Unknown Faces and Nonfaces

In the third series of experiments, the same types of stimuli were presented and described as in the previous section, but a memory search process was included followed by a decision process ("previously seen/not seen"). We tried to find out whether EPs depend on such memory search processes related to the three different stimulus categories. During the EEG recording session the subjects had to recognize nine slides (three of each category) that had been shown to them approximately 20 min before the recording experiment for approximately 10 sec each. These slides appeared in a random order within a set of 183 stimuli. The responses to these nine slides were excluded from averaging. In addition to the paradigm of the previous section, a fourth category of black and white photographs was added: every third to fifth slide, on the average, was one of a flower. The subjects were asked to press a button whenever a flower slide appeared immediately after a face, shoe, or vase slide known to them from the pretest inspection period. The curves obtained in this paradigm (Fig. 14) showed no significant differences during the first 400 msec as compared with the EPs described in the preceding section, but a very late positive wave appeared with a maximum at approximately 700 msec for faces, 792 msec for vases, and 698 msec for shoes. This wave was most prominent in the face responses and at electrode F_Z. Presumably it was related to the new

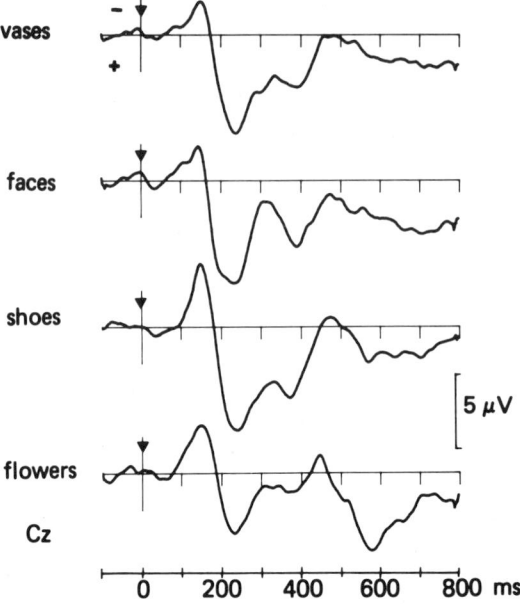

FIG. 14. EPs (grand averages) obtained at electrode C_z in 13 subjects (4 men, 9 women). Stimuli were black and white photographs of vases, faces, shoes, and flowers. A recognition task after presentation of a flower was included. Responses to unknown stimuli averaged. (From ref. 45.)

component in the experimental task, namely to store the necessary information for the decision required after a possibly appearing flower slide. Also the very pronounced positive wave peaking at approximately 580 msec after a flower slide was probably due to the cerebral mechanisms correlated with the decision required after the recognition of such a stimulus.

Learned and Unknown Faces Recognized in a Direct Response Task

In 15 subjects EEG responses were obtained during a face-recognition task, whereby the subjects had to press a key with the right hand whenever the face projected was known to them. The subjects inspected 11 face slides twice (6 and 4 secs) 10 min before the experiments and were first asked to rate the face as friendly, unfriendly, or neutral and then in the second run to recognize the neutral faces and signal this by pressing a bar. In the set of black and white photographs presented during the recording session approximately half of the faces were known, the other half unknown to the subjects. Figure 15 shows the responses obtained at electrodes T5, T6, and C_z for the two face categories. Under these stimulus conditions a left-right difference was present for

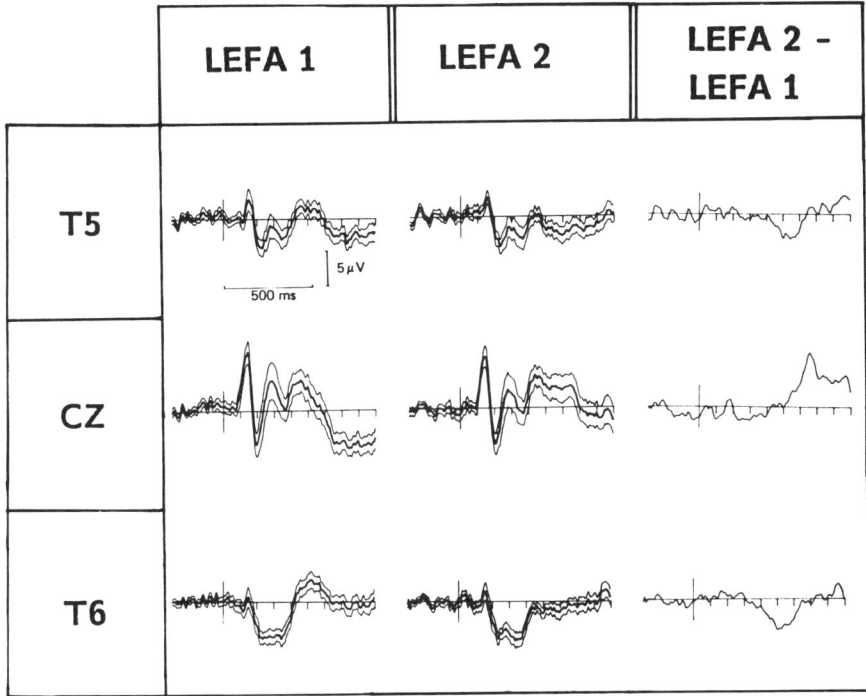

FIG. 15. Grand averages of the EPs of 15 subjects (8 men, 7 women). Recording examples from the electrodes T5, T6, and C_Z. In the middle column the responses to face photographs viewed before the tests (LEFA 2), in the left column the corresponding EPs to unknown face photographs (LEFA 1). In the right column, the difference between both curves is displayed. In the left and middle columns, the standard error is shown in addition to the grand average.

electrodes T4, T6, T3, and T5, but the most prominent responses were again recorded at C_Z. With known faces, the maintained negativity beginning approximately 400 msec after the stimulus change was of a longer duration than in the response to unknown faces.

Responses Evoked by Famous Faces as Compared with Unknown Faces

In the same group of 15 subjects (7 female, 8 male) 45 "famous" faces were intermingled with unknown faces (slides of black and white photographs), whereby the subjects were asked to press a key when a famous face known to them appeared. The average response time for this task was 750 msec, and the average "correct" response 74% (less than 6% "false positive" responses to unknown faces). The EPs are shown in Fig. 16. Again the most prominent responses were obtained at electrode C_Z, but the differences between the responses evoked by the two stimulus categories were small.

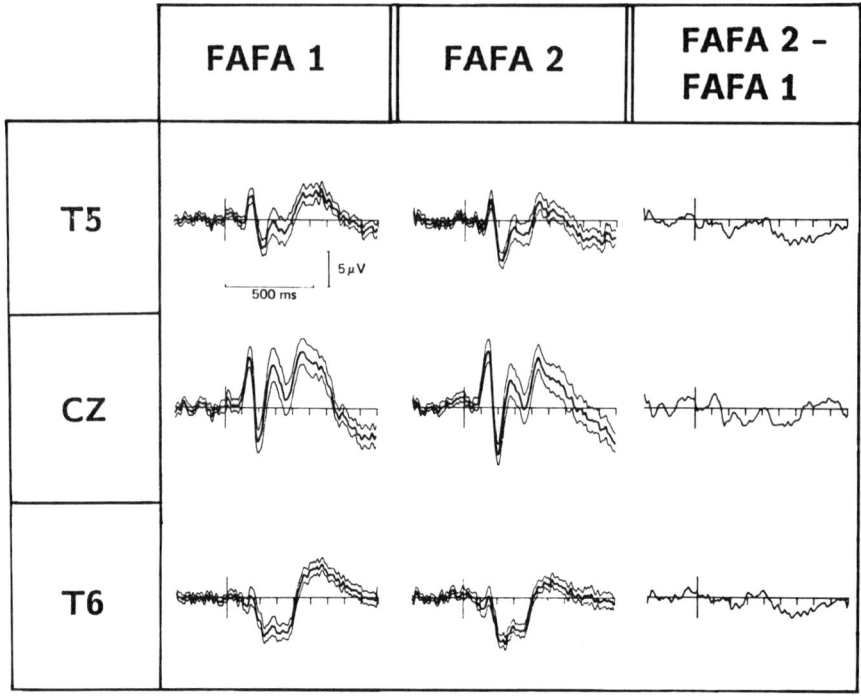

FIG. 16. Grand averages (±standard error) of EPs recorded at the electrodes T5, C_z, and T6. Same subjects as in Fig. 15. Stimuli were either famous faces (FAFA 2) or unknown faces (FAFA 1). In the right column, the subtraction curves are shown, indicating some differences, especially at the electrode C_z.

Responses to Learned and Unknown Flowers

To investigate the importance of known versus unknown stimuli, we applied the same general paradigm as described in a previous section of the same 12 subjects (5 female, 7 male), but instead of faces, black and white photographs of flowers were used. Figure 17 exhibits grand averages obtained for the EPs at electrodes T5, T6, and C_z in this paradigm. The positive waves occurring between 200 and 400 msec were significantly more pronounced and lasted longer with learned stimuli. These changes in EP components might be caused by a quasi-physiognomic quality attained by flower stimulus through the preceding learning procedure. When one compares the recordings, however, one recognizes that the face-evoked potentials—especially at electrode C_z—look quite different (with the pronounced negative peak at approximately 280 msec) from those evoked by flowers, despite the formal structural complexity of the stimuli being approximately the same for the two categories.

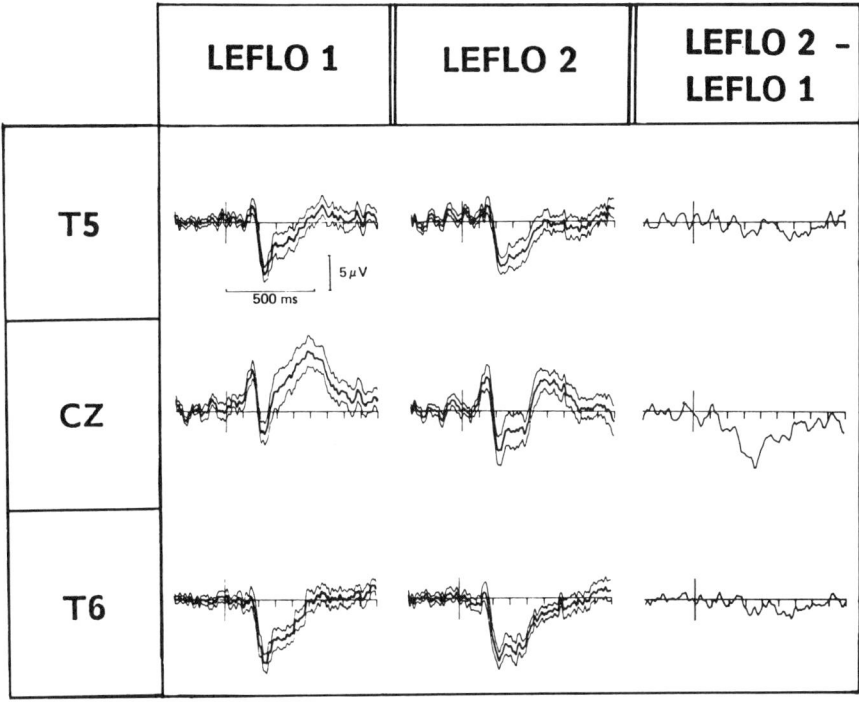

FIG. 17. Grand averages (±standard error) of the EPs of 12 adult subjects (7 men, 5 women). Stimuli were learned (LEFLO 2) and unknown flowers (LEFLO 1); otherwise the same paradigm as in Fig. 15. In the right column, the difference curves are shown, indicating a highly significant change in the EPs from learned to unknown flowers at the electrode C_z.

Potentials Evoked by Face Stimuli in Normal and Upside-Down Position

Recognition of faces in the upside-down position is considerably weaker than when the slides are seen in the normal position. Figure 18 demonstrates grand averages of EEG responses evoked by "pure" faces, i.e., face photographs restricted to the inner part of the face. The slides were projected either in the normal ("FACE 2") or upside-down ("FACE 3") position. It is evident that in general the EP shape is not considerably changed, at least not for the first 300 msec of the recordings, but the latency of the first positive peak at 215 msec is shifted to 220 msec when the face is presented upside-down (grand averages). The mean latencies computed from the 16 individual EPs at C_z were 210 and 221 msec, respectively (difference significant at $p < 0.05$). This increase in latency was also reported by Jeffreys and Musselwhite (43).

Conclusions

EP studies indicated that, in comparison to other complex visual stimuli (tree, chair, shoes, vases, flowers), the EEG responses evoked by face stimuli

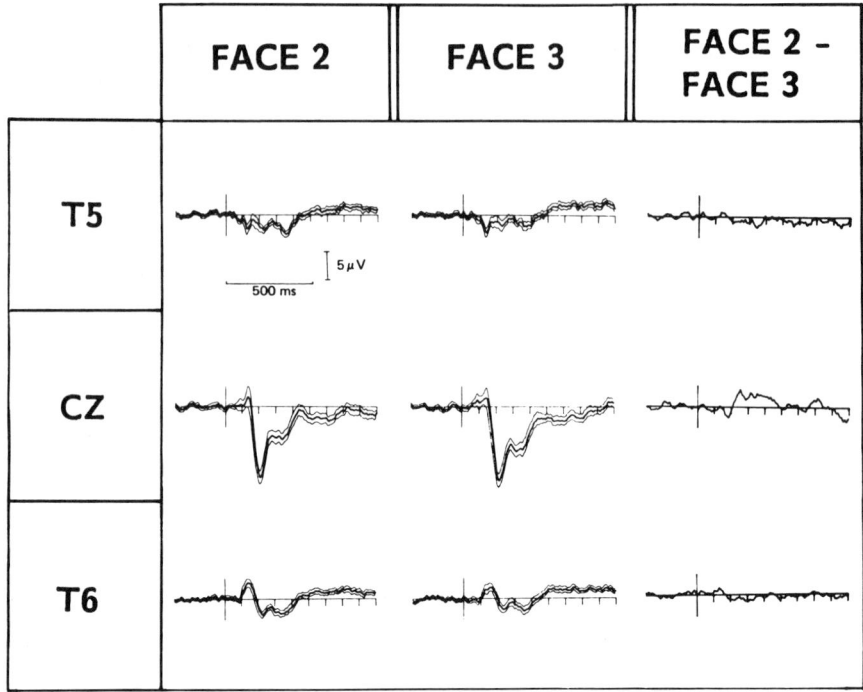

FIG. 18. Grand averages and standard deviation of EPs in 16 adult subjects (8 men, 8 women). Stimuli were photos of faces, restricted to the mouth, eye, and nose region. The faces were either in the normal upright position (FACE 2) or upside-down (FACE 3). Under the two conditions, only small differences were found at the electrode C_z. Note the less prominent face-responsive components at electrode C_z compared with Figs. 15 and 16, in which the stimuli were full photographs.

contain components denoting that face-specific responses might be measureable in the human brain. The most prominent face-responsive EP components were not evoked in the temporal or temporo-occipital region, however, but with midline recordings at electrode C_z. Thus, it seems probable that these face-specific response components do not originate in the temporo-occipital cortical face region but rather in symmetrically organized deep limbic structures, in basal parts of the temporal lobe, or in the gyrus cinguli. The latter structures are known to receive input from the amygdala, which contain a considerable amount of face-specific neurons in primates (27,28). The data presented in the preceding sections give further support to the concept that when recognizing a face and distinguishing it from nonface complex visual stimuli, structures widely distributed in the brain may be activated. Consequently, brain lesions outside of the prosopagnosia region might indeed lead to an impairment in recognition of faces and facial expression as described in the clinical studies presented in previous sections.

GENERAL CONCLUSIONS

The experimental data described here demonstrate that, in our opinion, the recognition and understanding of averbal communicative signals represented by faces, facial expressions, and gestures are not simple tasks, when one regards the underlying brain functions involved. Faces, facial expression, and gestures not only form a specific class of visual signals of a certain formal pictorial complexity (as expressed by the spatial frequency contents and phase relations and the changes in these parameters during the movie scenes), but also the stimuli contain meaningful social information that depends on prior subject experience and can be characterized by the following components:

1. elementary perception of the stimulus (as opposed to nonstimulus or "noise");
2. recognition of a face versus nonface, i.e., recognition of a human partner as opposed to any other visual stimulus;
3. recognition of the sex of the partner;
4. categorization of the partner as unknown or known;
5. categorization of the partner as friendly or unfriendly, important/unimportant, higher/lower rank on the social scale, etc.;
6. attributing a name to the face;
7. recognition of the averbal signals generated by the partner and conveying information in a larger social and/or circumstantial context;
8. interpretation of these messages as meaningful (or not) with respect to the behavior of the "receiver."

A similar categorization, of course, can be made in the motor or vegetative responses of the receiver of a face stimulus or a facial or gestural message, but we have only gained knowledge so far on the perceptive and cognitive aspects of this problem. This knowledge, as presented in the preceding schematic categories, is rather complex, however, and the same is true for the brain mechanisms involved in face- and expression-recognition tasks. Hereby, not only are the brain structures necessary for the formal analysis of the stimulus and its cognitive components important, but also the brain mechanisms encoding the emotional evaluation of the stimulus. This factor presumably leads to a strong involvement of the limbic structures and many other regions of the brain concerned with memory tasks and the individual experiences of the "receiving" subject. These conditions responsible for the recognition of faces, expression, and gestures seem to be viable to brain lesions in any part of neocortical associative or integration regions and the limbic system. The same is true for the impact of diseases on brain functions in a nonlocalized manner, such as in schizophrenia. The involvement of many different brain regions in face-recognition tasks might help us to understand why the evoked responses to face stimuli were recorded over a large part of the brain but were most pronounced in a fairly nonspecific way at the midline electrode C_Z. Perhaps our findings are explained by the increased electrical activity of limbic structures in the temporal lobe and of the gyrus cinguli, lying symmetrically below the midline electrodes.

SUMMARY

The perception and recognition of faces and nonface stimuli were investigated by means of EP techniques in normal subjects. Neuropsychological studies on recognition of faces, facial expression, and gestures were performed in normal subjects, brain-lesioned patients, and schizophrenic patients.

1. Two neuropsychological tests investigating recognition of faces, mimic expression, and gestures were applied in normals and brain-lesioned patients. In the first test, the recognition of faces and vases was tested 1 hr and 1 week after an inspection series. It was found that the size rather than the location of the lesion (excluding occipital lobe lesions) was an important determinant of the error score. No significant differences were found between patients suffering from RH and LH lesions.

In general the same observation was true when recognition of faces, expression, and gestures was studied by means of a movie test consisting of 12 10-sec movie scenes and 10 multiple-choice tests following inspection of each scene. A slight tendency to higher error scores appeared in patients suffering from right temporo-occipital lesions compared with other RH lesions.

2. Impairment in the perception and recognition of faces, facial expression, and gestures was also found in schizophrenic patients. Their error score, especially in the movie tests, was on the average higher than in brain-lesioned patients, indicating a major perceptual or cognitive deficit in this disease. This observation is consistent with some clinical symptoms of schizophrenia. It is remarkable that in the slide test, schizophrenic patients had a significantly higher error score in the easy tasks (recognition of upright faces) than normals, whereas in the difficult tasks (involving upside-down faces) their performance was not significantly different from that of an age- and socially matched group.

3. The degree of schizophrenic defect and acute psychotic symptoms had some effect on the impairment in schizophrenics performing these tests. When the error scores of adolescent and middle-aged schizophrenics were compared to corresponding control group error scores, the relative impairment of adolescent schizophrenic patients was found to be somewhat stronger than that of adult schizophrenics. This supports the hypothesis that the impairment in face and mimic recognition found in schizophrenic patients is caused by the disease and not by other factors such as duration of illness or hospitalization. It is conjectured that a component very specific to schizophrenia leads to the dramatic cognitive defect found in our tests in these patients.

4. Applying different stimulus paradigms, some evidence is presented that

face-responsive components appeared in the EPs when schematic drawings or black and white photographs of unknown, known, or famous faces were the stimuli. These face-specific responses were most prominent through the electrode C_z and only slight left-right differences were found in the EPs recorded with electrodes located on the skull above the temporal lobe of the cerebral cortex. It is conjectured that the gyri cinguli responses might contribute to the EPs recorded from midline electrodes.

5. The neuropsychological data obtained in brain-lesioned or schizophrenic patients as well as the EP studies in normals indicate that in addition to the face-specific areas in occipito-temporal cortical regions, limbic structures are involved in tasks concerning perception or recognition of faces and mimic expressions.

ACKNOWLEDGMENTS

This work was supported in part by a grant of the Deutsche Forschungsgemeinschaft (Gr 161). The senior author (O.-J.G) was supported by an "Akademie-Stipendium" of the Volkswagen Foundation. A.N. was supported by a NaFög-Fellowship. We thank Ms. D. Klingele for technical assistance, Dipl.-Ings. H. Nitert, J. Petsch, and L.-R. Weiss for their valuable help in setting up electronic equipment, Mr. J. Lerch for skillful construction of the stimulation equipment, and Mrs. J. Dames for her help in the English translation of the manuscript.

Some of the clinical studies were performed at the Bezirkskrankenhaus Kaufbeuren. The generous hospitality of the Director, Dr. M. von Cranach, is gratefully acknowledged.

REFERENCES

1. Cusanus N. *Compendium,* Latin-German. Decker B, Bormann K, eds. Hamburg: Meiner, 1982.
2. Bodamer J. Die Prosop-Agnosie. *Arch Psychiatr Nervenkr* 1948;179:6–53.
3. Hecaen H, Angelergues R. Agnosia for faces. *Arch Neurol* 1962;7:92–100.
4. Gloning I, Gloning K, Hoff H, Taschabitscher H. Zur Prosopagnosie. *Neuropsychologie* 1966;4:113–132.
5. Hecaen H. The neuropsychology of face recognition. In: Davies G, Ellis H, Shepherd H, eds. *Perceiving and remembering faces.* London: Academic Press, 1981;39–54.
6. Meadows JC. The anatomical basis of prosopagnosia. *J Neurol Neurosurg Psychiatry* 1974; 37:485–501.
7. Damasio AR, Damasio H, Hoesen GW van. Prosopagnosia: anatomical basis and neurobehavioral mechanisms. *J Neurol* 1982;32:331–341.
8. Landis T, Cummings, JL, Christen L, Bogen JE, Imhof HG. Are unilateral right posterior cerebral lesions sufficient to cause prosopagnosia? Clinical and radiological findings in six additional patients. *Cortex* 1986;22:243–252.
9. Landis T, Regard M, Bliestle A, Kleihnes P. Prosopagnosia and agnosia for non-canonical views: an autopsied case. *Brain* 1988;111:1287–1297.
10. Bliestle A, Regard M, Landis T. Prosopagnosia: an autopsied case. *J Clin Exp Neuropsychol* 1986;8:127.

11. Wolff W. The experimental study of forms of expression. In: *Char Pers* 1933 (as quoted by Milner 1979);168–176.
12. Gilbert C, Balkan P. Visual asymmetry in perception of faces. *Neuropsychologia* 1973;11: 355–362.
13. Lawson NC. Inverted writing in right- and left-handers in relation to lateralization of face recognition. *Cortex* 1978;14:207–211.
14. Milner B. Complementary functional specializations of the human cerebral hemispheres. *Pontif Acad Sci Scripta Var* 1979;45:601–620.
15. Campbell R. Asymmetries in the interpretation and expression of opposed expression. *Cortex* 1978;14:327–342.
16. Sackheim HA, Gur RC, Saucy MC. Emotions are expressed more strongly on the left side of the face. *Science* 1978;202:434–435.
17. Moscowitch M, Scullion D, Christie D. Early versus late stages of processing and their relation to functional hemispheric asymmetries in face recognition. *J Exp Psychol* 1976; 2:401–416.
18. Bradshaw JL, Sherlock D. Bugs and faces in the two visual fields: the analytical/holistic processing dichotomy and task sequencing. *Cortex* 1982;18:211–226.
19. Anderson E, Parkin AJ. On the nature of the left visual field advantage for faces. *Cortex* 1985;21:453–459.
20. Levy J, Sperry R, Trevarthen C. Perception of bilateral chimeric figures following hemispheric deconnexion. *Brain* 1972;95:61–78.
21. Marzi CA, Tassinari G, Tressoldi PE, Barry C, Grabowska A. Hemispheric asymmetry in face perception tasks of different cognitive requirement. *Human Neurobiol* 1985;4:15–20.
22. Perret DI, Rolls ET, Caan W. Visual neurons responsive to faces in the monkey temporal cortex. *Exp Brain Res* 1982;47:329–342.
23. Perret DI, Smith PAJ, Potter DD, et al. Neurones responsive to faces in the temporal cortex: studies of functional organization, sensitivity to identity and relation to perception. *Hum Neurobiol* 1984;3:197–208.
24. Desimone R, Albright TD, Gross C, Bruce C. Stimulus-selective properties of inferior temporal neurons in the macaque. *J Neurosci* 1984;4:2051–2062.
25. Baylis GC, Rolls ET, Leonard CM. Selectivity between faces in the responses of a population of neurons in the cortex in the superior temporal sulcus of the monkey. *Brain Res* 1985; 342:91–102.
26. Rolls, ET, Baylis GC. Size and contrast have only small effects on the responses to faces of neurons in the cortex of the superior temporal sulcus of the monkey. *Exp Brain Res* 1986;65:38–48.
27. Rolls ET. Neurons in the cortex of the temporal lobe and in the amygdala of the monkey with responses selective for faces. *Hum Neurobiol* 1984;3:209–222.
28. Leonard CM, Rolls ET, Wilson FAW, Baylis GC. Neurons in the amygdala of the monkey with responses selective for faces. *Behav Brain Res* 1985;15:159–176.
29. Creutzfeldt O. Gibt es eine Mechanik des Denkens? *Forsch Med* 1987;2:7–19.
30. Kendrick KM, Baldwin BA. Cells in temporal cortex of conscious sheep can respond preferentially to the sight of faces. *Science* 1987;236:448–450.
31. Grüsser OJ, Selke T, Zynda B. A developmental study of face recognition in children and adolescents. *Hum Neurobiol* 1985;4:33–39.
32. Berndl K, Grüsser OJ. Wahrnehmungsstörungen bei Schizophrenen. *Münch Med Wschr* 1986;128:768–773.
33. Berndl K, Dewitz W, Grüsser OJ, Kiefer RH. A test movie to study elementary abilities in perception and recognition of mimic and gestural expression. *Eur Arch Psychiatry Neurol Sci* 1986;235:276–281.
34. Berndl K, von Cranach M, Grüsser OJ. Impairment of perception and recognition of faces, mimic expression and gestures in schizophrenic patients. *Eur Arch Psychiatry Neurol Sci* 1986;235:282–291.
35. Berndl K, Grüsser OJ, Martin M, Remschmidt H. Comparative studies on recognition of faces, mimic and gestures in adolescent and middle-aged schizophrenic patients. *Eur Arch Psychiatry Neurol Sci* 1986;236:123–130.
36. Grüsser OJ, Kirchhoff N. Face recognition in brain-lesioned patients (*submitted*).

37. Dumas R, Morgan A. EEG-asymmetry as a function of occupation task, and task difficulty. *Neuropsychologia* 1975;13:219–228.
38. Small M. Asymmetrically evoked potentials in response to face stimuli. *Cortex* 1983;19: 441–450.
39. Sobotka S, Pizlo Z, Budohoska W. Hemispheric differences in evoked potentials to pictures of faces in the left and right visual field. *Electroencephalogr Clin Neurophysiol* 1984;58:441–453.
40. Neville H, Snyder E, Woods D, Galambos R. Recognition and surprise alter the human visual evoked response. *Proc Natl Acad Sci USA* 1982;79:2121–2123.
41. Srebro R. Localization of visually evoked cortical activity in humans. *J Physiol (Lond)* 1985;360:233–246.
42. Srebro R. Localization of cortical activity associated with visual recognition in humans. *J Physiol (Lond)* 1985;360:247–259.
43. Jeffreys DA, Musselwhite MJ. A face-responsive visual evoked potential in man. *J Physiol (Lond)* 1987;36.
44. Häussler B. Visuell evozierte Potentiale bei schematischen Gesichterstimuli. Dr. med.-Thesis, Freie Universität Berlin 1988.
45. Bötzel K, Grüsser OJ. Electrical brain potentials evoked by pictures of faces and nonfaces. A search for "face-specific" EEG-potentials. *Exp Brain Res (in press)*.
46. Oldfield RC. The assessment and analysis of handedness: the Edinburgh inventory. *Neuropsychologia* 1971;9:97–113.
47. Jasper HH. The ten-twenty electrode system of the international federation. *Electroencephalogr Clin Neurophysiol* 1958;10:371–375.
48. Grüsser OJ. Face recognition within the reach of neurobiology and beyond it. *Hum Neurobiol* 1984;3:183–190.

Vision and the Brain,
edited by B. Cohen and I. Bodis-Wollner.
Raven Press, Ltd., New York © 1990.

The Role of the Frontal Eye Field and Its Corticotectal Projection in the Generation of Eye Movements

Michael E. Goldberg and Mark A. Segraves

Laboratory of Sensorimotor Research, National Eye Institute, National Institutes of Health, Bethesda, Maryland 20892

Since Ferrier's original demonstration (1) that electrical stimulation of the monkey's prearcuate frontal cortex produced conjugate eye movements, it has been postulated that this region, named the frontal eye field, participates in the guidance of eye movements. However, the nature of this participation has not been clear. Both humans (2) and monkeys (3) with lesions that include the frontal eye field cortex are capable of making saccades in all directions, and the original single neuron studies of monkey frontal eye field function showed that neurons in this region do not discharge reliably before spontaneous saccades made in the dark (4,5). Although it was later shown that neurons in the frontal eye field discharge in response to visual stimuli (6), not all saccades are visually guided, and the question of whether the frontal eye field guides other than visually guided saccades remained an open one.

CELL TYPES IN THE MONKEY FRONTAL EYE FIELD

More recently, it has become clear that neurons in the frontal eye field discharge before all purposive saccades, not only visually guided ones. This was shown in a series of experiments that studied neurons in the frontal eye field of awake, behaving, rhesus monkeys who were trained to perform a number of different oculomotor tasks (7). The tasks are shown in Fig. 1. The first task is a fixation task (no saccade) in which a monkey looks at a spot of light (S1) and does not make a saccade to fixate a second spot (S2) when it appears. The second is a saccade task (saccade to visual target) in which the fixation point (S1) disappears when the target (S2) appears, and the monkey makes a saccade. The third is a learned saccade task, in which the monkey learns to make a saccade of particular amplitude and direction by making saccades to visual targets that appear for shorter and shorter periods of time. Ultimately the monkey makes the proper saccade in response to the disappearance of the fixation point without the monkey's ever seeing a target. By

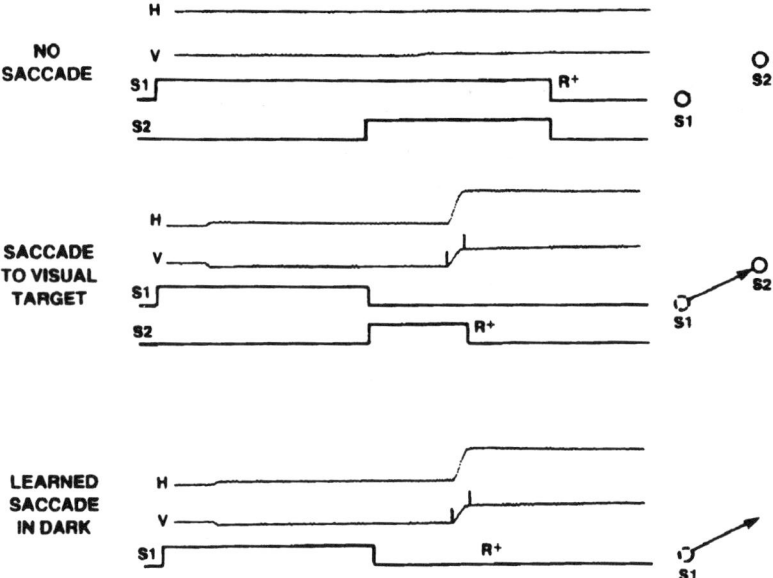

FIG. 1. Behavioral tasks. Horizontal and vertical eye position (H,V) and stimulus traces (S1, S2) are shown for each of three tasks. In the no saccade task S1 appears and remains on. Monkey fixates S1 and does not break gaze to look at S2 when it appears (upward deflection in S2 trace) or disappears (downward deflection). He is rewarded (R+) for either releasing a bar at the dimming of S1 or merely for maintaining proper eye position. Cartoon at the right shows that no eye movement is made. In the saccade to visual target task, S1 disappears when S2 appears and monkey makes saccades to fixate S2, as indicated by *arrow* in cartoon. *Ticks* at saccade beginning and end in vertical eye trace signal computer's on-line recognition of the saccade. The monkey is rewarded after having made a correct saccade to the position of S2. In the learned saccade in dark task, monkey makes a saccade to where S2 had been in previous saccade to visual target trials. The signal to make eye movement is disappearance of S1. Cartoon shows that saccade is made in absence of a target. The monkey is again rewarded after having made a saccade of appropriate amplitude and direction. (Modified from ref. 7.)

comparing the cell's discharge in the various tasks it is possible to understand what role the cell might have in the generation of saccadic eye movements.

In a survey of 752 neurons, 409 discharged before visually guided saccades. Forty percent of these neurons were visual cells: they discharged in the fixation task but not in the learned saccade task, as is shown in Fig. 2. The visual neuron gave a brisk discharge to the appearance of the stimulus in the fixation task (Fig. 2A), an even brisker discharge to the same stimulus when it became a target for a saccade (Fig. 2B, which shows the activity synchronized on the appearance of the target, and Fig. 2C, which shows the same activity synchronized on the end of the saccade), but no activity in relation to a learned saccade of the same amplitude and direction (Fig. 2D). This cell could provide a visual input to an oculomotor mechanism, but, because it does not discharge before the learned saccade and it does in response to visual stimuli, it is not likely by itself to be important in driving saccades.

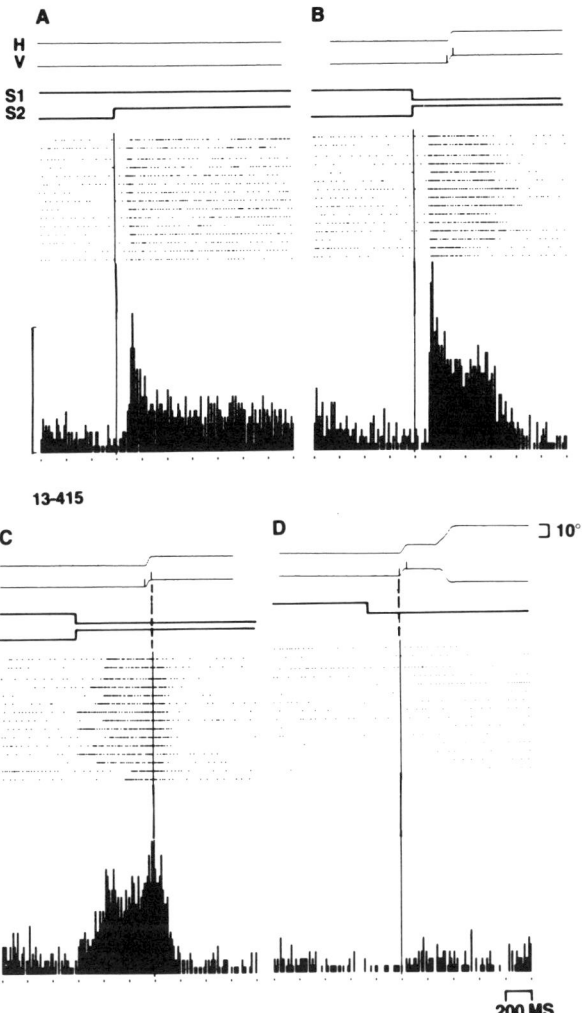

FIG. 2. Visual cell. **A** shows activity in no saccade task, synchronized on onset of receptive-field stimulus, S2. **B** shows an enhanced response in visual saccade task, with *raster* synchronized on the onset of S2. **C** shows same trials as B with raster synchronized on end of saccade. **D** shows an absence of response in learned saccade task. Each portion of this figure includes sample eye movement traces for the paradigm employed, a raster, and a histogram. The abbreviations and conventions for the eye movement and stimulus traces at the top of each raster are the same as those of Fig. 1. Each raster dot represents one neuron spike (sampled at 250 Hz), every raster line includes the neuron activity from a 2-sec interval of a single trial. Each histogram is the summation of the raster illustrated above it with 4 msec bin width. The calibration mark to the left of each histogram represents a firing rate of 100 spikes per second. The vertical line passing through both raster and histogram is the point of alignment for the activity. (From ref. 7.)

Many visual neurons in the frontal eye field have their visual responses modulated by nonvisual factors. The cell illustrated in Fig. 2 gives an example of one of these modulatory effects, presaccadic enhancement of a visual response. Note that the activity of the neuron is considerably brisker during the trials in which the stimulus in the receptive field is a target for a saccade (Fig. 2 B and C) than it is when the monkey does not make a saccade to the stimulus (Fig. 2A). This enhancement of activity is both spatially selective and task specific (8). It does not occur when the monkey makes a saccade to a stimulus outside the receptive field even though there is a stimulus in the receptive field. It does not occur when the monkey is going to use the stimulus in the receptive field for some reason other than to make a saccade to it, for example, to reach out and touch it or to signal a change in its luminance by pressing a bar. The second nonvisual influence on frontal visual neurons is the cancellation of visual activity by an eye movement. Figure 3 shows an example of a neuron that gives a tonic discharge, lasting well over a second, to the appearance of a stimulus flashed for 50 msec in its receptive field (Fig. 3A). The neuron does not discharge in the learned saccade task (Fig. 3B). When the monkey makes a saccade to where the flashed stimulus had been, the tonic discharge is truncated (Fig. 3C), and the truncation is well synchronized to the eye movement (Fig. 3D). Both of these activities could be used in channeling visual information to the oculomotor system: the enhancement in selecting targets and the truncation in eliminating false targets by erasing the trace of stimuli once an eye movement has occurred.

Twenty percent of the neurons discharging before visually guided saccades were movement neurons. They had weak or absent responses to visual stimuli and discharged strongly before saccades to visual stimuli and learned saccades in total darkness. Most discharged weakly if at all before spontaneous saccades of the optimum amplitude and direction. Figure 4 shows an example of a movement cell.

Another 40% of the presaccadic cells were visuomovement neurons. They discharged best before visually guided eye movements and less well to visual stimuli but also less well before learned saccades in the dark. In particular, visuomovement cells tended to discharge when a stimulus appeared and maintained discharge until the saccade took place. One can easily postulate a processing chain for visually guided saccades that begins with the response to the stimulus by the visual cells, continues with activity in the visuomovement cells, and ends with the discharge of the movement cells. Such a chain of discharge is shown in Fig. 5.

Seven percent (53/752) of the frontal eye field neurons discharged in relation to visual fixation. Most of these neurons could be driven by the appearance or disappearance of the foveal fixation point but discharged best during active fixation. Figure 6 shows an example of a foveal neuron. The neuron responds to a foveal fixation point and stops discharging during a temporary disappearance of the fixation point (Fig. 6A). It gives a transient burst when

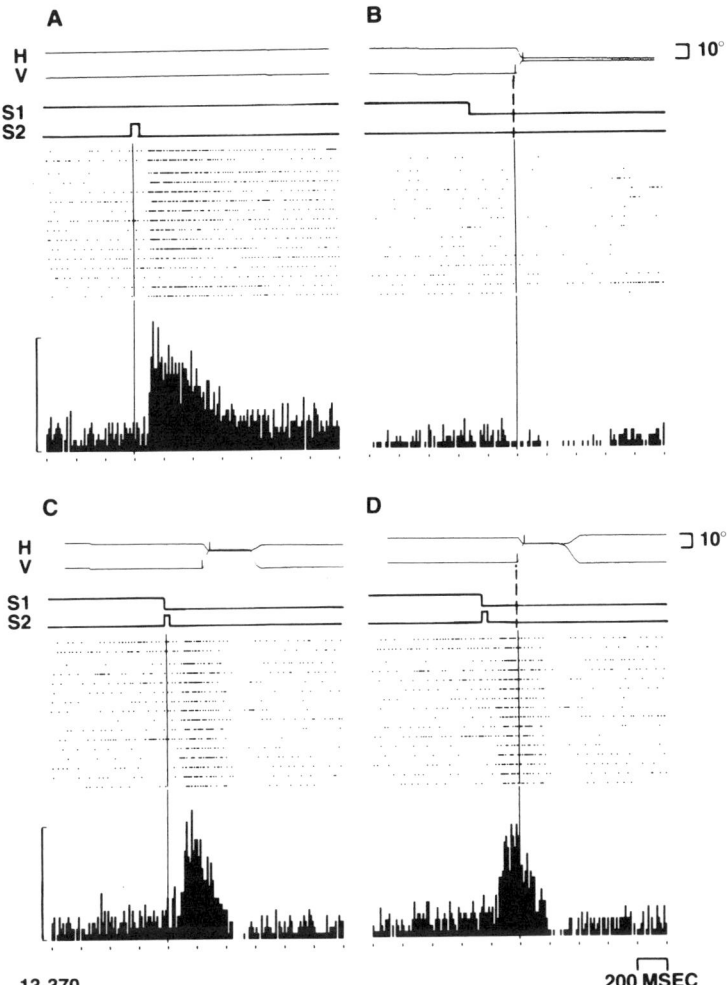

FIG. 3. Saccade-induced cancellation of a tonic visual response. **A** shows maintained discharge of a tonic visual cell to briefly (50 msec) flashed stimulus in the no saccade task. *Raster* and *histograms* aligned on the onset of stimulus, signified by the *vertical line*. **B** shows response of same neuron in learned saccade task. Trials are aligned on beginning of saccade. There is no presaccadic movement activity, but a suppression of base-line activity follows the saccade. **C** shows the truncation of visually evoked discharge when monkey made a saccade to same target that elicited a sustained response in the no saccade task. Raster and histogram aligned on onset of stimulus. **D** shows same trials shown in C aligned on beginning of saccade. (From ref. 7.)

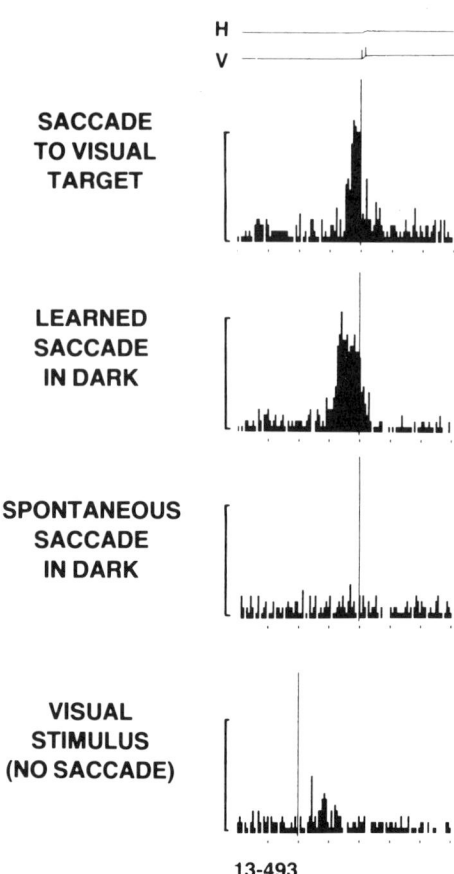

FIG. 4. Movement cell. Histograms of movement cell's discharge in several tasks. This cell gave brisk discharges before saccades to visual targets and to learned saccades made in the dark. It did not fire before saccades of optimal dimensions made spontaneously in total darkness. It had a very weak visual response. H, horizontal; V, vertical. (Modified from ref. 7.)

the fixation point reappears (Fig. 6B). It also ceases firing when the fixation point disappears as a signal to make a saccade (Fig. 6C). However, it begins to discharge again at the beginning of the saccade rather than at a visual latency after the resumption of fixation (Fig. 6D). This indicates that the neuron is likely to be more involved in the process of fixation than merely signaling a foveal event.

Other classes of frontal eye field neurons include postsaccadic neurons that discharge after all saccades (19%), miscellaneous nonsaccadic neurons (13%), and neurons whose discharge could not be affected by our techniques (7%). Miscellaneous neurons included smooth pursuit neurons, orbital position neurons, auditory neurons, and neurons that combined various nonsaccadic properties.

Before the discovery of the diversity of saccade-related activity in the frontal eye field, it was frequently postulated that eye movements evoked from this region were the result of antidromic excitation of the afferents responsible

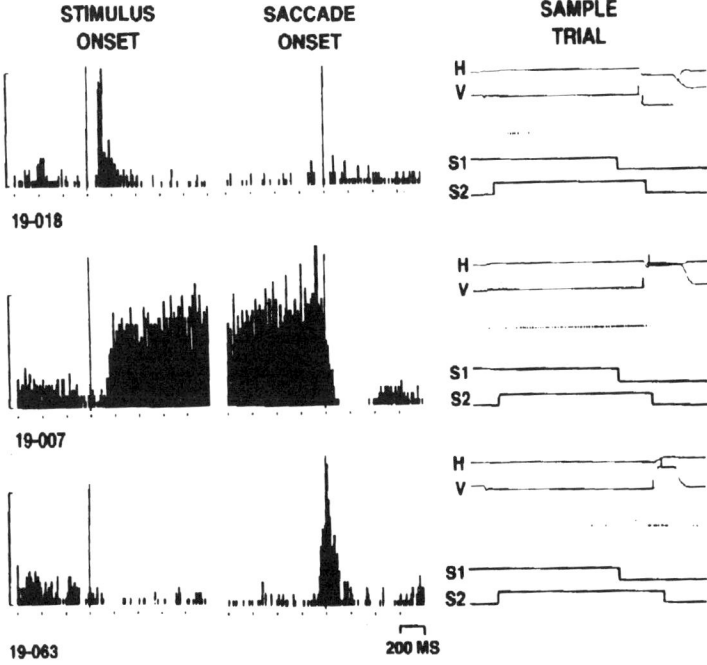

FIG. 5. A processing chain for visually guided saccades. Timing of responses to stimulus onset and eye movement in visual saccade task. Each row contains histograms aligned on target and saccade onsets and a representative record of a single trial showing eye position (H, horizontal; V, vertical), stimulus position (S1, the original fixation point; S2, the saccade target), and cell discharge (*dots* between the position and stimulus traces). **Top row** shows a visual cell that discharged in response to stimulus onset but not to movement. **Middle row** shows a visuomovement cell discharging in response to onset of stimulus and maintaining discharge until an eye movement triggered by the disappearance of the fixation point. **Bottom row** shows response of a movement cell that discharged in a burst around movement and not at all to stimulus. All calibration lines signify a discharge rate of 100 Hz. (From ref. 7.)

for the postsaccadic activity described by Bizzi (4,9). This now seems unlikely, since electrical stimulation through a recording microelectrode evoked saccades with the same amplitude and direction as saccades associated with the optimal cell discharge at the stimulation site (10). Moreover, thresholds for stimulation were as low as 10 μA. In general, movement cells were found at sites from which eye movements could be evoked at thresholds lower than 50 μA, and visual cells were rarely found at low threshold sites. Finally, at sites where cells have both presaccadic activity in one direction and postsaccadic activity in the opposite direction, the eye movements evoked by electrical stimulation were inevitably in the presaccadic direction. These results strongly suggest that the presaccadic activity that we have demonstrated in the frontal eye field participates in the neural events involved in the initiation of saccadic eye movements.

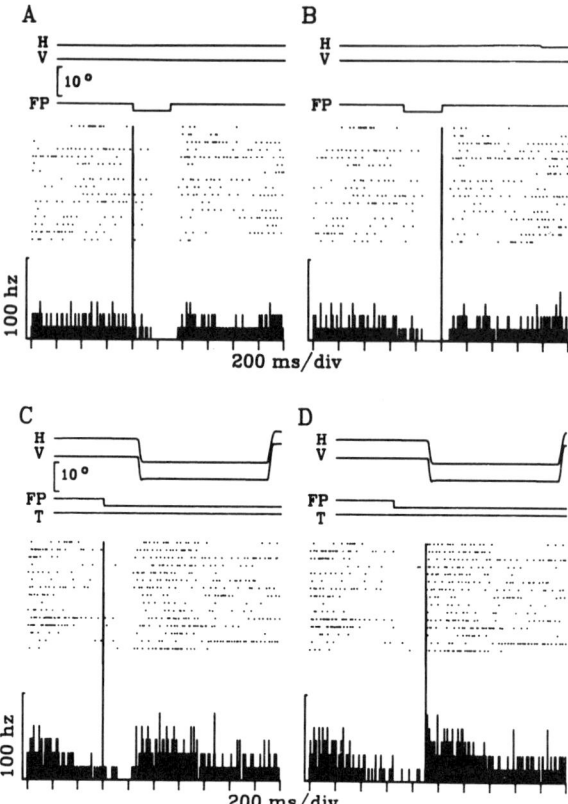

FIG. 6. Response of a foveal/fixation neuron in the fixation (**A, B**) and saccade (**C, D**) tasks. A, aligned on disappearance of fixation light during fixation task trial. B, reappearance of fixation light. C,D activity in a variation of the visually guided saccade task where the peripheral target is always on. C, aligned on disappearance of fixation light. D, aligned on the beginning of the saccade. Note that in C and D, the target light status line begins and ends in the on condition since the target light was never turned off in this task. The monkey was trained to always fixate the central light whenever it was present and make a saccade to and fixate the peripheral target light only when the central light was turned off. (From ref. 13.)

THE FUNCTIONAL SIGNIFICANCE OF THE FRONTOTECTAL PROJECTION

The frontal eye field has a direct projection to the intermediate layers of the superior colliculus (11). Neurons in this region of the colliculus discharge before all saccades of appropriate magnitude and direction (12), and the frontal projection could provide a powerful input to the collicular movement activity. However, to understand how the cerebral cortex controls a specific behavior it is insufficient to know the types of activity in the cortex and the anatomical projections of that region. One must also know what information is carried by the corticofugal signals. It is possible that all of the neuronal activity types found in the frontal eye field are found in the corticofugal signal. But this is unlikely, because one would assume that the cortical architecture is devoted to information processing and the generation of specific signals from the input to the region. It is probable that some of the neuronal signals found in the cortex are devoted to the development of the output signal, but that there is no trace of these component messages in the final signal. The output population, therefore, will be enriched for some signal types and lack others. To begin to answer this question, we identified corticotectal projection neurons by antidromic excitation from the superior colliculus, and then characterized these neurons in awake behaving animals according to the scheme described above (13).

To demonstrate antidromic excitation we first found neurons in the frontal eye field that could be excited by single current pulses to the superior colliculus. To ascertain that such excitation occurs antidromically, e.g., that the tectal electrode is exciting the very neuron recorded in the cortex, we used the collision technique shown in Fig. 7 (14,15). In this technique we used the occurrence of the cortical neuron spike to trigger the collicular current pulse. In Fig. 7 A and C, a collicular pulse was triggered 2.5 msec after the cortical neuron spike. The collicular stimulation antidromically excited the cortical neuron with a latency of 1.5 msec. When the interval between the neuronal spike originating in the cortex and the collicular stimulation is reduced to 0.6 msec (Fig. 7 B and D), the orthodromic and antidromic axon potentials collide at a point between the frontal eye field and superior colliculus, and the antidromic spike is not seen by the cortical electrode. Two smaller neuron spikes, indicated by arrows in Fig. 7 C and D, were excited by the collicular stimulation but did not collide with the neuron spike that was used to initiate the collicular stimulation.

We isolated 51 neurons in the frontal eye field that could be antidromically excited from an electrode in the superior colliculus, at thresholds from 6 μA to 1.2 mA. The lowest thresholds occurred when the optimal saccades represented at the collicular stimulation and frontal eye field recording sites were of equal amplitude and direction. There was a significant correlation between threshold and the degree of correspondence of saccade vectors represented at the stimulation and recording sites. Although the thresholds were sometimes high, the most effective site for antidromic stimulation was inevitably in the superior colliculus, primarily in the intermediate layers. This could be ascertained by stimulating at different sites along an electrode penetration in the colliculus and correlating antidromic threshold with electrode depth and the nature of the cells recorded. Figure 8 gives an example of such a penetration. The corticotectal cell's highest threshold was at the point of transition from superficial to intermediate layers. As the electrode moved deeper into the intermediate layers, the threshold decreased and reached a minimum of 25 μA at a depth of 2.5 mm, the transition between intermediate and deep layers

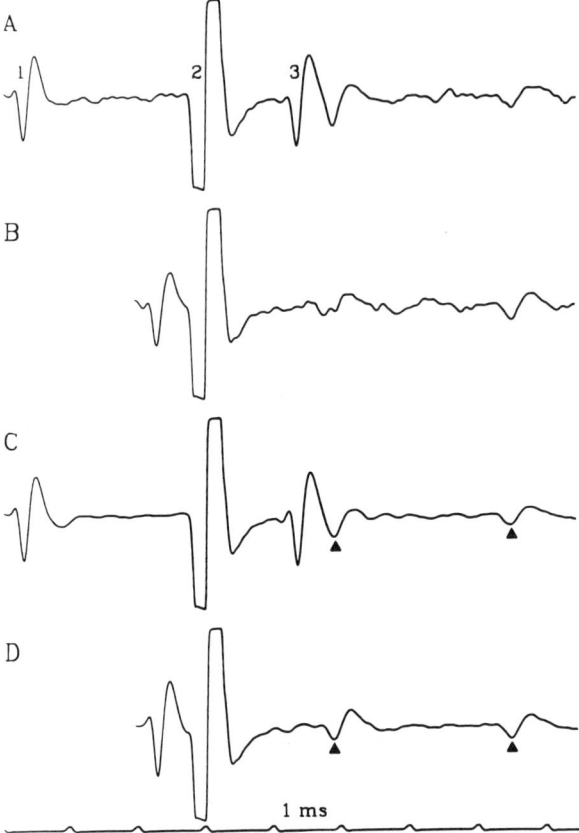

FIG. 7. Example of antidromic excitation and collision. Each trace begins with the occurrence of a spontaneous spike generated by a neuron isolated in the frontal eye field. Traces are aligned on the superior colliculus stimulus artifact. **A,B:** single traces of 8.5 msec in duration digitized by a high-speed analog to digital converter; **C,D:** averages of 10 consecutive traces. In A, 1 marks the spontaneous neuronal spike; 2, the superior colliculus stimulus artifact; and 3, the antidromically excited neuronal spike. When the spontaneous spike and superior colliculus stimulation were separated by 2.5 msec (A,C), the isolated neuron was excited antidromically with a latency of 1.5 msec. However, when the separation between spontaneous spike and stimulus was reduced to 0.6 msec, the antidromically evoked spike collided with the spontaneous spike and was not seen at the frontal eye field electrode (B,D). Note that two smaller neuron spikes evoked at constant latencies of 2.0 and 4.6 msec (*arrows* in C,D) were not affected. Time between ticks in lowest trace was 1 msec. Stimulus intensity, 50 µA. (From ref. 13.)

of the superior colliculus. Such threshold minima provided good evidence that the antidromic responses were arising from fibers in the superior colliculus.

Of the 51 antidromic neurons, 27 were movement neurons, 11 were fovealfixation neurons, three were visuomovement, eight were of miscellaneous types, one was postsaccadic, and one was nonresponsive. Figure 9 compares the distribution of antidromically activated neurons with the population of all

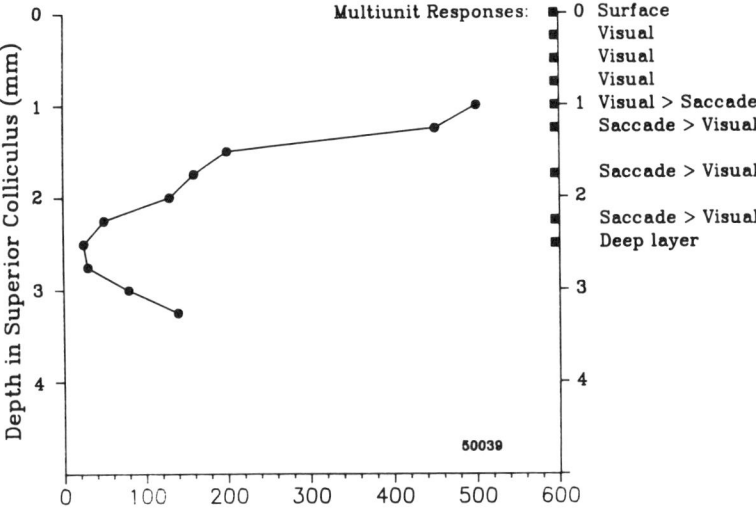

FIG. 8. Threshold for antidromic excitation compared with depth from collicular surface. Based on multineuron activity indicated on the right side of the figure, the transition between superficial and intermediate layers was at a depth of 1 mm from the collicular surface. The border between intermediate and deep layers was at 2.5 mm. The minimum threshold for antidromic excitation occurred at the transition point between intermediate and deep layers. Antidromic excitation thresholds increased both above and below this depth. (From ref. 13.)

frontal neurons. Several striking results emerge: there is an enrichment in the corticotectal population for movement and foveal-fixation neurons, whereas two of the most common frontal classes, visual and postsaccadic cells, were hardly represented at all. We were disturbed by our failure to drive antidromically visual neurons with nonfoveal receptive fields. We isolated more than 100 of these neurons during the course of our experiments and were never able to drive one antidromically. We made specific searches for visual corticotectal neurons, and although we frequently studied visual neurons close to antidromically excited neurons, we never found one that we could drive. Because visual neurons were common and antidromic excitation technically feasible in our hands, we think that it is unlikely that the frontal eye field sends a significant visual signal to the superior colliculus.

CONCLUSIONS

These results contribute to the growing evidence that the arcuate frontal eye field is important in the initiation of purposive saccadic eye movements. We have now established that the oculomotor region of the superior colliculus, the intermediate layers, receives a distinct oculomotor message from

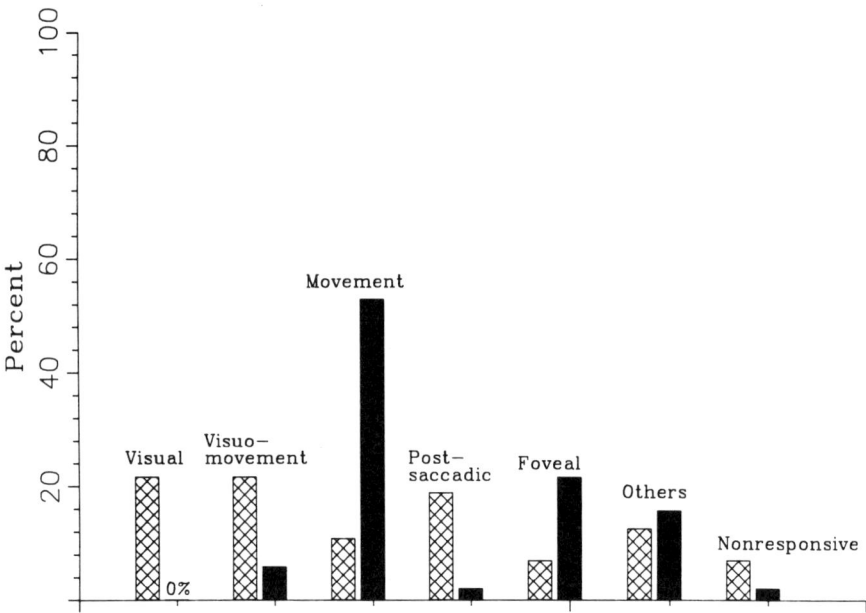

FIG. 9. Comparison of distribution among activity categories of frontal eye field neurons excited antidromically from the superior colliculus (■) ($n = 51$) to the distribution of all frontal eye field neurons ($n = 752$) reported by Bruce and Goldberg (7) (⌧). (From ref. 13.)

the frontal eye field. The message is twofold: it tells about the state of fixation and foveal stimulation, and sends a command to make a movement of certain dimensions.

The superior colliculus and the frontal eye field can act independently in the generation of saccades. Lesions of the superior colliculus do not affect the evocation of saccades by electrical stimulation of the frontal eye field (16), and monkeys can make visually guided saccades in the absence of either the frontal eye field or the superior colliculus, although they cannot make visually guided saccades at all when both are ablated (3). Recent results suggest that some types of saccades do in fact require the frontal eye field. We have shown that monkeys with unilateral frontal eye field lesions have difficulty learning to make saccades to remembered targets, and when they do learn, the motor performance of memory-guided but not visually guided saccades is impaired (17). Bruce and Borden (18) have shown that although normal monkeys can make predictive saccades, monkeys with frontal lesions cannot. Guitton and colleagues (2) have shown that humans with frontal lesions have difficulty making saccades away from a visual target and instead make inappropriate saccades toward the target. Thus, there is a repertory of saccades characterized by behavioral complexity that require the presence of the frontal eye field.

Our results suggest that in normal monkeys the signals for saccades guided by cognitive processes as well as visually guided saccades progress from the frontal eye field to the intermediate layers of the superior colliculus, which in normal monkeys then serve as a final common path (19). Neurons in the superior colliculus discharge before all saccades (12,19) and the region has a monosynaptic projection to the long-lead bursters in the brainstem reticular formation (20). The arcuate frontal eye field can affect this presaccadic final common path in several ways. One kind of control could be exerted by the foveal-fixation neurons, which could directly trigger or suppress a collicular saccadic signal. The movement neurons could exert control over the saccadic system by three separate pathways that are illustrated in Fig. 10. The first is through the direct targeting signal to the colliculus, which we have demonstrated here. The second is by a direct projection to perioculomotor regions in the midbrain and pons (21). The third is by a projection to the caudate nucleus, where eye movement-related activity has recently been discovered (22). The caudate presaccadic signal is similar in quality but reversed in sign

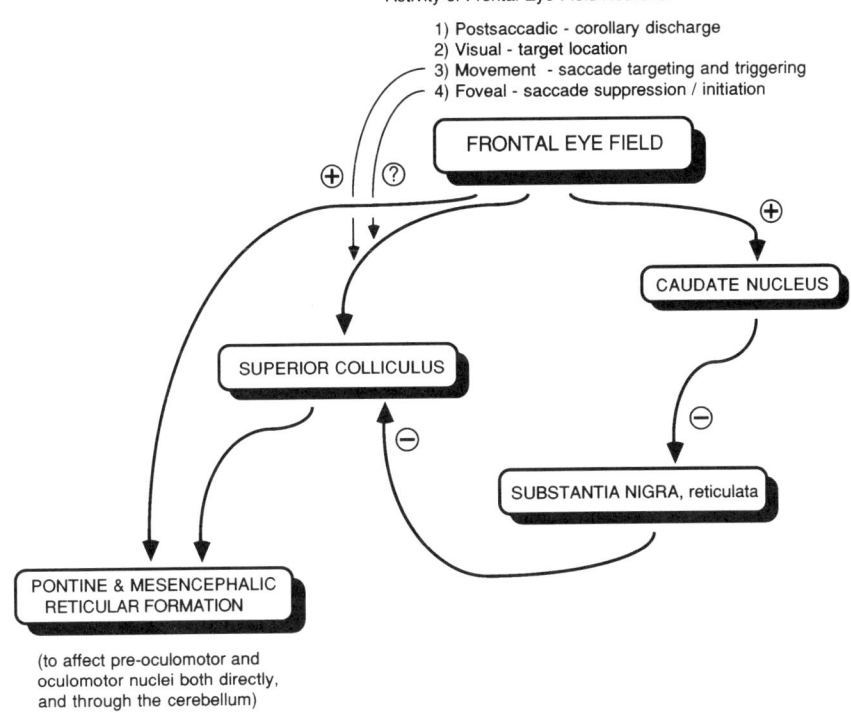

FIG. 10. Frontal eye field pathways to effect the saccade generation process in the brainstem. See text for description.

from that of the substantia nigra, which has been shown to exert a tonic suppression on the superior colliculus except before and during saccades (23). This frontal-caudate signal could inhibit the substantia nigra and result in a presaccadic release of the nigral suppression of the superior colliculus. Thus, the frontal movement command to the colliculus would be exceedingly powerful because it combines an excitatory signal with the release of a suppressive one. When a monkey is actively fixating, thresholds for evoking saccades from the superior colliculus (24) are elevated. Presumably this is true because saccades that occur without changes in frontal and nigral activity must overcome the suppression that inhibits them. Since monkeys and humans can make normal saccades after lesions of the frontal eye field, the colliculus must be able to function on its own, and under certain circumstances, e.g., in spontaneous saccades made in total darkness, there is little or no frontal signal (4,7). Presumably such spontaneous saccades originate in the superior colliculus without concurrent cortical activity. However, when a monkey, or by inference a human, makes a purposive saccadic eye movement, that movement is driven by the frontal eye field, which drives both the superior colliculus as well as midbrain and pontine perioculomotor regions directly and the substantia nigra indirectly, thereby releasing an inhibition of the colliculus. Such a powerful and redundant signal must ensure that the oculomotor system does what the cortex wants it to do. The elimination of activity, which may contribute to the cortical signal but by itself is inadequate to drive a saccade, e.g., visual and postsaccadic activity, insures that the only activity that reaches the colliculus is the actual command to make the saccade. A brainstem apparatus for generating eye movements to visual stimuli, the "visual grasp reflex" exists at many levels of evolutionary development, including fish, amphibians, reptiles, and birds, as well as monkeys and humans. It is intriguing to note that along with the development of a very sophisticated cortex that can direct eye movements in response to many different cues, of both internal and external origin, there has been a parallel development of the primate cortex's ability to take control of lower oculomotor centers, giving its own desires precedence.

ACKNOWLEDGMENTS

The authors are grateful to the technical staff of the Laboratory of Sensorimotor Research for their invaluable help: Al Ziminsky for electronic support, Chuck Crist and Tom Ruffner for machining, George Creswell and Laurie Cooper for histology, Geraldine Snodgrass and John Pellegrini for animal care and surgical assistance, Art Hays for computer hardware support, Jean Steinberg for manuscript preparation, and Nita Hight for facilitating everything. We thank the photographic staff of the National Eye Institute for preparation of figures.

REFERENCES

1. Ferrier D. The localization of function in the brain. *Proc R Soc* 1874;22:229–232.
2. Guitton D, Buchtel HA, Douglas RM. Disturbances of voluntary saccadic eye movement mechanisms following discrete unilateral frontal lobe removals. In: Lennerstrand G, Zee DS, Keller EL, eds. *Functional basis of ocular motility disorders.* Oxford: Pergamon Press, 1982;497–500.
3. Schiller PH, True SD, Conway JL. Deficits in eye movements following frontal eye field and superior colliculus ablations. *J Neurophysiol* 1980;44:1175–1189.
4. Bizzi E. Discharge of frontal eye field neurons during saccadic and following eye movements in unanesthetized monkeys. *Exp Brain Res* 1968;6:69–80.
5. Bizzi E, Schiller PH. Single unit activity in the frontal eye fields of unanesthetized monkeys during head and eye movement. *Exp Brain Res* 1970;10:151–158.
6. Mohler CW, Goldberg ME, Wurtz RH. Visual receptive fields of frontal eye field neurons. *Brain Res* 1973;61:385–389.
7. Bruce CJ, Goldberg ME. Primate frontal eye fields: I. Single neurons discharging before saccades. *J Neurophysiol* 1985;53:603–635.
8. Goldberg ME, Bushnell MC. Behavioral enhancement of visual responses in monkey cerebral cortex. II. Modulation in frontal eye fields specifically related to saccades. *J Neurophysiol* 1981;46:773–787.
9. Roucoux A, Crommelinck M. Influence of supranuclear structures on brainstem neurons. In: Berthoz A, ed. *Control of gaze by brain stem neurons.* New York: Elsevier/North Holland, 1977;487.
10. Bruce CJ, Goldberg ME, Stanton GB, Bushnell MC. Primate frontal eye fields. II. Physiological and anatomical correlates of electrically evoked eye movements. *J Neurophysiol* 1985;54:714–734.
11. Kunzle H, Akert K. Efferent connections of cortical area 8 (frontal eye field) in Macaca fascicularis. A reinvestigation using the autoradiographic technique. *J Comp Neurol* 1977;173:147–164.
12. Wurtz RH, Goldberg ME. Activity of superior colliculus in behaving monkey: III. Cells discharging before eye movements. *J Neurophysiol* 1972;35:575–586.
13. Segraves MA, Goldberg ME. Functional properties of corticotectal neurons in the monkey frontal eye fields. *J Neurophysiol* 1987;58:1387–1419.
14. Bishop PO, Burke W, Davis R. Single-unit recording from antidromically activated optic radiation neurones. *J Physiol (Lond)* 1962;162:432–450.
15. Fuller JH, Schlag JD. Determination of antidromic excitation by the collision test: problems of interpretation. *Brain Res* 1976;112:283–298.
16. Schiller PH. The effect of superior colliculus ablation on saccades elicited by cortical stimulation. *Brain Res.* 1977;122:154–156.
17. Deng S-Y, Goldberg ME, Segraves MA, Ungerleider LG, Mishkin M. The effect of unilateral ablation of the frontal eye fields on saccadic performance in the monkey. In: Keller E, Zee DS, eds. *Adaptive process in the visual and oculomotor systems.* Oxford: Pergamon Press, 1986;201–208.
18. Bruce CJ, Borden JA. The primate frontal eye fields are necessary for predictive saccadic tracking. *Soc Neurosci Abstr* 1986;12:1086.
19. Schiller PH, Koerner F. Discharge characteristics of single units in superior colliculus of the alert rhesus monkey. *J Neurophysiol* 1971;34:920–936.
20. Raybourn MS, Keller EL. Colliculo-reticular organization in primate oculomotor system. *J Neurophysiol* 1977;40:861–878.
21. Leichnetz G, Smith DJ, Spencer RF. Cortical projections to the paramedian tegmental and basilar pons in the monkey. *J Comp Neurol* 1984;228:388–408.
22. Hikosaka O, Sakamoto M. Cell activity in monkey caudate nucleus preceding saccadic eye movements. *Exp Brain Res* 1986;63:659–662.
23. Hikosaka O, Wurtz RH. Visual and oculomotor functions of monkey substantia nigra pars reticulata. IV. Relation of substantia nigra to superior colliculus. *J Neurophysiol* 1983;49:1285–1301.
24. Guthrie BL, Porter JD, Sparks DL. Corollary discharge provides accurate eye position information to the oculomotor system. *Science* 1983;221:1193–1195.

Vision and the Brain,
edited by B. Cohen and I. Bodis-Wollner.
Raven Press, Ltd., New York © 1990.

Cortical Visual Motion Processing for Oculomotor Control

Robert H. Wurtz, Hidehiko Komatsu, Dwayne S. G. Yamasaki, and Max R. Dürsteler

Laboratory of Sensorimotor Research, National Eye Institute, National Institutes of Health, Bethesda, Maryland 20892

Humans and monkeys move their eyes in remarkably similar ways. They make rapid or saccadic eye movements in order to shift the fovea from one object of interest to another within the visual field. They make smooth pursuit eye movements to keep moving targets on the fovea. They both benefit from the optokinetic and vestibular systems that maintain the stability and clarity of vision in spite of movements of the head and body. Monkeys, therefore, offer an ideal model for the investigation of the neural basis of these sophisticated control systems within the brain.

These systems cannot be regarded as just output or movement systems, however, but instead they represent complete circuits through the brain from sensory input to movement output. An essential part of such circuits is the visual processing that in many cases governs the eye movement. In this chapter we concentrate on this visual processing and on those eye movements that depend on one type of visual processing, that for visual motion. Such motion processing has been investigated intensively in the cerebral cortex during the past several years, and several areas apparently devoted to motion processing have been identified. We first indicate where in the cerebral cortex visual motion processing is concentrated and the relation of cells in these areas to visual input and eye movement output. We then consider the contribution of these areas to the generation of pursuit eye movements, to the generation of saccades to moving stimuli, and to the generation of optokinetic nystagmus. This brief presentation is based largely on several experimental reports (1–6) and a recent summary article (7).

LOCALIZATION OF VISUAL MOTION PROCESSING

Response to a moving stimulus alone is an inadequate criterion for relating cellular discharge to motion processing since many cells throughout the monkey's central visual pathways respond to such motion. Instead, it is a property referred to as "directional selectivity" that is generally taken as an indication that a neuron is involved in visual motion processing. Neurons are regarded as directionally selective if they respond to motion in one direction but not to motion in the opposite direction. Use of this criterion allows us to identify the areas along the visual pathways where such processing is performed. In the Old World monkey such directional selectivity is seen for the first time along the geniculocortical pathway in the striate or primary visual cortex (8). In contrast, in the monkey superior colliculus little such directional selectivity is evident (9). Some subcortical motion processing is found in the accessory optic system, but exploration of this area in the primate is only beginning (10; Cohen, *this volume*).

The striate cortex, however, is only the start of visual processing in the cerebral cortex. A dramatic increase in our knowledge of these extrastriate areas has occurred in the past two decades, and Fig. 1, modified from a recent review by Maunsell and Newsome (11), indicates these areas. Many areas are

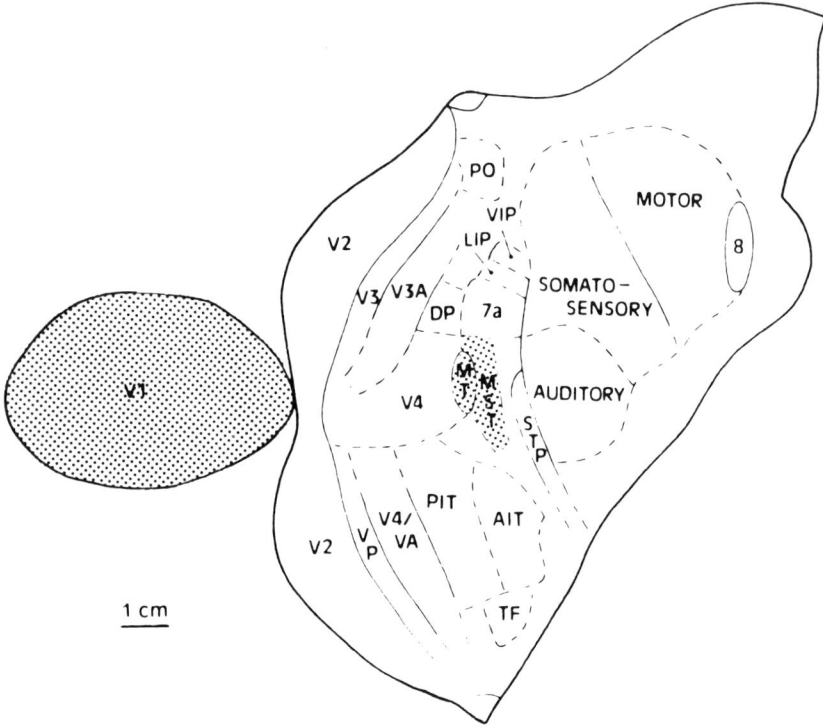

FIG. 1. Cortical areas related to visual motion processing as modified from Maunsell and Newsome (11). The areas are indicated on a flat map of cerebral cortex that shows both the cortical surface and the cortex within the unfolded sulci. Caudal areas are to the left, rostral to the right, with the oval area protruding on the left representing striate cortex (V1). Shading indicates areas concerned with visual motion processing that are emphasized in this chapter: primary visual cortex (V1), middle temporal area (MT), and the medial superior temporal area (MST). Other visual areas are indicated by their letter designations.

buried in sulci, but using a mapping procedure detailed by Van Essen and Maunsell (12) the sulci can be laid out in a flat plane, and it is such a flattened map that Fig. 1 shows. Among the multiple extrastriate visual areas, two have been identified as being largely devoted to visual motion processing, i.e., they have a high proportion of directionally selective cells. These areas are the middle temporal (MT) area and the medial superior temporal (MST) area, and these areas are indicated in Fig. 1 by shading as is striate cortex (V1). These areas might represent a sequence of visual processing since area MT receives a direct anatomical projection from V1, and area MST, in turn, receives a direct projection from area MT (11,13). Other extrastriate areas have directionally selective cells, but the proportion of such cells is small when compared with the proportion of such cells in the MT and MST areas. Pathways through these other areas are also available for information flow from V1 to area MT.

RESPONSE OF MT AND MST CELLS

Examples of the visual response of an MT neuron and an MST neuron are shown in Fig. 2A and B, respectively. While the rhesus monkey (*Macaca mulatta*) looked at a fixation point at the center of a screen in front of it (FP on the schematic drawing in Fig. 2A), we moved a spot of light at 16°/sec across the visual receptive field of the cell. In Fig. 2A, upward motion was followed by an increase in the discharge rate of the cell, whereas motion downward was not, indicating the directional selectivity of the cell. The MST neuron (Fig. 2B) also showed such directional selectivity, as has been reported previously (4,14–16). In contrast to MT, however, MST has large receptive fields, that frequently include both the contralateral and ipsilateral visual field (4), as illustrated by the large area of the upper visual field included in the receptive field shown in Fig. 2B.

In addition to a visual response, many cells in MT and MST also discharged during pursuit eye movements. Cells in the superior temporal sulcus (STS) that discharged during pursuit have been found previously by Sakata and collaborators (17), and we determined the location of these cells with respect to the identified visual areas. Within both MT and MST areas we found cells that discharged continuously during pursuit, and we refer to these cells simply as pursuit cells (4). The cell shown in Fig. 3, for example, had a visual receptive field and a directionally selective response to downward motion (as indicated by the schematic drawing in Fig. 3). To test the response of the cell during pursuit, the fixation target the monkey was looking at was turned off, and it reappeared at another point above the location of the fixation point (for example), and then moved downward with a constant speed, usually of 16°/sec. For the cell response shown in Fig. 3, during pursuit of a target moving downward the cell discharged continuously (Fig. 3, top) but not with pursuit upward (Fig.

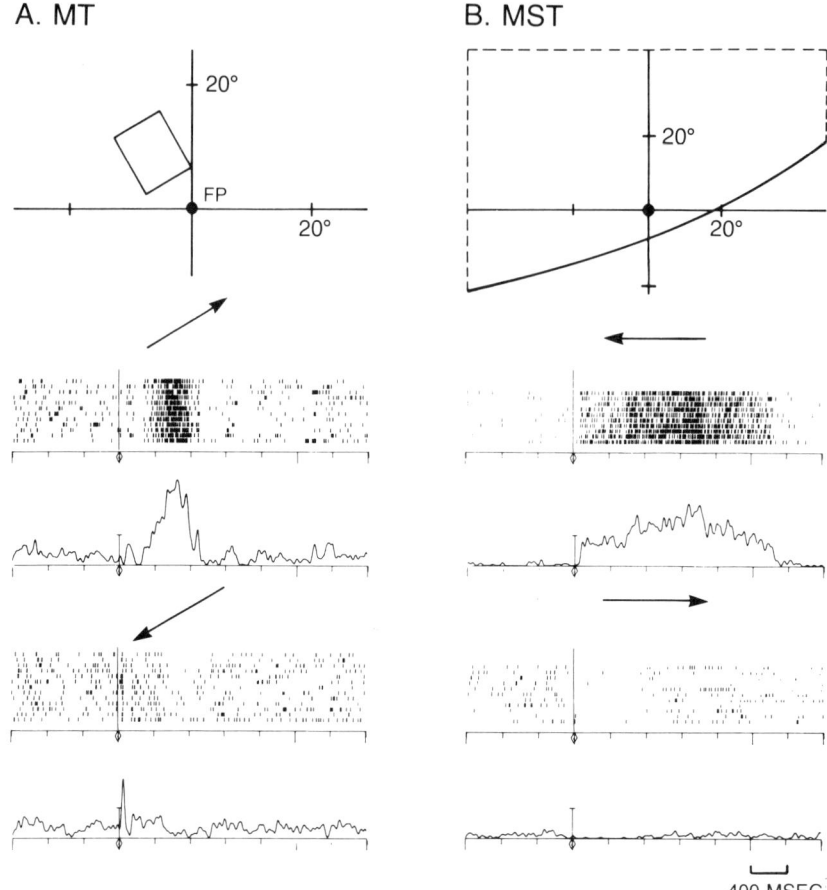

FIG. 2. Directionally selective responses of MT and MST cells. **A:** Outline of the receptive field of an MT cell (*top*), its response in the preferred direction of visual motion (up and to the right, *middle*), and in the opposite direction (down and to the left, *bottom*). The responses are indicated by a dot pattern or raster that shows individual trials and the spike density averaged over the individual trials. Both are aligned with the onset of stimulus motion. In this and subsequent rasters, *dots* indicate cell discharges, *solid lines* indicate successive stimulus presentations. In the spike density displays, the sigma was 15 msec. For details of method, see (53). The height of the vertical bar indicates 50 spikes/sec/trial. Tick marks on the abscissa indicate 400 msec. **B:** Receptive field and directionally selective response of an MST area cell. This receptive field included much of the upper visual field (*dashed lines* indicate that the edge of the mapped field extended beyond the tangent screen). (From ref. 7.)

3, bottom). The pursuit cells almost always showed this type of directional selectivity for pursuit; they discharged with pursuit movement in one direction but failed to do so with pursuit in the opposite direction. The response of these cells does not depend on motion of the visual background across the receptive field of the cell, because we obtained pursuit responses when the monkey was in a room that was totally dark except for the target spot. These cells are similar to

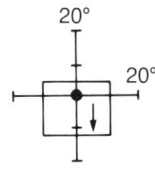

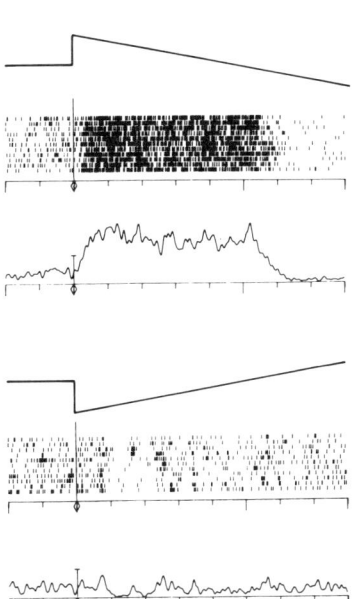

FIG. 3. Discharge of a pursuit cell during smooth pursuit eye movements. The drawing **(top)** shows the size of the receptive field of an MSTl area cell and indicates that the preferred direction for motion of a visual stimulus is downward. The responses below show the cell discharge during pursuit in the preferred downward direction (at 16°/sec, middle records) and in the opposite upward direction (top records). The rasters and spike densities are aligned on onset of the target motion, indicated schematically by the step and ramp of the target above each record. The preferred direction of pursuit was the same as for visual stimulation. (From ref. 7.)

the "true pursuit cells" identified by Sakata et al. (17). The relationship of the direction of the pursuit response and the visual response is an important one, but one that we consider in detail elsewhere (6).

We have found pursuit cells both in areas MT and MST, but the cells were not evenly distributed. The pursuit cells were concentrated in three areas: the lateral MT area (MTf) representing the fovea, the dorsal-medial MST area (MSTd) on the anterior bank of the STS, and the lateral-anterior MST area (MSTl) on the posterior bank and floor of the STS. Pursuit cells had a directionally selective response to visual stimuli, and all cells were in areas of MT or MST, where visual receptive fields included the region of the visual field near the fovea. Cells in MT fovea always had small receptive fields whereas those in the dorsal-medial MST area always had large receptive fields—fields that included an entire quadrant or hemifield and that frequently extended far into the ipsilateral visual field. In addition, cells in MT fovea preferred small spots of light as stimuli, but those in the dorsal-medial MST area preferred large moving fields of stimuli. Cells in the lateral-anterior MST area had either small or large receptive fields. Some cells in MSTl preferred spots and some preferred large field stimuli. Therefore, MT fovea formed a group of homogeneous cells as did cells in the dorsal-medial MST area, but cells in the lateral-anterior MST area had a mixture of the cell types found in the two other areas. A discussion of the relationship of these areas to each other and to other subdivisions within the STS has been previously presented (4).

The response of these cells during pursuit could result from the visual motion or slip of the target on the retina that is an inevitable concomitant of imperfect pursuit or from an extraretinal signal related to the generation of the pursuit movement itself. We next attempted to distinguish between pursuit inputs of retinal and extraretinal origin and to see if there was a difference between MT and MST area cells (5). The distinction between retinal and extraretinal input was made by reducing visual input during pursuit, i.e., by reducing the retinal slip signal. We did this first by "blinking" off the target briefly during pursuit, thereby removing the visual stimulation from the cell. Figure 4 shows the results of these experiments for a cell in the foveal region of area MT and for one from the lateral-anterior MST area. Figure 4 (top) shows the response of a cell during pursuit in the optimal direction made in total darkness except for the pursuit target. When we blinked off the target, momentarily removing the visual stimulus, there was a brief pause in the discharge for the MT foveal cells (Fig. 4, left middle). In a second experiment, we removed motion information during pursuit by stabilizing the image of the pursuit target on the retina. After the monkey had established pursuit, the target was moved each time the eye moved, thus largely removing the retinal slip of the target. Such a stabilization procedure also reduced the discharge rate of an MT area foveal cell (Fig. 4, left bottom). Therefore, either blink or stabilization reduced the response of this and other MT foveal cells, indicating that the response of these cells depended on visual motion information.

For MST area cells, the results of these tests were frequently very different (Fig. 4, right). In spite of a reduction of retinal slip, by either blinking off or stabilizing the target, the cell continued to discharge, indicating that the cell was receiving an extraretinal input. Many cells with large visual fields in the medial-dorsal MST area received this extraretinal input, but in lateral-anterior MST only a subset received such input. Although not all MST area cells receive an extraretinal input, *none* of the MT area cells we studied received a significant extraretinal input. We therefore see a transition from area MT to MST: the introduction of an extraretinal signal in area MST related to pursuit eye movements.

PURSUIT INITIATION FOLLOWING AREA MT LESIONS

Initiation of pursuit to a moving target depends on information about target direction and speed. Furthermore, since pursuit can be initiated to a target moving in any part of the visual field, motion analysis in any part of the visual

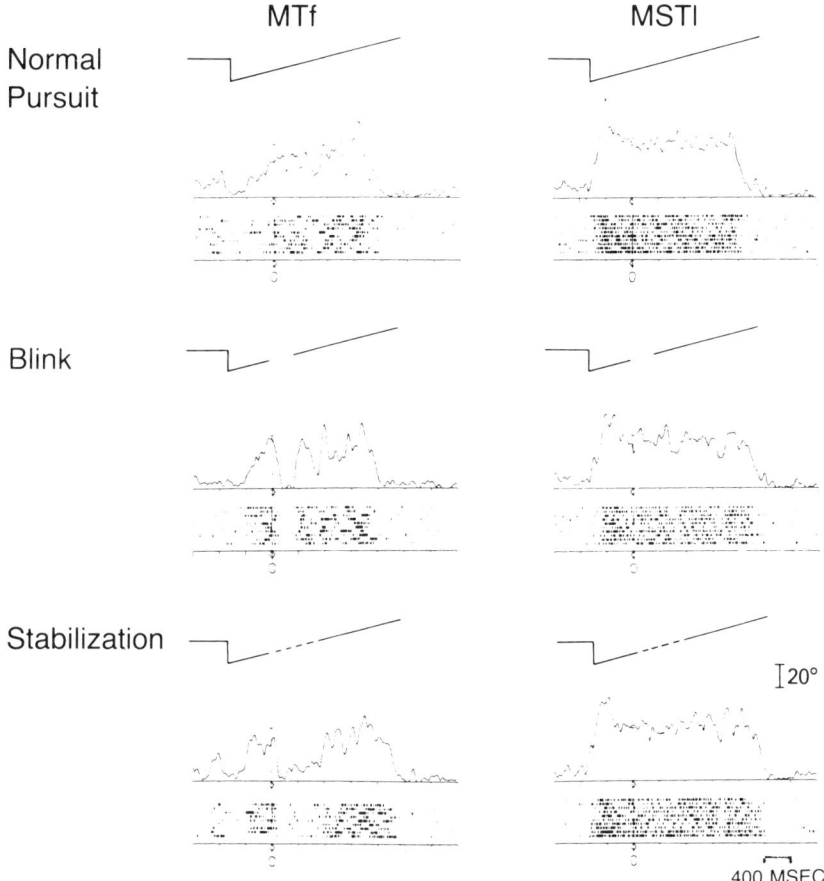

FIG. 4. Two types of pursuit cells, one dependent on retinal input, the other independent of retinal input. All cells in the foveal region of area MT depend on retinal input and an example of such a cell is illustrated in the left column. Cells that received an extraretinal input were all in area MST and the right column shows an example of such an MST area cell. The labels above the two columns indicate that cells with the retinal input are found in areas MTf and MSTl, whereas cells with extraretinal input are located in areas MSTd and MSTl. Top records during normal pursuit show the response of the cells with pursuit in the optimal direction. Middle records show blink of the target (break in the target line) during pursuit. The MT cell showed a pause in discharge, the MST cell did not. Bottom records show stabilization of the target (*dashed target line*) during pursuit. Again, the MT cell showed reduced discharge as a result of the stabilization whereas the MST cell did not. Rasters and spike density displays are aligned on the blink (middle), the stabilization (bottom), or at a comparable time in normal pursuit (top). (From ref. 7.)

field must be available to the pursuit system. Area MT, like striate cortex, has a retinotopic map for the contralateral visual field and so has motion information available that is required by the pursuit system. Previous work has shown that area MT cells convey information about the speed and direction of visual motion (14,18–21).

Area MT would seem to be the appropriate structure to provide information for guiding pursuit eye movements since it also has appropriate efferent anatomical connections. The STS, including areas MT and MST, projects directly to the dorsolateral pontine nucleus of the brainstem (22). Cells in this area in turn have been shown to respond to visual motion and to discharge during pursuit eye movements (23,24). This pontine area then projects to the contralateral cerebellar flocculus (25). Cells in the flocculus discharge during pursuit eye movements (26–28), and projections from the flocculus to brainstem oculomotor areas in the pons could complete the pathway for the generation of eye movements. We know the pathway from the retina through the lateral geniculate nucleus, striate cortex, and MT area, so that we have an outline of the entire circuit from visual input to eye movement output.

We tested the possibility that these cells do provide the motion information needed for initiating pursuit movements by removing the MT cells related to one part of the visual field and then determining the monkey's ability to initiate pursuit to target motion in that part of the visual field. The sequence of stimulus motions and eye movements in our test of pursuit is shown on the graph in Fig. 5A. The step of the target from the fixation point and the ramp away is indicated by the dotted line, and the subsequent movement of the eye is indicated by the solid line. The monkey first made a rapid or saccadic eye movement to bring the target near the fovea and then followed this with a smooth pursuit eye movement that kept the target on or near the fovea. By using the step-ramp stimulus illustrated in Fig. 5A, we could shift target motion to any area of the visual field. In the experiment we randomly shifted the target on successive trials to different points along the horizontal meridian in either the contralateral or ipsilateral visual field (1).

Since we were considering initiation of pursuit, we concentrated on the initial speed of the eye after the monkey made a saccade to the target. Because the latency of the pursuit system is 80 to 100 msec (29), the monkey's initial velocity must depend on the motion of the target approximately 100 msec earlier—when it was still looking at the original fixation point. Therefore, the motion information derived from the peripheral retina *before* the initial saccade provides the motion information for programming the first 100 msec of the pursuit movement. By changing the location of the target step, we could use the target motion in different areas of the visual field as a probe of the efficiency of visual motion processing in that part of the visual field (30).

To remove area MT, we used a neurotoxin that killed cells but left fibers of passage intact (1,31). We injected microliter quantities of the neurotoxin ibotenic acid into an area where single-cell recording had indicated that the location of the receptive fields of the cells were extrafoveal, on the horizontal meridian, and usually 5° to 15° from the center of gaze. Figure 6A shows an example of one of these lesions on a sagittal section stained for cells, and Fig. 6B shows the area affected by one of these injections plotted on a flattened

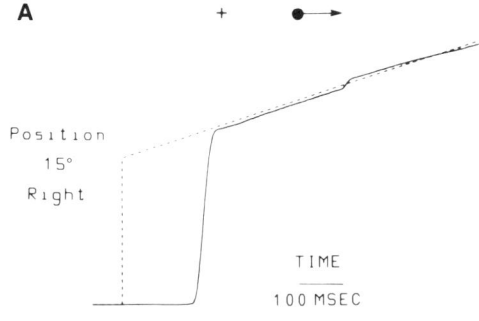
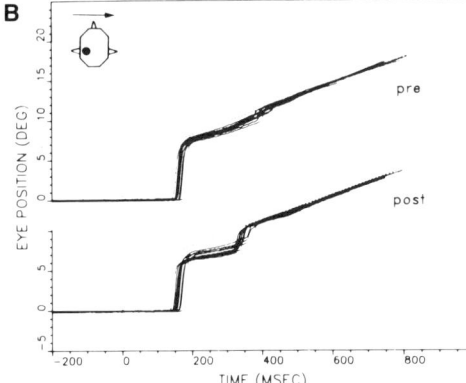
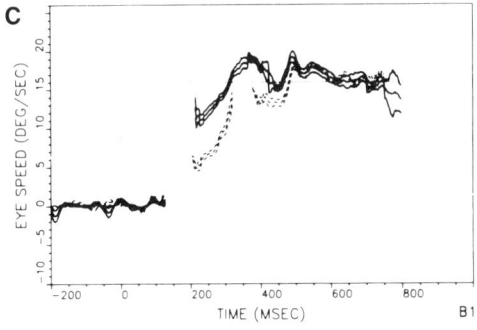

FIG. 5. Effect of a chemical lesion in area MT on the initiation of pursuit eye movements. **A:** Paradigm used to study pursuit eye movements. On the diagram at the top, the initial position of fixation is indicated by the *cross;* this target goes off as a spot of light comes on to the right and moves away as is indicated by the *dot* and *arrow.* On the graph, this "step" of the target 15° to the right and the subsequent "ramp" away at 16°/sec are indicated by the *dotted line.* Time is on the abscissa, position on the ordinate. The eye movement (*solid line* on the graph) follows the step with a rapid or saccadic eye movement to correct the position error and then a smooth pursuit eye movement that keeps the fovea near the visual target. **B:** Comparison of pursuit initiation prelesion (pre) and 24 hr after (post) injection of 1 µl of ibotenic acid into the left MT. The schematic drawing in the upper left indicates a lesion in the left hemisphere with target motion to the right: the target stepped 5° to the right and moved smoothly at 16°/sec away from the center of gaze. Ten superimposed trials are shown. **C:** Mean and standard error of eye speed before (*solid lines*) and after (*dashed lines*) the injection. Breaks in the traces are at the points where the high velocity of saccades interrupted the records. The deficit following the injection is both a reduction in the speed of pursuit and a failure to adjust the amplitude of the saccade to compensate for target motion. (Modified from ref. 1.)

map comparable to that of Fig. 1. The damaged region is contained entirely within area MT.

We made such an injection after having trained the monkey to make a smooth pursuit eye movement to the step-ramp target already described. The effect of one of these lesions is shown in Fig. 5B. The graph shows the position of the eye over time following the step and ramp of the target. The 10 superimposed prelesion traces show an accurate saccade to the location of the moving target and a close match of eye speed to target speed. The day after the ibotenic acid injection, the speed of eye movement just after the target was

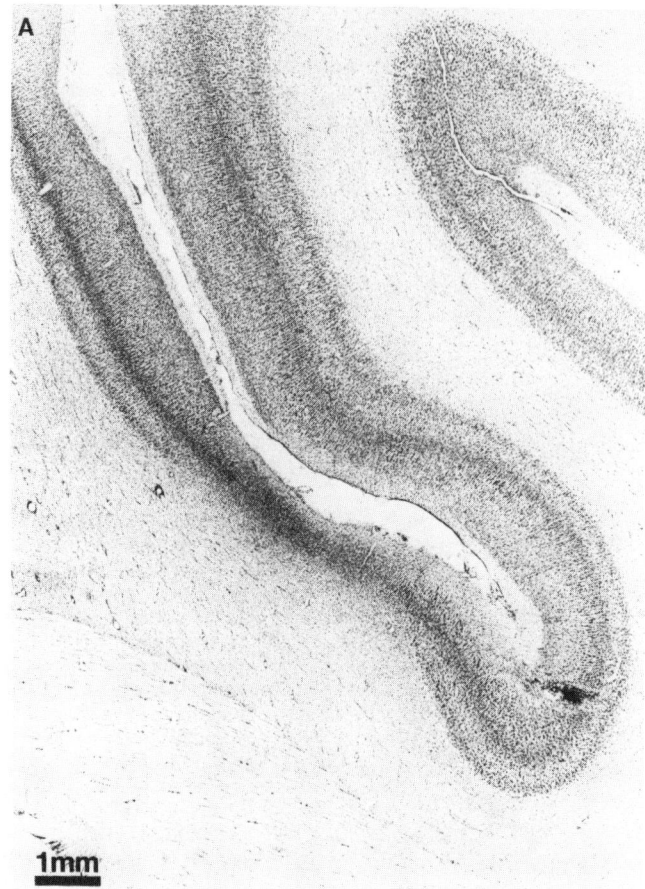

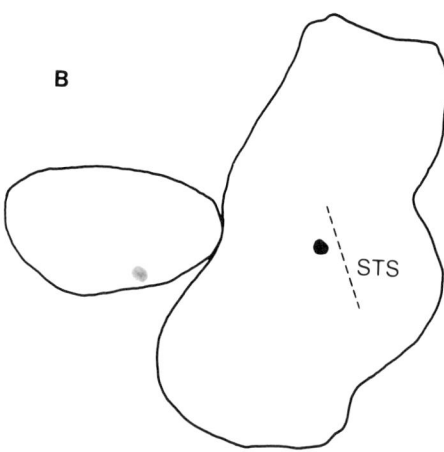

FIG. 6. A: Example of an ibotenic acid lesion shown on a sagittal section stained for cells with cresyl violet. The superior temporal sulcus (STS) runs through the center of the figure and the lesion is in area MT, which lies on the posterior bank (to the left on the figure). **B:** Size of the area damaged by an ibotenic acid injection in area MT shown on a flattened map similar to that of Fig. 1. This lesion is the one that produced the deficit shown in Figs. 5 and 7.

acquired was reduced. Figure 5C shows this initial deficit in eye speed more clearly. Once the fovea was brought near the target, the affected area of the visual field had been moved away from the target, and normal pursuit would be expected to resume, as it did. In addition to the deficit in pursuit speed, the monkey failed to adjust the amplitude of the saccade to match the position of the moving target, the saccade fell short of the moving target (Fig. 5B).

These two deficits in the use of motion information, a failure to match the speed of the eye to the speed of the target and a failure for the amplitude of the saccade to compensate for the motion of the target, were present only for saccades to one part of the contralateral visual field. Within this part of the visual field, however, the deficit was clear for any direction of target motion, either away from the center of gaze or toward the center of gaze.

The localization of this deficit is shown on the graph in Fig. 7 (top), which plots the amplitude of the saccadic error before and after the lesion. Target steps were 1°, 5°, 10°, and 15° into the contralateral visual field and to the same points in the ipsilateral visual field. For both sides of Fig. 7, target motion was away from the center of gaze. The deficit was limited to an area of approximately 5° eccentricity in the contralateral visual field. This was the same area that showed a deficit in the initial speed of eye movement. It was also the location of the visual receptive fields of cells recorded at the site of the ibotenic acid injection, as indicated by the arrow in Fig. 7 (top). This dependence of the deficit on the part of the visual field where the target motion occurred led us to characterize this deficit as a *retinotopic* deficit; it is related to one area of the retinotopically organized contralateral visual field.

The error in the amplitude of the saccade made to a moving target was not found when saccades were made to stationary targets (Fig. 7, bottom). This indicates that the monkey was able to use the *position* information of a stationary target to control the amplitude of a saccade but was unable to use the *motion* information from a moving target to adjust the amplitude of the saccade to compensate for this motion. These experiments suggest that area MT is contributing information on motion and not on position to the oculomotor system. A similar conclusion has been drawn from a recent study by Newsome and Pare (32) in which a monkey's ability to make a discrimination based on motion was reduced by an ibotenic acid lesion of area MT, whereas the monkey's ability to perform contrast discriminations was minimally affected.

Taken together, these experiments on the relation of area MT to pursuit eye movements and to perception of motion are consistent with the hypothesis that the area is selectively related to visual motion processing. The deficit in both initiation of movement (for pursuit eye movements) and perception of motion (discrimination and detection of moving targets) suggests in addition that motion processing in area MT is not committed to a specific function such as control of movement or perception. Rather, the output of the area, although selective for motion processing, is available for any use of that motion

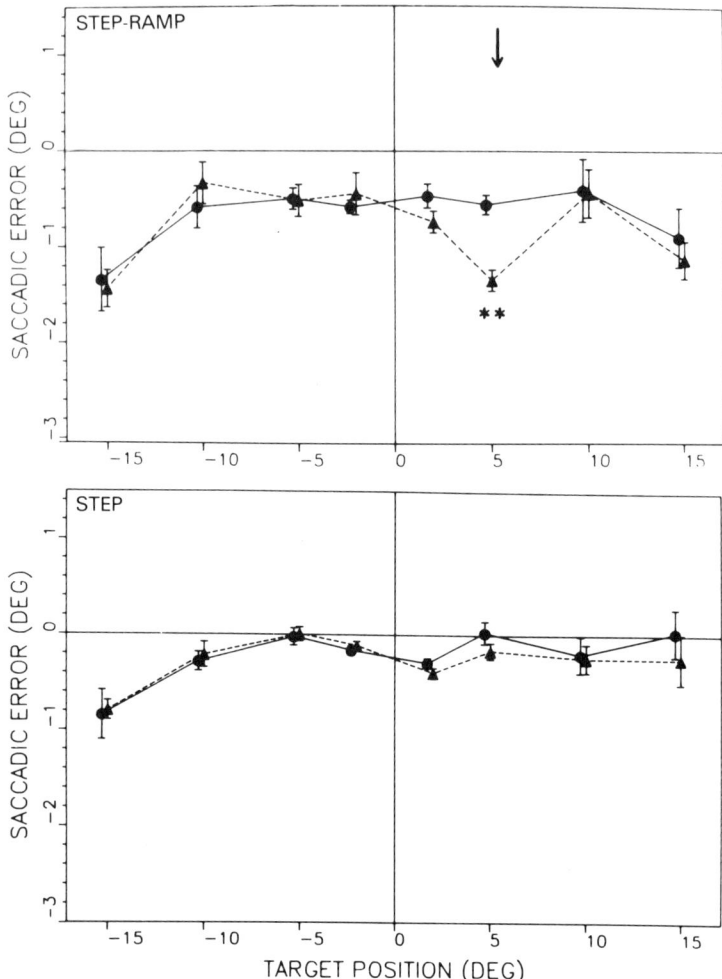

FIG. 7. Spatial localization of the pursuit deficit and the relation of the deficit to motion not position. Each graph shows the saccadic error—the difference between eye position and target position at the end of a saccade made to acquire the target—plotted against each of the target step positions. The top graph shows the saccadic error for a series of positions to the left with motion toward the left (− numbers) and to the right with motion to the right (+ numbers) for prelesion (●) and postlesion (▲) conditions for the experiments illustrated in Fig. 5. Mean and standard errors are shown, with (**) indicating a significance at the 0.001 level (*t*-test). The deficit is limited to the area of the contralateral visual field centered on 5° to the right. The *arrow* at the top of the figure indicates the center of the visual receptive fields recorded at the site of the injection and corresponds to the visual field area showing the deficit. The bottom graph shows the lack of deficit and saccadic error when a saccade was made to a stationary rather than a moving target. The lack of an amplitude error here indicates that the deficit is one related to loss of visual motion information, not the loss of position information. (Modified from ref. 1.)

processing. Area MT might be regarded as the extrastriate area where motion processing is concentrated.

RECOVERY FROM MT LESIONS

Pursuit recovered largely within a week and almost completely within two weeks of the lesion. With larger lesions, however, deficits usually last longer (2,32), but the lasting deficit is never as substantial as the initial deficit. We do not think that this recovery compromises our basic conclusion that in the normal monkey, the cells removed by lesion were an essential part of the neuronal processing underlying pursuit. Our conclusion is based on the specificity of the deficits, not on their duration; the lesions alter performance on tasks dependent on motion but not on those independent of motion. We interpret the recovery of function as indicating that other cells can eventually provide the necessary pursuit-related information.

One possible mechanism for recovery following MT area lesions is that other cells within this area take over the function of damaged cells. For example, the receptive fields of cells that are adjacent to the lesion area in MT might expand to functionally cover the area of the visual field affected by the lesion. Such an expansion of the visual fields toward that area of the field previously served by the ablated cells is suggested by recent experiments on somatosensory cortex showing expansion of tactile receptive fields into areas once occupied by the receptive fields of amputated fingers (33). To investigate such an effect, we (34) recorded from cells adjacent to the lesion site before and after punctate chemical lesions of the MT area. The receptive fields of some cells did expand after the injection and the large size of some receptive fields was beyond any seen before the lesion. This indicated a dynamic control of the receptive fields of these visual cells, as has been suggested by Merzenich and his collaborators (33). However, the expansion of the receptive fields was in all directions, both toward and away from the area of the visual field affected by the lesion. There was no indication that the changes specifically compensated for lesion deficit. Furthermore, the expansion of the receptive fields was observed on the day following the lesion, at a time when the deficit in pursuit was maximal. Thus, although the expansion of the receptive fields of adjacent cells within area MT might contribute to the recovery of function, we think that it is unlikely to account for the recovery by itself.

The eventual recovery following larger lesions that virtually eliminate area MT (2) indicates that information from areas outside it can be used in the course of recovery. Since monkeys with unilateral removal of striate cortex do not show such recovery (35), it seems likely that this recovery depends on visual motion information provided through striate cortex. We have already noted that a number of extrastriate areas are known to convey visual motion information, and these areas might well provide the needed visual motion information. The effect of damage to these other extrastriate areas, either alone or in conjunction with area MT lesions, has not been tested.

The recovery of the pursuit system following area MT lesions is reminiscent of the recovery of the saccadic system after superior colliculus lesions. The discharge characteristics of collicular neurons suggested that this structure played a role in the generation of saccades, yet the amplitude of saccades was nearly normal on the day following an electrolytic lesion of the structure—only the latency of saccades was increased (36). Schiller and collaborators (37) later demonstrated, however, that damage to the frontal eye fields in conjunction with lesions of the superior colliculus eliminated the ability to make these saccades. These structures would therefore seem to act in parallel, and it would be incorrect to conclude that either one is not involved in the generation of saccades just because the deficits following damage to either are transient. Furthermore, Hikosaka and Wurtz (38) recently found substantial deficits after chemical lesions of the superior colliculus when saccades were tested immediately after the lesion before compensation can occur. This series of experiments emphasizes the importance of assessing the behavioral consequences of lesions immediately after alteration of brain areas and the risks of inferring that a brain structure is not involved in a given function because recovery occurs after damage.

For critical behavioral functions such as the control of eye movements in primates, it is not surprising, given the rich interconnections between visual-motor areas, that compensation can occur for damage to even major areas. Many of the otherwise puzzling multiplicity of connections between these areas might serve this purpose and might effectively provide a built-in resistance to the deleterious effects of localized lesions. Furthermore, once the potential for the rapid recovery in these systems is recognized, it becomes obvious that the functions of an area can only be inferred before the compensatory mechanisms obscure or compound the deficit.

PURSUIT FOLLOWING MST AREA LESIONS

Area MST differs from area MT in having large visual fields and an extraretinal input. We next investigated whether restricted lesions of the MST area would produce deficits that also differ from those following lesions of area MT. We again used the chemical lesion technique to remove limited groups of cells. We made injections in selective areas in and around area MST (3) as well as the foveal region of area MT (2) where cells discharge during the maintenance of pursuit.

Figure 8A shows an example of the deficit we observed following an injection of ibotenic acid into area MST. The target stepped into the left visual field and moved to the left, and after the lesion (lower of the two position traces), this placed the target in the field ipsilateral to the lesion (as indicated by the

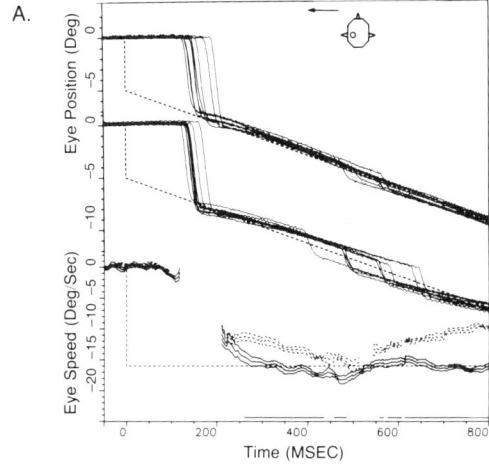

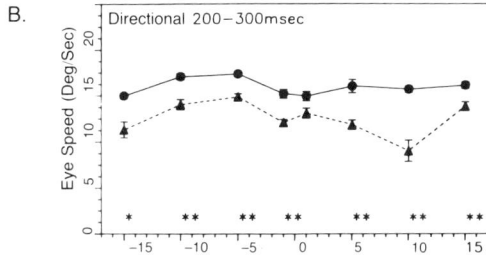

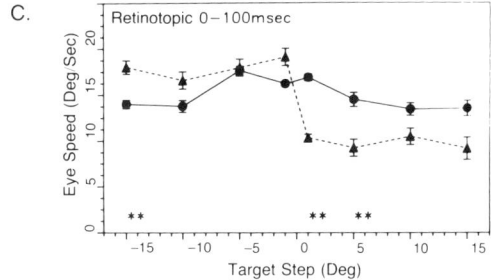

FIG. 8. Directional pursuit deficit following ibotenic acid lesion of area MST. **A:** Position and speed of the pursuit eye movement. The lesion was in the left hemisphere, as indicated on the drawing in the upper right corner. The target stepped 5° to the left and moved away at 16°/sec. Records are shown for eye position both prelesion (*upper*) and postlesion (*lower*). For eye speed (with periods of high velocity saccades removed), *solid lines* indicate mean and standard error prelesion, *dashed lines* indicate the same for postlesion trials. The pursuit shows a reduced speed throughout the duration of the trial. **B:** Speed of pursuit for targets moving toward the side of the lesion (*left*). The directional deficit is evident as reduced pursuit speed for target steps throughout the visual field tested, both to the left (− numbers) and to the right (+ numbers). Pursuit speed was taken in the period 200 to 300 msec after the saccade to the target in order to minimize the effect of the retinotopic deficit in the field contralateral to the lesion. Mean and standard errors with *t*-test significance indicated at the 0.01 (*) and 0.001 level (**). (●) prelesion; (▲) postlesion. **C:** Pursuit speed for targets moving away from the side of the lesion which shows the retinotopic deficit in the contralateral (right) visual field. Eye speed here was taken 0–100 msec after the initial saccade. (Modified from ref. 3.)

schematic drawing at the top of the figure). The monkey's ability to maintain the pursuit eye movement was impaired since pursuit speed remained lower than target speed for the duration of the trial. The records of eye speed below the two position traces indicate the reduction in pursuit speed after the lesion.

The deficit following the MST lesion differs from that following an MT lesion in that even when the monkey's eye was near the target, the eye never matched the target speed. Furthermore, this deficit was present for any step at any point in the visual field as long as the target motion was *toward* the side of the lesion. Figure 8B shows the magnitude of this *directional* deficit. This graph shows pursuit of target steps to the left and to the right but with target motion always to the left, i.e., *toward* the side of the lesion. In nearly every case there was a highly significant pursuit deficit, and this deficit persisted throughout the period in which the target was pursued by the monkey. For target motion in the visual field contralateral to the lesion, there was also a retinotopic deficit. Like that seen following MT lesions, this retinotopic deficit was independent of the direction of target motion. Figure 8C shows pursuit of targets moving away from the side of the injection so that only the retinotopic deficit was evident. Following injections in area MST, the retinotopic deficit frequently extended throughout the contralateral visual field (right side of Fig. 8C).

Although the chemical lesions are not as precisely localized as the single-cell recording, they do give some information about the contribution of the different regions we have considered within areas MT and MST to the generation of pursuit. We have found that the retinotopic deficits followed all of the injections in area MT or MST, and it therefore seems clear that the visual information related to pursuit initiation can be derived from any of these areas. In contrast, we did not see the directional deficit with all lesions in the MST area. Lesions on the anterior bank of the STS that are centered on the dorsal-medial MST area produced minimal directional deficits. Lesions more closely related to the lateral-anterior MST area have a more profound directional effect. At this point we do not know whether damage to the MT fovea area alone produces the directional deficit, but we do know that lesions that include this area and spread to the adjacent MST areas definitely do produce the directional deficit.

OPTOKINETIC DEFICITS FOLLOWING MST AREA LESIONS

Another oculomotor mechanism dependent on visual motion information is the optokinetic (OKN) system that acts to stabilize the eye in spite of motion of the head. This mechanism for stabilization is usually tested in the clinic or laboratory by moving visual patterns in front of the subject. This produces slow eye movements that follow the moving pattern, interrupted by fast movements that rapidly return the eye closer to the center of the orbit. The slow phase of OKN in turn consists of two components: an immediate rise, which might share common neural mechanisms with the pursuit system, and a slow buildup of response, which depends on a velocity storage mechanism (39,40). We found deficits following MST area lesions in both responses.

Figure 9 shows the results of a lesion that produced a decrease primarily in the slow buildup of OKN. The records in Fig. 9 indicate the mean and standard error of 100-msec periods of the slow phase of nystagmus averaged over five trials. The solid lines show prelesion values, and the dashed lines show

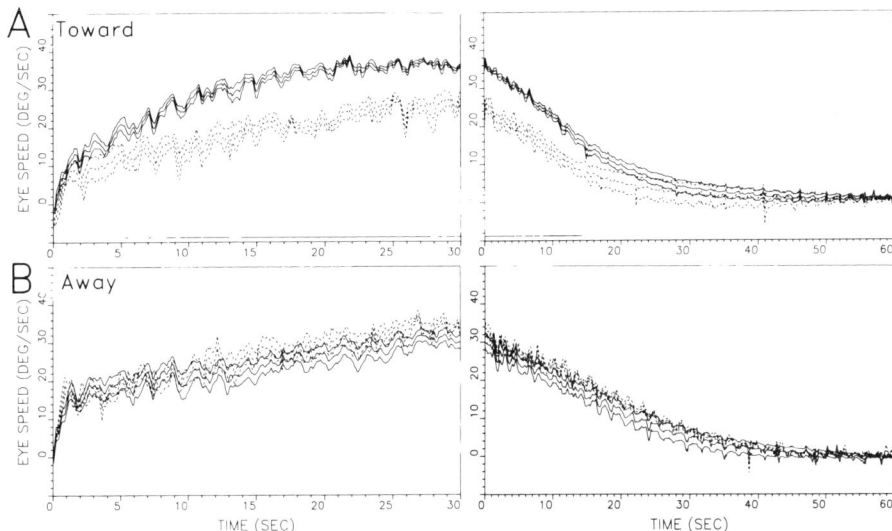

FIG. 9. Deficits in OKN and OKAN for stimulus motion toward the side of the lesion that showed prominent direction pursuit deficit. In **A**, drum motion was toward the side of the lesion (right is up) and in **B** it was away from the side of the lesion (left is up). OKN is shown on the left; 0 on the abscissa is time of drum illumination. OKAN is on the right; 0 is the time drum illumination was turned off. The *solid* and *dashed lines* represent the mean and standard error of the *slow phase* eye speed (see [54]) for 10 superimposed prelesion trials and five superimposed postlesion trials, respectively. Solid lines on the abscissa indicate a significant difference at the $p < 0.01$ level between the mean pre- and postlesion means (Student's *t*-test). Such differences were clear in the slower buildup of OKN with stimulus motion toward the side of the lesion in the right hemisphere (A, left) and in the lower OKAN level (A, right), but not with stimulus motion away from the side of the lesion (B). The experiment was done binocularly with drum rotation of 36°/sec and a period of stripes of 15.6 cycles/degree.

postlesion values. The records on the left show the slow rise in OKN during a 30-sec period after illumination of the drum rotating around the monkey at 72°/sec toward the side of the lesion (Fig. 9A) or away from the side of the lesion (Fig. 9B). The records on the right show the immediately following 60-sec period of OKN afternystagmus (OKAN) in the dark. Figure 9A shows a decrease in the buildup of OKN in the 30-sec period of stimulation with drum motion toward the side of the lesion; the difference was consistently significant after the first 8 sec of OKN stimulation. Similarly, the initial OKAN was reduced and the decrease was statistically significant throughout the entire period. In contrast, for drum motion away from the side of the lesion (Fig. 9B), we saw no difference between pre- and postlesion records.

The deficit in OKN buildup was more severe for motion toward the side of the brain with the lesion than for motion away from that side. Furthermore, this directional OKN deficit tended to be associated with a directional pursuit deficit. This overlap of the two deficits in the same area of the cortex raises the possibility that the same mechanism underlies both deficits, but this overlap might be fortuitous and requires verification using more restricted lesions within the STS.

A second type of deficit was a decrease in the rapid rise in eye speed seen in the first few seconds of OKN. This deficit was usually seen for motion both toward and away from the side of the brain with the lesion, and tended to be associated with lesions that produced a prominent retinotopic pursuit deficit. One possible reason for this association of deficits might be that the same visual motion processing stage that underlies the initiation of pursuit also serves the initial rapid rise of OKN. A relationship between pursuit and initial OKN has been suggested previously (39,41–44).

CONCLUSION

Our goal in these experiments has been to investigate the neuronal mechanisms underlying eye movements that depend on visual motion processing. To do this we have explored the contribution of two areas of cerebral cortex known to have a high proportion of cells sensitive to visual motion.

At a cellular level, we have been able to analyze the discharge of neurons in areas MT and MST to both visual motion input and pursuit eye movement output. We have seen a shift from a clear retinotopic organization in the first of these visual areas, MT, to a more complex organization in what can be regarded as a second or higher area, MST. Furthermore, the MST areas studied have been related to movement of the eye in addition to motion of the visual stimulus, indicating the presence of an extraretinal input. What we might be seeing in these shifts between areas MT and MST is a crossover from an area devoted to visual processing that has a clear retinotopic map but no dedicated relationship to a particular function, either movement or perception, to an area devoted to specific functions. In this case, area MST could be regarded as devoted to different functions, possibly concentrated in different subregions. Furthermore, we think our experiments show that localization of function is strengthened by an approach that considers both the visual input and the movement output of an area. This emphasizes the importance of considering the neuronal processing in an area of cortex in relation to the functional contribution the cells in the area make to a behavioral system within the brain.

We have also shown that the effect of highly localized lesions of these different groups of cells leads to different deficits in pursuit, either a retinotopic pursuit deficit in areas MT and MST or an additional directional pursuit deficit in area MST. The directional deficits we have seen following punctate lesions in the monkey are also very similar to a directional deficit seen in humans following large parietal lesions or hemispherectomy. This directional deficit was seen in the slow phase of OKN, as first described by Fox and Holmes (45) and then by others (46,47). The deficit was subsequently described for pursuit as well (48–51). The deficit in humans is one of inadequate pursuit or slow phase when the target moves toward the side of the brain containing the cerebral cortical damage. Recent experiments by Leigh and his collaborators (52) have shown that the distinctions between a retinotopic and a directional deficit can be seen following cortical lesions in humans. Since the brain area damaged is known in a number of these cases, it is also possible to develop hypotheses about the location of pursuit-related areas in humans. In the near future, however, our understanding of the underlying mechanisms controlling pursuit is likely to continue to be derived from growing knowledge of the monkey visual and oculomotor systems.

REFERENCES

1. Newsome WT, Wurtz RH, Dursteler MR, Mikami A. Deficits in visual motion processing following ibotenic acid lesions of the middle temporal visual area of the macaque monkey. *J Neurosci* 1985;5:825–840.
2. Dursteler MR, Wurtz RH, Newsome WT. Directional pursuit deficits following lesions of the foveal representation within the superior temporal sulcus of the macaque monkey. *J Neurophysiol* 1987;57:1262–1287.
3. Dursteler MR, Wurtz RH. Pursuit and optokinetic deficits following chemical lesions of cortical areas MT and MST. *J Neurophysiol* 1988;60:940–965.
4. Komatsu H, Wurtz RH. Relation of cortical areas MT and MST to pursuit eye movements. I. Localization and visual properties of neurons. *J Neurophysiol* 1988;60:580–603.
5. Newsome WT, Wurtz RH, Komatsu H. Relation of cortical areas MT and MST to pursuit eye movements. II. Differentiation of retinal from extraretinal inputs. *J Neurophysiol* 1988;60:604–620.
6. Komatsu H, Wurtz RH. Relation of cortical areas MT and MST to pursuit eye movements. III. Interaction with full field visual stimulation. *J Neurophysiol* 1988;60:621–644.
7. Wurtz RH, Komatsu H, Yamasaki DSG, Dursteler MR. Motion to movement: cerebral cortical visual motion processing for pursuit eye movements. In: Einer Gall W, ed. *Signal and sense: local and global order in perceptual maps.* New York: John Wiley (*submitted*).
8. Hubel DH, Wiesel TN. Receptive fields and functional architecture of monkey striate cortex. *J Physiol (Lond)* 1968;195:215–243.
9. Goldberg ME, Wurtz RH. Activity of superior colliculus in behaving monkey: I. Visual receptive fields of single neurons. *J Neurophysiol* 1972;35:542–559.
10. Hoffmann K-P, Distler C. The role of direction selective cells in the nucleus of the optic tracts of cat and monkey during optokinetic nystagmus. In: Keller E, Zee DS, eds. *Adaptive processes in the visual and oculomotor systems.* Oxford: Pergamon Press, 1986;261–266.
11. Maunsell JHR, Newsome WT. Visual processing in monkey extrastriate cortex. *Annu Rev Neurosci* 1987;10:363–401.
12. Van Essen DC, Maunsell JHR. Two-dimensional maps of the cerebral cortex. *J Comp Neurol* 1980;191:255–281.
13. Van Essen DC. Functional organization of primate visual cortex. In: Peters A, Jones EG, eds. *Cerebral cortex,* vol. III. New York: Plenum, 1985;259–329.
14. Van Essen DC, Maunsell JHR, Bixby JL. The middle temporal visual area in the macaque: myeloarchitecture, connections, functional properties and topographic organization. *J Comp Neurol* 1981;199:293–326.
15. Tanaka K, Hikosaka K, Saito H-A, Yukie M, Fukada Y, Iwai E. Analysis of local and wide-field movements in the superior temporal visual areas of the macaque monkey. *J Neurosci* 1986;6:134–144.
16. Desimone R, Ungerleider LG. Multiple visual areas in the caudal superior temporal sulcus of the macaque. *J Comp Neurol* 1986;248:164–189.
17. Sakata H, Shibutani H, Kawano K. Functional properties of visual tracking neurons in posterior parietal association cortex of the monkey. *J Neurophysiol* 1983;49:1364–1380.

18. Baker JF, Petersen SE, Newsome WT, Allman JM. Visual response properties of neurons in four extrastriate visual areas of the owl monkey (*Aotus trivirgatus*): a quantitative comparison of the medial, dorsomedial, dorsolateral, and middle temporal areas. *J Neurophysiol* 1981;45:397–416.
19. Felleman DJ, Kaas JH. Receptive-field properties of neuron in middle temporal visual area (MT) of owl monkeys. *J Neurophysiol* 1984;52:488–513.
20. Maunsell JHR, Van Essen DC. Functional properties of neurons in middle temporal visual area of the macaque monkey. I. Selectivity for stimulus direction, speed, and orientation. *J Neurophysiol* 1983;49:1127–1147.
21. Mikami A, Newsome WT, Wurtz RH. Motion selectivity in macaque visual cortex. I. Mechanisms of direction and speed selectivity in extrastriate area MT. *J Neurophysiol* 1986;55:1308–1327.
22. Glickstein M, Cohen JL, Dixon B, et al. Corticopontine visual projections in macaque monkeys. *J Comp Neurol* 1980;190:209–229.
23. Mustari MJ, Fuchs AF, Wallman J. The physiological response properties of single pontine units related to smooth pursuit in the trained monkey. In: Keller E, Zee DS, eds. *Adaptive processes in the visual and oculomotor systems.* Oxford: Pergamon Press, 1986;253–260.
24. Suzuki DA, Keller EL. Visual signals in the dorsolateral pontine nucleus of the alert monkey: their relationship to smooth-pursuit eye movements. *Exp Brain Res* 1984;53:473–478.
25. Langer T, Fuchs AF, Scudder CA, Chubb MC. Afferents to the flocculus of the cerebellum in the rhesus macaque as revealed by retrograde transport of horseradish peroxidase. *J Comp Neurol* 1985;235:1–25.
26. Lisberger SG, Fuchs AF. Role of primate flocculus during rapid behavioral modification of vestibuloocular reflex. I. Purkinje cell activity during visually guided horizontal smooth-pursuit eye movements and passive head rotation. *J Neurophysiol* 1978;41:733–777.
27. Miles FA, Fuller JH. Visual tracking and the primate flocculus. *Science* 1975;189:1000–1002.
28. Noda H, Suzuki DA. The role of the flocculus of the monkey in fixation and smooth pursuit eye movements. *J Physiol (Lond)* 1979;294:335–348.
29. Lanman J, Bizzi E, Allum J. The coordination of eye and head movement during smooth pursuit. *Brain Res* 1978;153:39–53.
30. Lisberger SG, Westbrook LE. Properties of visual inputs that initiate horizontal smooth pursuit eye movements in monkeys. *J Neurosci* 1985;5:1662–1673.
31. Newsome WT, Wurtz RH, Dursteler MR, Mikami A. Punctate chemical lesions of striate cortex in the macaque monkey: effect on visually guided saccades. *Exp Brain Res* 1985;58:392–399.
32. Newsome WT, Pare EB. MT lesions impair discrimination of direction in a stochastic motion display. *Soc Neurosci Abstr* 1986;12:1183.
33. Merzenich MM, Kaas JH, Wall JT, Nelson RJ, Sur M, Felleman DJ. Topographic reorganization of somatosensory cortical areas 3b and 1 in adult monkeys following restricted deafferentation. *Neuroscience* 1983;8:33–55.
34. Yamasaki DSG, Wurtz RH. Recovery of function following chemical lesions of cortical area MT. *Soc Neurosci Abstr* 1987;13:625.
35. Segraves MA, Goldberg ME, Deng SY, Bruce CJ, Ungerleider L, Mishkin M. The role of striate cortex in the guidance of eye movements in the monkey. *J Neurosci* 1987;7:3040–3058.
36. Wurtz RH, Goldberg ME. Activity of superior colliculus in behaving monkey: IV. Effects of lesions on eye movements. *J Neurophysiol* 1972;35:587–596.
37. Schiller PH, True SD, Conway JL. Deficits in eye movements following frontal eye field and superior colliculus ablations. *J Neurophysiol* 1980;44:1175–1189.
38. Hikosaka O, Wurtz RH. Modification of saccadic eye movements by GABA-related substances. I. Effect of muscimol and bicuculline in monkey superior colliculus. *J Neurophysiol* 1985;53:266–291.
39. Cohen B, Matsuo V, Raphan T. Quantitative analysis of the velocity characteristics of optokinetic nystagmus and optokinetic afternystagmus. *J Physiol (Lond)* 1977;270:321–344.
40. Raphan T, Matsuo V, Cohen B. Velocity storage in the vestibulo-ocular reflex arc (VOR). *Exp Brain Res* 1979;35:229–248.
41. Lisberger SG, Miles FA, Optican LM, Eighmy BB. Optokinetic response in monkey: underlying mechanisms and their sensitivity to long-term adaptive changes in vestibuloocular reflex. *J Neurophysiol* 1981;45:869–890.

42. Robinson DA. Linear addition of optokinetic and vestibular signals in the vestibular nucleus. *Exp Brain Res* 1977;30:447–450.
43. Waespe W, Henn V. Neuronal activity in the vestibular nuclei of the alert monkey during vestibular and optokinetic stimulation. *Exp Brain Res* 1977;27:523–538.
44. Zee DS, Yamazaki A, Butler PH, Gücer G. Effects of ablation of flocculus and paraflocculus on eye movements in primate. *J Neurophysiol* 1981;46:878–899.
45. Fox JC, Holmes G. Optic nystagmus and its value in the localization of cerebral lesions. *Brain* 1926;49:333–371.
46. Cogan DG, Loeb DR. Optokinetic response and intracranial lesions. *Arch Neurol Psychiatr* 1949;61:183–187.
47. Baloh RW, Yee RD, Honrubia V. Optokinetic nystagmus and parietal lobe lesions. *Ann Neurol* 1980;7:269–276.
48. Sharpe JA, Lo AW, Rabinovitch HE. Control of the saccadic and smooth pursuit systems after cerebral hemidecortication. *Brain* 1979;102:387–403.
49. Leigh RJ, Thurston SE. Recovery of ocular motor function in humans with cerebral lesions. In: Keller E, Zee DS, eds. *Adaptive process in the visual and oculomotor systems*. New York: Elsevier, 1986;231–238.
50. Troost BT, Daroff RB, Weber RB, Dell'Osso LF. Hemispheric control of eye movements. II. Quantitative analysis of smooth pursuit in a hemispherectomy patient. *Arch Neurol* 1972;27:449–452.
51. Leigh RJ, Tusa RJ. Disturbance of smooth pursuit caused by infarction of occipitoparietal cortex. *Ann Neurol* 1985;17:185–187.
52. Thurston SE, Leigh RJ, Kennard C. Two distinct deficits of visual tracking caused by unilateral lesions of cerebral cortex in man (*submitted*).
53. Richmond, BJ, Optican LM, Podell M, Spitzer H. Temporal encoding of two-dimensional patterns by single units in primate inferior temporal cortex: I. Response characteristics. *J Neurophysiol* 1987;57:132–146.
54. Dursteler MR, Wurtz RH, Yamasaki DSG. Pursuit and OKN deficits following ibotenic acid lesions in the medial superior temporal area (MST) of monkey. *Soc Neurosci Abstr* 1986;12.

Vision and the Brain,
edited by B. Cohen and I. Bodis-Wollner.
Raven Press, Ltd., New York © 1990.

Contribution of the Nucleus of the Optic Tract to Optokinetic Nystagmus and Optokinetic Afternystagmus in the Monkey: Clinical Implications

*Bernard Cohen, *Daniel Schiff, and †Jean Buettner

*Department of Neurology, Mount Sinai School of Medicine,
New York, New York 10029; †Department of Physiology, University of Munich,
Munich, West Germany

The nucleus of the optic tract (NOT) and the dorsal terminal nucleus of the accessory optic system (DTN) have been implicated in producing optokinetic nystagmus (OKN) in the monkey, cat, rabbit, and rat (1–12). Until recently, there has been little information about subcortical processing for OKN in the NOT of subhuman primates or humans. In this chapter we summarize results of two studies reported in greater detail elsewhere (10,11). We electrically stimulated the pretectum of the monkey in the NOT region to determine whether eye movements could be evoked and whether the dynamics of the induced eye movements were related to those of OKN and optokinetic afternystagmus (OKAN) (13,14). We also made lesions of NOT, DTN, and the surrounding region. From the results we conclude that NOT plays an important role in processing activity related to the slow component of horizontal OKN and OKAN in the monkey.

DEFINITION OF THE NOT AND THE DTN

There has been controversy as to the location of NOT in the monkey (12). We define NOT as a pretectal nucleus, interstitial to the brachium of the superior colliculus (BSC). DTN lies ventral to BCS (15). NOT and DTN contain small, medium, and large cells that receive direct input from the retina (16,17). The large fusiform cells of NOT project to the dorsal cap of Kooy and the beta nucleus of the ipsilateral inferior olive (7,18). DTN and NOT are interconnected, and DTN also projects to the contralateral NOT (12,19,20).

Figure 1A shows the location of NOT and DTN and the surrounding nuclei of the upper mesencephalon, as determined by the criteria of direct

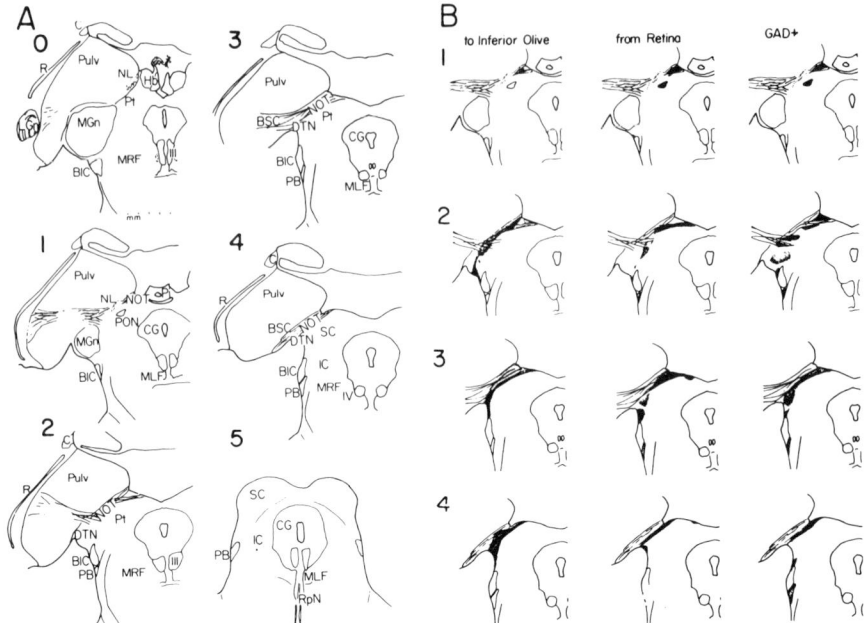

FIG. 1. Upper brainstem, including NOT, DTN, and the pretectum. The sections are 300 μm apart and extend from rostral **(0)** to caudal **(5)** in this and in subsequent figures. The location of NOT cells that project to the inferior olive is shown in **B, left;** the site of termination of direct input from the retina in **B, center;** and the location of GAD staining in **B, right.** (A is from Fig. 1 of ref. 11; B, left and right, are drawn from material provided by A. K. E. Horn and K.-P. Hoffmann and B, center, from material supplied by R. Spencer.)

retinal input, projection to the inferior olive, and GAD staining (Fig. 1B).[1] NOT extends caudally, laterally, and ventrally in BCS to the lateral edge of the brainstem (sections A.1–4), where NOT lies dorsal to DTN (sections A.2–4). This corresponds to the spatial coordinates of the region from which nystagmus was produced by electrical stimulation (Fig. 8 of [10]). According to these criteria NOT and DTN are differentiated primarily by their location. Nucleus limitans (NL), shown by the heavy dots in sections A0 and A1 of Fig. 1 and the pretectal olivary nucleus (PON) (section A1) are largely rostral to NOT.

---

[1] Figure 1B was reconstructed from primate material that was kindly lent to us by Drs. Anja Horn, Klaus-Peter Hoffmann, and Robert Spencer. Projections to the inferior olive, shown on the left, were drawn from an experiment by Dr. Hoffmann. Horseradish peroxidase (HRP) was injected into the inferior olive. The shaded areas show the location of retrogradely labeled NOT neurons. Retinal projections to the region of NOT, labeled by Dr. Spencer with tritiated leucine, are shown by the shaded areas in the middle. GAD-positive staining in the region of NOT, taken from experiments of Drs. Horn and Hoffman, is shown on the right.

In the rat both NOT and DTN have a dense plexus of cells that stain for glutamate decarboxylase (GAD) (20,21). It has been suggested that the γ-aminobutyric acid (GABA) neurons are both local circuit and projection neurons (20). In NOT of the monkey neither the retinal terminals in NOT nor the large neurons that project to the inferior olive have terminals that stain histochemically for GABA (22). This suggests that the GABAergic terminals may not end on cells that form the NOT-olivary pathway.

THEORETICAL BASIS FOR OKN AND OKAN

OKN, elicited by movement of the entire surrounding visual field, occurs naturally under two circumstances. When the head is moving with regard to the body, if the vestibulo-ocular reflex (VOR) does not exactly compensate for head movement, there is retinal slip of the visual surround in the direction opposite to head movement. Such full-field retinal slip is a powerful stimulus for the production of OKN (23,24). There is also movement of the entire visual surround and production of OKN during walking or running, particularly when the subject is moving with an angular trajectory (25). From the point of view of the vestibular system and for visual-vestibular interactions, therefore, OKN, elicited by full-field stimulation, can be considered as the response of the oculomotor system to movement of the visual surround that occurs during head on body movement or during locomotion.

In the monkey, OKN and OKAN can be modeled in one dimension as the interaction of two processes (13,14,26–28). One process produces rapid changes in eye velocity, such as occur at the onset and end of OKN and during visual suppression of VOR. This has been called the "direct" visual-oculomotor pathway. (The term derives from modeling and does not imply monosynaptic or oligosynaptic connectivity.) A second process causes only slow changes in eye velocity. It has been labeled the "indirect" visual-oculomotor pathway. It contains an integrator that is capable of storing activity related to slow-phase eye velocity.

Because it is relevant to the data to be presented, the characteristics of the response of the one-dimensional model to visual surround movement will be described (Fig. 2.1C). This can be compared with normal OKN and OKAN shown in Fig. 2.1A. At the onset of OKN the direct pathway produces an initial jump in slow-phase velocity, whereas the indirect pathway, activated by retinal slip, charges the velocity storage integrator to cause a slow rise in OKN. The two pathways combine to produce steady-state OKN. The discharge of the velocity storage integrator at the end of stimulation produces OKAN. Thus, OKAN is a direct measure of the activity in the storage integrator. Factors that influence the rate of rise of activity in the velocity storage

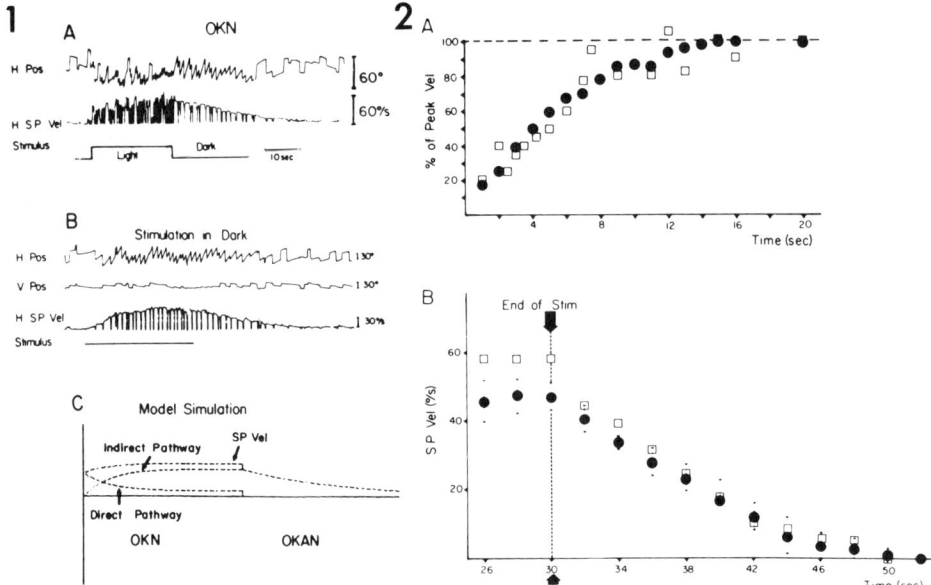

FIG. 2. 1A: OKN and OKAN of a normal monkey responding to visual field motion of 60°/sec. **1B:** Stimulation of the right NOT of the same monkey in darkness. Eye movements were recorded with a scleral magnetic search coil. The top trace is horizontal eye position (H Pos), the second trace is vertical eye position (V Pos), and the third trace is horizontal slow-phase velocity (H SP Vel). The quick phase velocities have been removed. The period of stimulation is shown by the *solid bar* under the slow-phase velocity trace. The stimulus frequency was 250 Hz. Movements to the right were associated with upward trace deflections in this and subsequent figures. Note that stimulation in darkness caused brisk nystagmus with ipsilateral (right) slow phases. This was followed by afternystagmus in the same direction. **1C:** Simulation of OKN and OKAN by the model of Waespe et al. (27). The initial jump in slow-phase velocity is due to activation of the indirect pathway, followed by a slow rise to a steady-state level. At the end of stimulation there is a rapid initial fall due to the drop in activity of the direct pathway. This is followed by a slower fall to zero as the velocity storage integrator discharges. **2A:** Comparison of the charging time course of OKAN (□) with the slow rise in stimulus-induced nystagmus (●). **2B:** Comparison with OKN and OKAN (□) with stimulus-induced nystagmus and afternystagmus (●). The time course and magnitude of the stimulus-induced nystagmus and of afternystagmus are the same as those of the slow component of OKN and of OKAN. (Adapted from ref. 10.)

integrator include the gain of the direct pathway, the time constant of the velocity storage integrator, and the characteristics of the coupling between the visual system and the indirect pathway. This coupling, which is a nonlinear function of retinal slip, determines the time constant of charge of the storage integrator at different velocities of stimulation (14,26,27). The ability of the integrator to store charge is determined by its dominant or falling time constant and is reflected in the peak or saturation velocity of OKAN. The falling time constant is subject to habituation and is under control of circuitry in the nodulus and uvula (29).

Anatomical correlates have been found for processing represented in the direct and indirect pathways of the model at various locations in the central nervous system. Activity of floccular Purkinje's cells is related to the rapid rise in OKN and to rapid suppression of vestibular nystagmus (30–32), suggesting that at least part of the direct pathway lies in the flocculus. In accord with this, floccular and parafloccular lesions disrupt the rapid rise in OKN and visual suppression of the VOR without affecting the slow rise in OKN or OKAN (27,33). On the other hand, the velocity storage integrator appears to be represented in the activity of cells in the vestibular nuclei. Type I and II neurons, which receive input from the lateral semicircular canals, have firing rates that parallel the slow rise in OKN slow-phase velocity and OKAN, not the rapid rise in OKN (34,35). Moreover, OKAN is lost after labyrinthectomy (36–38), semicircular canal nerve section (39), or midline section of the medulla (40,41), lesions that do not affect the rapid rise in OKN. Separate representations of activity in the direct and indirect pathways are found at other levels of the nervous system as well.

The eye velocity envelope during OKN and OKAN with a large initial jump in eye velocity, shown in Fig. 2.1C, is characteristic of the monkey. In the cat, rabbit, and rat there is only a small jump in eye velocity at the onset of OKN, and slow-phase velocity develops much more slowly (6,42–44). This suggests that OKN is produced primarily by activation of the indirect pathway in these animals. In each of these species activity related to retinal image motion in the horizontal plane is found in NOT (1,4,5,45). Thus, NOT processes information about retinal slip in the animal's horizontal or yaw plane. In agreement with this, horizontal nystagmus and afternystagmus can be elicited by stimulation of NOT in the rabbit, whereas NOT lesions cause a loss of OKN (2). Whether the indirect pathway is also located in NOT in the monkey is not known, although it would seem consistent with the finding of Kato et al. (8,9) that OKN and OKAN were lost after lesions in the region of NOT.

ELECTRICAL STIMULATION OF NOT, DTN, AND THE SURROUNDING REGION

Stimulation of the pretectum in light, at sites located in and around NOT, had no effect in the alert monkey. In contrast, stimulation of these same regions in darkness induced horizontal conjugate nystagmus with slow phases toward the side of stimulation (Fig. 2.1B) (10). The slow-phase velocity of the induced nystagmus rose slowly to a peak value that was maintained for the duration of stimulation. Regardless of stimulus frequency there was no initial jump in slow-phase velocity. At the end of stimulation eye velocity fell smoothly to zero, and there was no rapid drop in velocity, as after OKN. This suggests that the response evoked by electric stimulation was produced by the indirect and not the direct pathway (Fig. 2.1C). In accord with this, the rising time course of the velocity of the induced nystagmus (Fig. 2.2A, circles) was similar to the buildup or "charge" of OKAN during optokinetic stimulation (Fig. 2.2A, squares) (13), and the fall in slow-phase eye velocity of the afternystagmus (Fig. 2.2B, circles) paralleled the time course of OKAN (Fig. 2.2B, squares). Peak slow-phase eye velocities attained during the induced nystagmus ranged from 60 to 80°/sec and were close to the peak velocities of OKAN.

Thus, the general characterstics of the stimulus-induced nystagmus were similar to those of the slow component of OKN, i.e., to that component that is attributable to excitation of the velocity storage integrator in the vestibular system.

INTERACTION OF NOT STIMULATION WITH NATURALLY EVOKED OKN AND VESTIBULAR NYSTAGMUS

If NOT stimulation had activated the indirect pathway and the velocity storage integrator, it should be possible to affect naturally evoked optokinetic and vestibular nystagmus by electrical stimulation of NOT. Such interactions are shown in Fig. 3. The control stimulus-induced nystagmus is shown in Fig. 3A. Activation of NOT during OKAN with slow phases toward the side of stimulation (Fig. 3C) caused only a prolongation of the nystagmus for the duration of stimulation. This shows that the induced nystagmus was limited by the characteristics of OKAN, i.e., by its saturation velocity and its falling time constant.

When NOT stimulation was combined with OKN with contralateral slow phases (Fig. 3D), there was a rapid rise in slow-phase velocity at the onset of stimulation but no subsequent slow rise above this level, and the nystagmus was irregular. At the termination of OKN and electric stimulation, there was a sudden fall of eye velocity back to zero and no afternystagmus. The maximum steady-state slow-phase velocity of the OKN elicited by surround movement at 60°/sec during combined stimulation was similar to that of the initial jump of OKN slow-phase velocity in response to a 60°/sec step of velocity (37.5 ± 4.3°/sec during combined stimulation versus 36 ± 3.1°/sec for the initial jump during OKN). Similar nystagmus, due only to activation of the direct pathway, is found after bilateral labyrinthectomy or lateral semicircular canal nerve section when velocity storage is lost (36,39). This demonstrates that activity elicited by NOT stimulation can counteract oppositely directed OKAN and the slow rise in OKN, leaving the direct pathway response intact. Thus, activity elicited by NOT stimulation supports OKN in a manner similar to OKAN when the slow-phase velocities are in the same direction and counteracts the slow component of OKN as well as OKAN when they are in opposite directions.

The same stimulus-induced nystagmus (Fig. 3A) was also combined with per- and postrotatory nystagmus produced by rotation of the animal at a

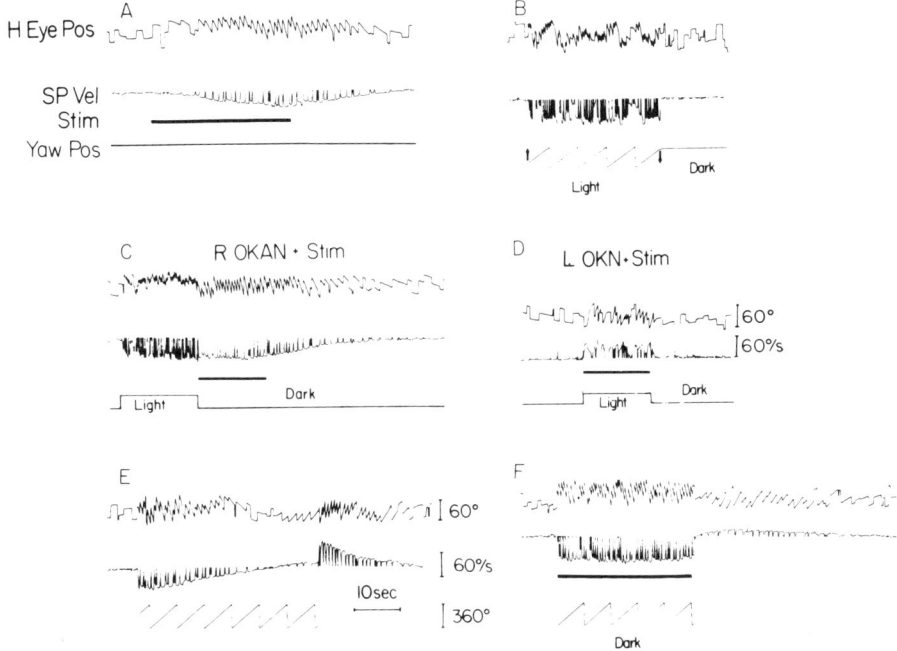

FIG. 3. A: Nystagmus induced by stimulation at 250 Hz for the period shown by the *black bar* (Stim) under the eye velocity trace. The top trace in each panel is horizontal eye position (H Eye Pos); the second trace is slow-phase velocity (SP Vel). **B:** Nystagmus induced by rotation in light with a stop in darkness. The third trace is a potentiometer recording of yaw position that reset every 360° during rotation, creating the sawtooth appearance. **C–D:** Interaction of OKN and stimulus-induced nystagmus. See text for details. **E:** Per- and postrotatory nystagmus induced by rotation at constant velocity around a vertical axis in darkness. **F:** Summation of stimulation-induced nystagmus with per-rotatory nystagmus caused eye velocity to be maintained for the duration of stimulation. Note the reduction in the postrotatory nystagmus. The animal was in darkness throughout E and F. (Adapted from ref. 10.)

constant velocity about a vertical axis in darkness. Slow-phase velocity during per- and postrotatory nystagmus in darkness characteristically rises rapidly and then falls to zero over the dominant time constant of the VOR (Fig. 3E) (26). When the slow phases of the induced and per-rotatory nystagmus were ipsilateral to the side of stimulation (Fig. 3F), the velocity of the nystagmus was maintained for as long as stimulation continued, and there was only minimal postrotatory nystagmus. A similar velocity envelope is produced under natural circumstances by a step of rotation in light, followed by a stop in darkness (Fig. 3B). In this condition activity induced by optokinetic stimulation and velocity storage sustains eye velocity during rotation and counteracts the activity coming from the semicircular canals at the end of rotation (26,27,46). Thus, activity induced by electric stimulation of NOT could also interact with activity coming from the semicircular canals to sustain eye velocity when the slow phases of the per-rotatory response and the stimulation-induced nystagmus were in the same direction and to block the postrotatory response when the two were oppositely directed.

EFFECTS OF GRAVITY ON STIMULUS-INDUCED NYSTAGMUS

If horizontal OKN is elicited with monkeys upright, the subsequent OKAN is horizontal and has no vertical component. With animals on their side in a 90° roll position, however, OKN in the animal's horizontal or yaw plane is followed by OKAN, which develops a prominent vertical component. This causes the beating plane of the nystagmus to shift from the animal horizontal toward the spatial horizontal plane (47,48). We have referred to this as "cross-coupling," and shown that it is related to the influence of the otoliths on the three-dimensional structure of the velocity storage integrator (47,48).

Consistent with the analogy between stimulus-induced afternystagmus and OKAN, when NOT was electrically stimulated with the animal in the upright position in darkness, the evoked nystagmus was predominantly horizontal (Fig. 4A). When the same stimulus was applied with the animal tilted on its side, as shown by the stick figures at the right of Fig. 4B and C, the evoked nystagmus and afternystagmus had both horizontal and vertical components. The vertical components (arrows) tended to bring the stimulus-induced nystagmus and afternystagmus toward a spatial horizontal plane. Thus, the horizontal nystagmus induced by electric stimulation of NOT could be cross-coupled through velocity storage to produce afternystagmus in other planes, similar to OKAN. An interesting aspect of the cross-coupled nystagmus was that it was present from the onset of stimulation with the animal in tilted positions (Fig. 4B and C). This shows that cross-coupling takes place from the onset of the response. Frequently, with natural stimulation the presence of a structured visual field helps the animal hold the OKN in the plane of stimulation, suppressing the cross-coupled response until the lights are extinguished.

LOCATION OF STIMULATION SITES

Positive stimulus sites for eliciting nystagmus lay in NOT, interstitial to and slightly below BSC. The location of the positive sites from five tracks are shown projected onto the diagrams from Fig. 1 in Fig. 5 by the vertical bars. These sites extended caudally and laterally from the level of PON to the edge of the brainstem. Several tracks also extended ventrally into DTN, as defined by Lin and Giolli (15). Nystagmus was not evoked by stimulation anterior or medial to PON, from tracks in NL or from stimulation in the adjacent portions of the pretectum. However, it was possible to elicit nystagmus with similar characteristics by stimulation of a fiber bundle that emerges from the internal capsule dorsal to the lateral geniculate nucleus (LGN) and progresses medially and

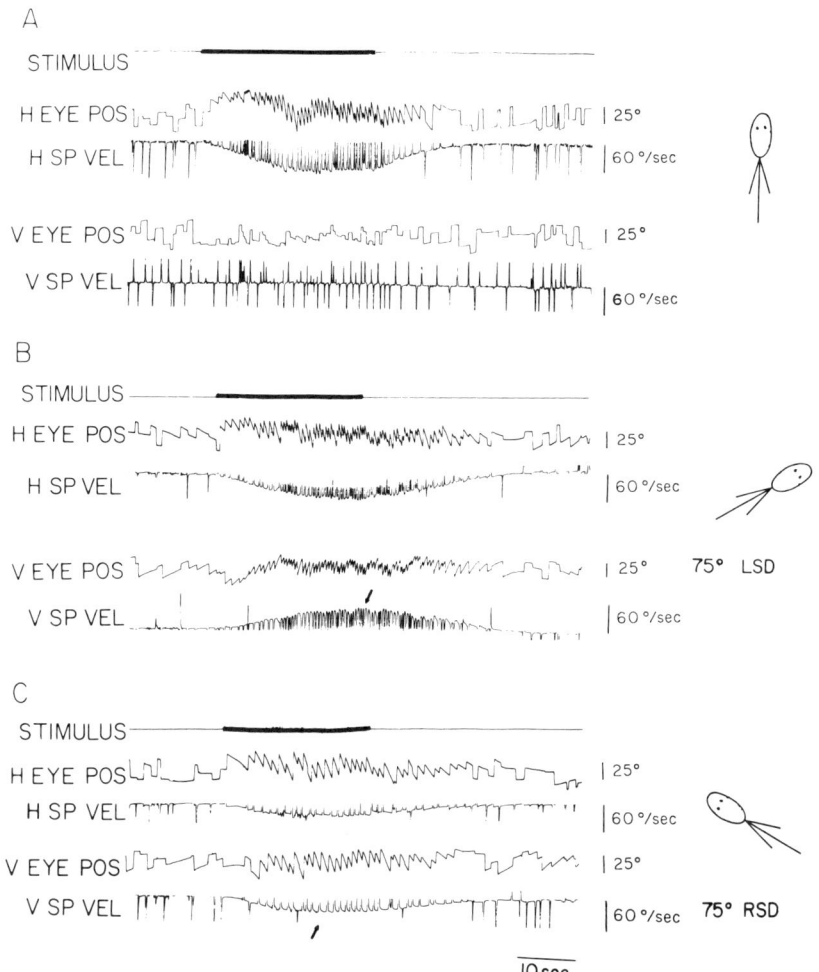

FIG. 4. Effect of head position with regard to gravity on stimulus-induced nystagmus (200 Hz, 40 µA). The traces are from top to bottom, period of stimulation, horizontal eye position (H EYE POS), horizontal slow-phase eye velocity (H SP VEL), vertical eye position (V EYE POS), and vertical slow-phase eye velocity (V SP VEL). The stick figures on the side of each panel show the position of the animal while receiving stimulation. The experiment was conducted in darkness. **A:** With the animal upright, stimulation induced pure leftward slow-phase velocity, and there was no vertical nystagmus. **B:** Stimulation given with the animal tilted 75° left side down (LSD) caused slow phases up and to the left. **C:** In the 75° right side down (RSD) position the induced slow phases were down and to the left. The vertical components are marked by *arrows*. In both C and D the vertical components tended to bring the induced nystagmus toward a spatial horizontal plane. (From ref. 10.)

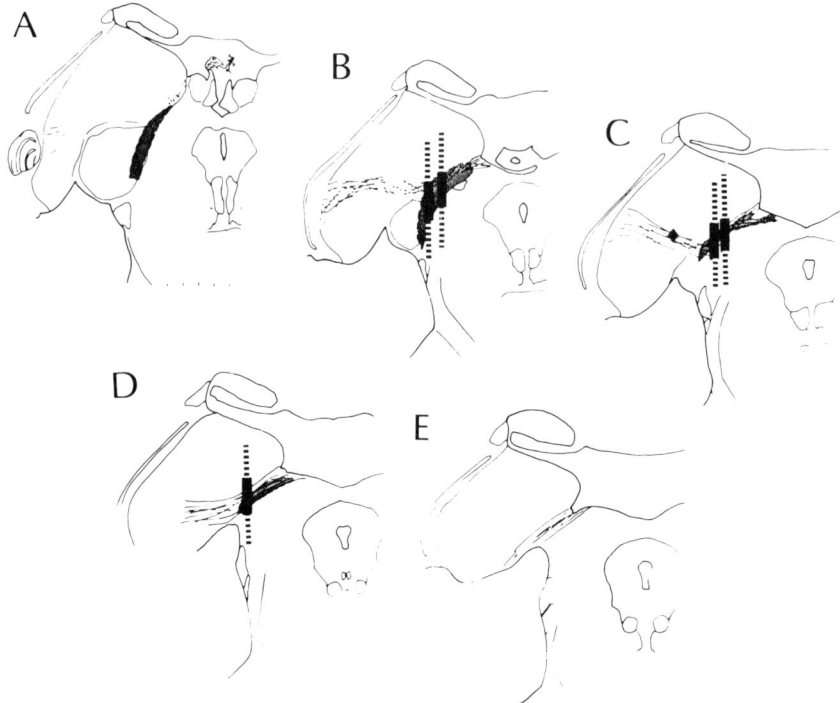

FIG. 5. A–D: Overlap of large kainic acid lesions of the pulvinar and MRF, respectively (*black areas*), and sites from which electrical stimulation induced horizontal nystagmus of the type shown in Figs. 2B and 3A. (See ref. 11 for full details of the kainic acid lesions in these animals.) Stimulus sites lay over the region that, when lesioned, produced a loss of OKAN and the slow component of OKN. **B–E** are the same as sections 1–4 in Fig. 1A. The areas shown in A–D overlap with the area that receives input from the retina, has GAD-staining cells, and projects to the inferior olive (Fig. 1B). The *diamond* in C shows a site where stimulation induced nystagmus and afternystagmus similar to that from NOT stimulation. Presumably, stimulation at this site activated fibers that input to NOT.

caudally through the pulvinar into NOT. One of these stimulus sites is shown by the dot in Fig. 5C. Presumably this bundle lies in the region of a fiber tract that carries projections from regions of the visual cortex where information related to motion and retinal slip is processed (49), such as the medial temporal (MT) and the medial superior temporal (MST) areas (50,51; Wurtz et al., *this volume*). Since stimulation of this fiber bundle elicited nystagmus with only a slow rise in slow-phase velocity, the cortical output responsible for OKN is probably split into pathways that carry activity for the slow and rapid components separately.

EFFECTS OF LESIONS OF NOT AND DTN

Electrolytic lesions were made in BCS in the region of NOT and DTN (11). In one animal, a small (1 mm) lesion destroyed the central, caudal, and lateral parts of NOT and most of DTN (Fig. 6A–C). Such a lesion would also interrupt the descending output pathways of the rostral medial NOT (Schiff, Buttner-Ennever, and Cohen, *unpublished data*). We also made larger kainic acid lesions that involved NOT and DTN in two animals. In both monkeys the lesions were large, extending in opposite directions into the mesencephalic reticular formation (MRF) and pulvinar (11). The common area of overlap of damage to NOT and DTN in these two animals is shown in black in Fig. 5 (11). Nystagmus was elicited from the same region by electrical stimulation (Fig. 5, bars) (10).

Each of the preceding lesions affected OKN and OKAN with slow phases toward the side of the lesion but caused no change in OKN and OKAN with contralateral slow phases. Immediately after lesion there was spontaneous

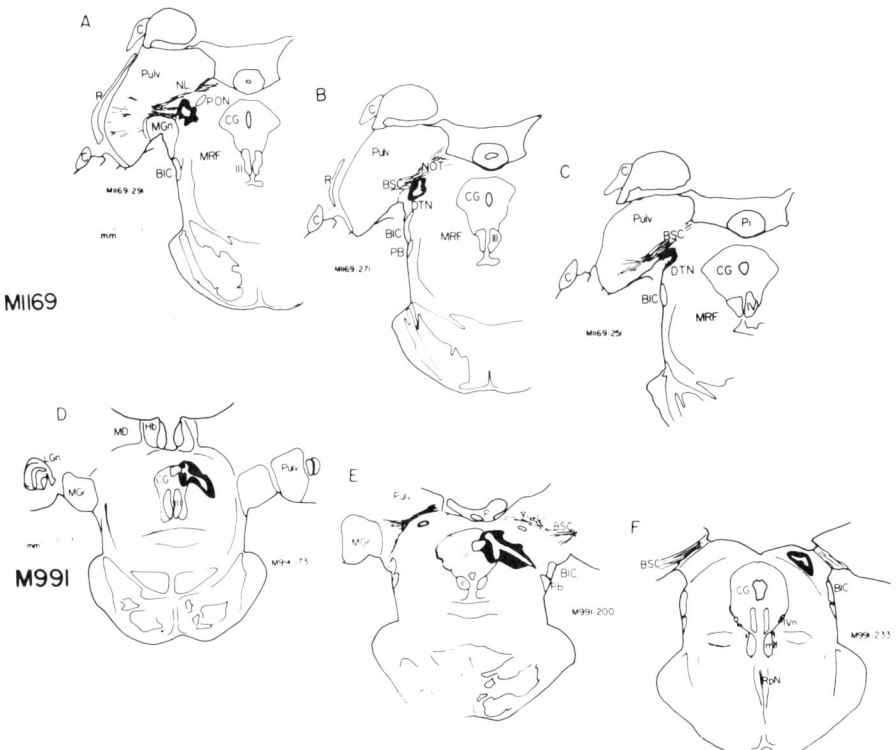

FIG. 6. A–C: Diagrams of an electrolytic lesion of NOT and DTN. The sections are separated by 300 μm. The lesion was approximately 1 mm in diameter. It lay in the caudal, lateral portion of NOT, in and under BSC, ventral and lateral to PON (A), and extended into DTN (C). This lesion caused the changes in OKN and OKAN shown in Fig. 8, i.e., a loss of the slow component of OKN and of OKAN. **D–F:** Vascular lesion involving the central gray, the caudal MRF, the medial pretectum, and the rostral superior colliculus. This lesion caused the deficit in the rapid rise in OKN shown in Fig. 9C. (Adapted from ref. 11.)

horizontal nystagmus with contralateral slow phases. This nystagmus subsided within several days. There was no obvious postural or behavioral modifications aside from a slight head tilt in one animal. The lesions did not affect vertical OKN or saccadic eye movements. Vestibular nystagmus was intact, and when tested 1 to 2 weeks after lesion, the slow-phase velocities of per- and postrotatory nystagmus were symmetrical and of normal gain.

OKN and OKAN after the electrolytic lesion of NOT and DTN of Fig. 6A–C is shown in Fig. 7. OKN with slow phases toward the side opposite the lesion was normal and was followed by OKAN whose peak velocity was close to 60°/sec (Fig. 7A). In contrast, OKN with ipsilateral slow phases was strongly affected (Fig. 7B). The eyes reached steady-state velocity immediately without a subsequent slow rise in velocity, and steady-state OKN was low, never exceeding 10°/sec. The initial jump was smaller than to the contralateral side. At the conclusion of OKN, there were only a few beats of OKAN.

Findings were similar after the kainic acid lesions. OKN and OKAN with slow phases to the contralateral side were unaffected. The preoperative OKN and OKAN with ipsilateral slow phases are shown in Fig. 8A. After lesion (Fig. 8B) the initial jump in OKN with slow-phase velocity toward the side of the lesion was lower than pre-operatively. Slow-phase eye velocity fluctuated irregularly during OKN, with peak velocities being held only for several beats. Steady-state eye velocities were lower than before lesion. At the end of stimulation there was no OKAN. Eye velocity fell abruptly and was followed by spontaneous nystagmus in the opposite direction.

In summary, steady-state OKN and OKAN with ipsilateral slow phases

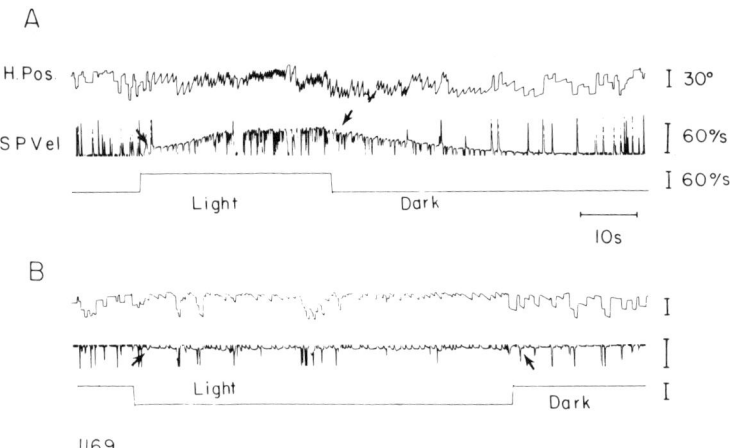

FIG. 7. OKN in response to movement of the visual surround at 60°/sec 18 days after the left-sided NOT lesion shown in Fig. 7A–C. *Arrows* show the onset and end of optokinetic stimulation. OKN and OKAN with contralateral slow phases were intact **(A)**. The slow rise in OKN with ipsilateral (left) slow phases was lost **(B)**, and there was little or no OKAN. Peak OKN velocity was less than 10°/sec toward the lesioned side (B).

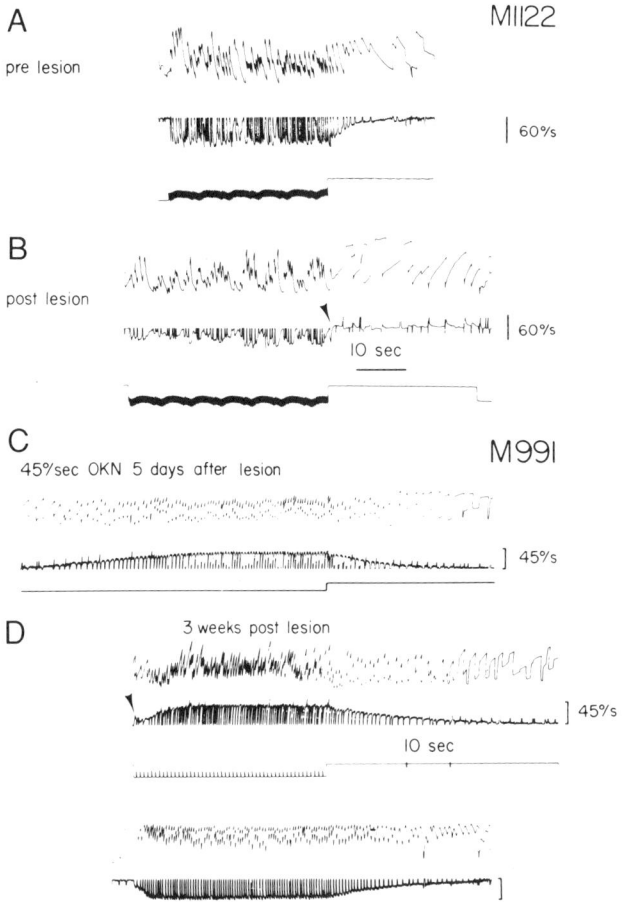

FIG. 8. A,B: Effects of destruction of NOT by kainic acid on OKN and OKAN. The preoperative OKN and OKAN are shown in A. After lesion (B), the rapid rise in slow-phase velocity at the onset of stimulation was somewhat reduced, OKN slow-phase velocities were not well maintained, and there was no OKAN at the end of stimulation. **C,D:** Alteration in OKN produced by the lesion of the MRF shown in Fig. 6D–F. After lesion (C), the initial jump in OKN was lost, and the rise in slow-phase eye velocity to a steady-state level was considerably prolonged. The OKAN was normal. The initial jump recovered several weeks later (D, *arrow*), so that the response was similar to OKN and OKAN to the contralateral side (lower panel). (From ref. 11.)

were strongly and permanently affected after NOT and DTN lesions. The initial jump in OKN was normal or was somewhat smaller. OKN and OKAN with contralateral slow phases were unaffected.

EFFECTS OF LESIONS OUTSIDE NOT AND DTN

Large bilateral electrolytic lesions in one monkey that destroyed the region designated as caudal MRF (cMRF) (52,53) had no effect on OKN or OKAN

(11). A kainic acid lesion of the superior colliculus also did not affect OKN or OKAN. However, a vascular lesion that involved the dorsal caudal MRF, the superior colliculus, and the adjacent central gray matter (Fig. 6D–F) altered OKN in a fashion that was quite different from the NOT and DTN lesions. The initial jump in velocity at the onset of optokinetic stimulation was lost, and slow rise in slow-phase velocity took much longer than before lesion (Fig. 8C). OKAN was unaffected. The loss of the rapid component of OKN in this monkey can be contrasted to the findings in the monkey whose results are shown in Fig. 8B where the predominant effect was on the slow component. Within a few weeks the animal had recovered its ability to accelerate its eyes rapidly at the onset of stimulation (Fig. 8D, arrow). OKN and OKAN with contralateral slow phases were not affected (Fig. 8D, bottom panel). Kainic acid injected into this region had no effect on OKN or OKAN. The failure of kainic acid to alter OKN or OKAN suggests that a fiber pathway located in the dorsal cMRF carries activity from the cortex to the brainstem for the initial jump in OKN.

The major input to NOT in the cat and monkey comes from the visual cortex (7), although NOT also gets activity directly from the retina (16,17). To provide a basis for comparison with NOT lesions, OKN and OKAN were studied in one monkey that had had bilateral removal of the occipital lobes (Fig. 9).[2] After the visual cortex was removed, the animal permanently lost its ability to produce rapid changes in slow-phase velocity during OKN. Maximum accelerations during optokinetic stimulation were approximately $2.5°/sec^2$ (Fig. 9B). Maximum velocities achieved during OKN were also limited to approximately $30°/sec$ (Fig. 9A and B). Rotation, which activated the vestibular system, caused a prompt rise in slow-phase velocity (Fig. 9C), showing that the peripheral oculomotor apparatus and the vestibulo-ocular pathways were functioning normally. Velocity storage was also intact since it could be charged by vestibular and optokinetic stimulation during rotation in light to reduce the postrotatory response when the animal was stopped in darkness (Fig. 9C, right). The difference in the maximum velocity of the per- and postrotatory step response in Fig. 10C was approximately $40°/sec$, which was the saturation velocity of OKAN in this animal.

This lesion demonstrates that when large areas of the visual cortex are removed and the main input to NOT is retinal, there is a limit to eye accelerations and maximal slow-phase eye velocity of OKN in response to movement of the full visual field. This supports the postulate of Hoffmann (4) that the major input to NOT in the normal monkey and cat is from the visual cortex and that direct input from the retina is of secondary importance in generating OKN. Zee et al. (54) came to a similar conclusion after occipital lobectomy.

---

[2] We thank Drs. Pedro and Tauba Pasik for allowing us to study this monkey from their series on effects of occipital lobectomy.

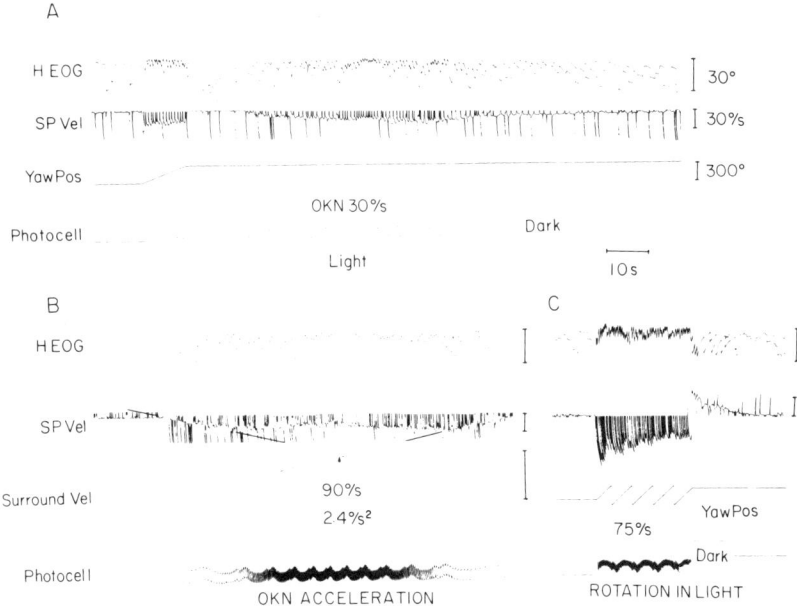

FIG. 9. Effects of removal of the occipital lobes on OKN and OKAN. The recordings were done several years after lesion. **A:** Movement of the visual surround at 30°/sec caused a slow increase in slow-phase velocity (SP Vel) to a peak value of 20°/sec. **B:** Peak acceleration of OKN was approximately 2.5°/sec^2, and peak velocities reached were approximately 15 to 20°/sec. **C:** Despite the deficit in visually induced nystagmus, the animal could rapidly change eye velocity during vestibular stimulation in light. The velocity storage mechanism was intact. (Compare the reduction in the postrotatory response at the end of rotation with the per-rotatory response at the onset of rotation. The two were of equal magnitude when elicited in darkness after the per-rotatory response had died away.)

Surprisingly, however, in the Zee et al. study the monkeys regained their ability to generate high velocity ocular pursuit after occipital lobectomy. This is evidence that there is considerable difference in the processing responsible for the rapid rise in OKN and for ocular pursuit.

DISCUSSION

We have demonstrated that the region of the brainstem that includes NOT and DTN contains that part of the visual-oculomotor pathway that produces the slow component of horizontal OKN and OKAN. Interpreted in terms of the model shown in Fig. 2.1C, NOT is the anatomical correlate of processing represented by the indirect pathway, and it drives the velocity storage integrator in the vestibular system. Support for this idea comes from the finding that stimulation of NOT could mimic many of the properties of velocity storage, including its ability to reduce or abolish postrotatory nystagmus (Fig. 3F). The implication of the latter is that activity in the velocity storage integrator that had originated in NOT is able to counteract activity originating in the semicircular canals.

Vestibular nuclei neurons that receive input from the lateral canals in the monkey respond to movement of the visual surround in the corresponding plane (34,35). However, their firing rates are related only to the slow rise in OKN and to OKAN, not to the rapid changes in eye velocity that occur at the beginning and end of OKN or when the VOR is suppressed visually. This suggests that these neurons get their visual input primarily from the velocity storage integrator and the indirect pathway. Taken together with the present results, this suggests that activity related to retinal slip in the animal's yaw plane that reaches the lateral semicircular canal-related neurons in the vestibular nuclei is channeled through NOT in the monkey as in the cat, rabbit, and rat (12). The target cells are likely to be neurons in the contralateral vestibular nuclei since they are responsible for producing eye movement to the contralateral side, which in this case would be ipsilateral to the NOT.

Only slow changes in eye velocity were produced by stimulation of NOT. This shows that the direct pathway, carrying activity for the rapid rise in OKN as well as pathways for ocular pursuit in the horizontal plane, are separate from the indirect pathway at the level of NOT. Pathways that carry activity related to retinal slip in planes other than an animal's yaw or horizontal plane are probably also located elsewhere.

A striking finding was that only slow phases toward the side of the lesion were induced by electrical stimulation or affected by NOT lesions and that contralatral and vertical OKAN slow phases were unaffected. The loss of ipsilateral slow phases during the slow component of OKN and during OKAN was permanent after unilateral NOT/DTN lesions and did not recover. This indicates that the pathways from the cortex to the oculomotor system that produce the rapid rise in OKN are not sufficient to excite velocity storage in the vestibular system. It also shows that pathways from NOT to the vestibular system carrying activity for producing horizontal OKAN and the slow component of OKN are strictly ipsilateral. Although push-pull activation has been described in neurons in NOT that process activity related to retinal slip (45), the animals did not appear to be able to utilize this activity to support OKN or to generate OKAN in the absence of the excitatory activity from NOT on the ipsilateral side.

Although the induced nystagmus from stimulation of NOT and DTN was predominantly horizontal when the animal was upright, vertical components of slow-phase velocity could be elicited when animals were tilted with regard to gravity (Fig. 4B and C). This shows that gravity plays an important role in determining how the signal coming from NOT is interpreted in a three-dimensional sense (47,48). It is unlikely that the vertical components of the nystagmus arose in NOT. Rather, they probably were elicited at the level of the vestibular nuclei, with information that arises in the otolith organs and possibly the somatosensory system, acting as a gating mechanism to distribute the velocity command signal to horizontal and vertical second-order vestibular nuclei neurons.

There was a striking congruence between the area identified by electric stimulation (10) and the region that, when lesioned, caused the greatest deficits in the slow component of OKN and OKAN (11) (Fig. 5). This supports the idea that the indirect pathway, responsible for the slow component of OKN and for OKAN, lies in NOT. From this it is possible to consider the characteristics of NOT projection neurons that carry activity for the slow component of OKN somewhat more closely. They should receive retinal slip information from the cortex and retina, and eventually project to the vestibular nuclei on the contralateral side. How the activity reaches the vestibular nuclei is not certain, although it could be directed through the prepositus nucleus (19,55).

In contrast to the preferential effect of NOT/DTN lesions on the slow component of OKN and on OKAN, a vascular lesion of the dorsal caudal MRF affected only the rapid component of OKN, leaving the slow component intact. The slow rise in velocity was prolonged after lesion (Fig. 8C), similar to the prolongation of the slow rise after the loss of the direct pathway after flocculectomy (27), ablation of the visual cortex (Fig. 9) (54), or destruction of the dorsolateral pontine nucleus (56). The long slow rise after removal of the direct pathway can be explained by increased retinal slip plus the effect of a nonlinear processing element that is present in visual-oculomotor pathways, probably at the level of NOT (27,54).

The effects of the vascular lesion of Fig. 6D–F can be contrasted with the effects of a kainic acid lesion of the same region that only destroyed cells. The latter did not alter either OKN or OKAN. This suggests that that activity responsible for the rapid component of OKN is probably carried in a fiber tract from the visual cortex that courses through MRF just at the lateral margins of the central gray, anterior to the superior colliculus. Presumably it reaches the dorsolateral pontine nucleus (56), before projecting to the region of the flocculus and paraflocculus. The transient nature of the deficit in the initial jump in OKN slow-phase velocity produced by the MRF lesion is consistent with the transient nature of the pursuit deficits reported by Newsome et al. (50) after MT and MST lesions (Wurtz et al., *this volume*).

One other class of lesions affected OKN and OKAN, although transiently, namely, partial lesions of the fiber tract in the lateral pulvinar that projects to BSC. Characteristic nystagmus with only a slow component and afternystagmus were induced by electrical stimulation at these locations. Two animals with incomplete lesions of this fiber tract had similar effects: the rising time constant of OKAN was slowed, and the maximum velocity of steady-state OKN was transiently reduced. The rapid rise in OKN was unaffected. It seems likely that cortical information, which makes a major contribution to NOT and to the indirect pathway in the cat and primate (45), reaches NOT and DTN through this fiber bundle.

CLINICAL IMPLICATIONS

The importance of the pathway through NOT and DTN to the vestibular system in the primate has not been widely appreciated. If movement of the entire visual field occurs mainly during head movement on the body or during body movement in space, then the pathway through NOT provides a major component of the visual input that signals yaw or horizontal head on body or body in space velocity to cells in the vestibular nuclei. One implication is that disruption of this input could affect spatial orientation, perception of motion, and balance and coordination. As we and Kato and colleagues (8,9) have shown, this pathway is of great importance for production of horizontal OKN in the monkey. The same is probably true in humans.

Spontaneous horizontal nystagmus is frequently observed after deep lesions of the cerebrum. This nystagmus has not been easy to explain, particularly in view of the finding that nystagmus is not readily induced by cortical, thalamic, or collicular stimulation (57,58). A zone was originally described in the upper brainstem of the rabbit that, when stimulated, cause brisk horizontal nystagmus with ipsilateral slow phases (nystagmogenic zone) (59,60). In the rabbit this zone lies in and around NOT (2). Given that NOT appears to function similarly in primates as in lateral-eyed animals in producing OKN and OKAN, the nystagmus observed after upper brainstem lesions could be due to involvement of NOT and DTN or to damage to their input and output pathways. Alternatively, such nystagmus could be caused by damage of pathways that carry information from the visual cortex to the brainstem for production of the initial jump in OKN.

Based on our results we would expect that several clinical syndromes might be present in humans after lesions of the mesencephalon in the region of the pretectum. Damage that involved NOT and DTN, which interrupted the slow or indirect pathway to the vestibular nuclei, initially should be associated with spontaneous horizontal nystagmus in darkness. This nystagmus should have contralateral slow phases with quick phases toward the side of the lesion. There should also be some reduction of steady-state OKN and a loss of OKAN with ipsilateral slow phases during nystagmus with quick phases away from the side of the lesion. We found a limited reduction in the initial rapid rise in horizontal OKN after lesions confined to NOT (11), but it is not clear whether the initial rapid rise would also be affected in humans. Vertical OKN and OKAN should be preserved, and vestibular function should be intact after the spontaneous nystagmus subsides. According to the results of Kato et al. (8,9), horizontal ocular pursuit should be normal if only NOT and DTN are involved, although Hoffmann et al. (18) recently suggested that the presence of cells sensitive to high velocities of retinal slip in NOT may imply a relationship between activity in NOT and ocular pursuit.

Lesions of the MRF, medial to the pretectum and just rostral to the superior colliculus, on the other hand, would interrupt the direct optokinetic pathway, carrying activity for the initial rapid rise in ipsilateral slow-phase velocity for

OKN and possibly for ocular pursuit. Velocity storage is considerably weaker in humans than in monkeys (61,62), and the direct pathway is responsible for the major portion of the response (61). Therefore, one would expect more drastic effects of a lesion of the direct pathway in the caudal MRF on horizontal OKN in humans than in monkeys. OKAN should be preserved, vertical OKN and OKAN should be normal, and vestibular function should be intact in these patients.

Given that the distance between NOT and the caudal MRF is small, it is not unlikely that upper brainstem lesions might involve both regions and produce effects on all components of the optokinetic response. This would result in an alteration of both the rapid rise and steady-state velocity of OKN and OKAN with ipsilateral slow phases and contralateral quick phases. Thus, the strong effects on OKN and OKAN of large lesions of the MRF of the monkey, noted by Komatsuzaki et al. (63) and Bender and Shanzer (64) are probably best explained by damage of both the direct pathways in MRF and of the indirect pathway in NOT. It should be stressed that the deficits under discussion would be in horizontal nystagmus and that the alterations in vertical eye movements that occur after lesions of the medial pretectum (65-67) would not be present after lesions confined to lateral portions of the brainstem at the junction of the superior colliculus and the caudal pulvinar, in the region of BSC.

In summary, we have shown that lesions that involve NOT and DTN strongly affect the slow component of horizontal OKN and OKAN, leaving vestibular nystagmus intact. We conclude that NOT and DTN process information for the slow component of OKN and for OKAN with ipsilateral slow phases via the indirect pathway. This pathway excites the velocity storage integrator in the vestibular system, allowing it to interact with activity arising in the semicircular canals. Functionally, this pathway supports slow-phase velocity during per-rotatory nystagmus and suppresses it during postrotatory responses. The target cells of NOT activity are likely to be neurons in the contralateral vestibular nuclei that receive input from the lateral semicircular canals, unless they are type II neurons in the ipsilateral vestibular nuclei. The input pathway to NOT and DTN from the visual cortex is probably carried through BSC. The direct pathway appears to be carried in a fiber tract through the dorsal caudal MRF, adjacent to the central gray and rostral superior colliculus. The physiological findings suggest that NOT and DTN may be important for processing visual information related to horizontal head movement and locomotion. The finding that NOT and DTN are of importance in subhuman primates suggests that similar syndromes of dysfunction related to interruption of direct and indirect pathways after NOT or MRF lesions may also be present in humans.

SUMMARY

1. The role of the pretectal NOT and the DTN in producing horizontal OKN and OKAN were studied using electrical stimulation and lesions. Posi-

tive stimulation sites lay in NOT, DTN, and in a fiber bundle in the pulvinar that is presumably a cortical input to NOT.

2. When the region of NOT was electrically stimulated in darkness, horizontal nystagmus was evoked with ipsilateral slow phases. Eye velocity rose slowly to a steady-state level and was followed by afternystagmus at the end of stimulation. The time constant of rise of stimulus-induced nystagmus was similar to the slow rise of slow-phase eye velocity during OKN. The saturation velocity of the induced nystagmus and the falling time constant of the stimulus afternystagmus were the same as those of OKAN. This suggests that electrical stimulation of NOT and DTN had elicited the slow component of OKN, i.e., that component produced by the velocity storage mechanism in the vestibular system.

3. Consistent with this postulate, activity induced by NOT stimulation could enhance, prolong, or block the slow component of OKN and OKAN depending on whether slow phases were to the same or opposite side. Stimulus-induced activity also interacted with vestibular nystagmus as would OKN and OKAN.

4. Unilateral lesions of NOT and DTN caused a loss of OKAN and the slow rise in OKN to the ipsilateral side. Steady-state velocities of OKN were reduced. The initial jump of OKN slow-phase velocity was the same or somewhat less after lesions but was not lost.

5. Partial lesions of a fiber bundle in the lateral pulvinar caused a transient change in OKN and OKAN, consistent with the idea that it carries activity for the slow component from the cortex to NOT. A lesion of the MRF, just rostral to the superior colliculus, caused a transient loss of the rapid component of OKN. This region appears to carry activity responsible for the initial jump in slow-phase velocity at the onset of stimulation.

6. We conclude that: (a) NOT and probably DTN lie in the indirect pathway that produces the slow component of horizontal OKN and OKAN to the ipsilateral side in the rhesus monkey. This pathway activates the velocity storage mechanism in the vestibular nuclei. (b) At the level of NOT, the pathway responsible for the slow component of OKN and OKAN is anatomically distinct from the pathway responsible for rapid changes in eye velocity at the onset of OKN. (c) The system is organized to produce ipsilateral changes in slow-phase velocity and does not rebalance itself when the input from one NOT is lost. (d) Clinical syndromes may be present in humans after lesions of NOT or of the MRF that are similar to those in the monkey.

ACKNOWLEDGMENTS

This work was supported by NEI grant EY02296, Core Center Grant EY01867, and Training Grants NS07245 and SFB 220/08. We gratefully acknowledge the help of Drs. Anja Horn, Klaus-Peter Hoffmann, Robert Spencer, Tauba Pasik, and Pedro Pasik in making experimental material available to us that was used in the preparation of this chapter.

REFERENCES

1. Collewijn H. Direction selective units in the rabbit's nucleus of the optic tract. *Brain Res* 1975;100:489–508.
2. Collewijn H. Oculomotor areas in the rabbit's midbrain and pretectum. *J Neurobiol* 1975;6:3–22.
3. Cazin L, Precht W, Lannou J. Pathways mediating optokinetic responses of vestibular nucleus neurons in the rat. *Pflugers Arch* 1980;384:19–29.
4. Hoffmann KP. Cortical versus subcortical contributions to the optokinetic reflex in the cat. In: Lennerstrand G, et al., eds. *Functional basis of ocular motility disorders.* Oxford: Pergamon Press, 1982;303–310.
5. Maekawa K, Takeda T, Kimura M. Responses of the nucleus of the optic tract neurons projecting to the nucleus reticularis tegmenti pontis upon optokinetic stimulation in the rabbit. *Neurosci Res* 1984;2:1–25.
6. Hess BJM, Precht W, Reber A, Cazin L. Horizontal optokinetic ocular nystagmus in the pigmented rat. *Neuroscience* 1985;15:97–107.
7. Hoffmann KP, Distler C. The role of direction selective cells in the nucleus of the optic tract of cat and monkey during optokinetic nystagmus. In: Keller EL, Zee DS, eds. *Adaptive processes in visual and oculomotor systems, vol 57.* Oxford/New York: Pergamon Press, 1986;261–266.
8. Kato I, Harada K, Hasegawa T, Igarashi T, Koike Y, Kawasaki T. Role of the nucleus of the optic tract in monkeys in relation to optokinetic nystagmus. *Brain Res* 1986;364:12–22.
9. Kato I, Harada K, Hasegawa K, Koike Y. Role of the nucleus of the optic tract of monkeys in optokinetic nystagmus and optokinetic-afternystagmus. *Brain Res* 1988;474:16–27.
10. Schiff D, Cohen B, Raphan T. Nystagmus induced by stimulation of the nucleus of the optic tract in the monkey. *Exp Brain Res* 1988;70:1–14.
11. Schiff D, Cohen B, Buettner-Ennever J, Matsuo V. Effects of lesions of the nucleus of the optic tract on optokinetic nystagmus and after-nystagmus in the monkey. *Exp Brain Res (in press).*
12. Simpson JI, Giolli RA, Blanks R. Anatomy of the accessory optic system. In: Buettner J, ed. *Anatomy of the oculomotor system. Progress in oculomotor research.* Amsterdam: Elsevier *(in press).*
13. Cohen B, Matsuo V, Raphan T. Quantitative analysis of the velocity characteristics of optokinetic nystagmus and optokinetic after-nystagmus. *J Physiol (Lond)* 1977;270:321–344.
14. Cohen B, Helwig D, Raphan T. Baclofen and velocity storage: a model of the effects of the drug on the vestibulo-ocular reflex. *J Physiol (Lond)* 1987;393:703–725.
15. Lin H, Giolli RA. Accessory optic system of rhesus monkey. *Exp Neurol* 1979;63:163–176.
16. Ballas I, Hoffmann KP, Wagner HJ. Retinal projection to the nucleus of the optic tract in the cat as revealed by retrograde transport of horseradish peroxide. *Neurosci Lett* 1981;26:197–202.
17. Hutchins R, Weber JT. The pretectal complex of the monkey: a reinvestigation of the morphology and retinal terminations. *J Comp Neurol* 1985;232:425–442.
18. Hoffman KP, Distler C, Erickson RG, Mader W. Physiological and anatomical identification of the nucleus of the optic tract and dorsal terminal nucleus of the accessory optic tract in monkeys. *Exp Brain Res* 1988;69:635–644.
19. Holstege G, Collewijn H. The efferent connections of the nucleus of the optic tract and the superior colliculus in the rabbit. *J Comp Neurol* 1982;209:139–175.
20. Giolli RA, Peterson GM, Ribak CE, McDonald HM, Blanks RHI, Fallon JH. GABAergic neurons comprise a major cell type in rodent relay visual nuclei: an immunocytochemical study of pretectal and accessory optic nuclei. *Exp Brain Res* 1985;61:194–203.
21. Mugnaini E, Oertel WH. An atlas of the distribution of GABAergic neurons and terminals in the rat CNS as revealed by GAD immunohistochemistry. In: Bjorklund A, Hokfelt T, eds. *Handbook of chemical neuroanatomy, vol 4: GABA and neuropeptide in the CNS.* 1985;436–605.
22. Horn AKE, Hoffmann KP. Combined GABA-immunochemistry and TMB-HRP histochemistry of pretectal nuclei projecting to the inferior olive in rats, cats and monkeys. *Brain Res* 1987;409:133–138.

23. Hood JD. Observations upon the neurological mechanism of optokinetic nystagmus with especial reference to the contribution of peripheral vision. *Acta Otolaryngol (Stockh)* 1967;63:208–215.
24. Dichgans J, Nauck B, Wolpert E. The influence of attention, vigilance and stimulus area on optokinetic and vestibular nystagmus and voluntary saccades. In: Zikmund V, ed. *The oculomotor system and brain functions: proceedings of the international colloquium.* London: Butterworths, 1973;280–294.
25. Solomon D, Cohen B. Relative contributions of compensatory head and eye movements to visual stabilization during circular locomotion in light. *Soc Neurosi Abstr* 1988;14(pt 1):332.
26. Raphan T, Matsuo V, Cohen B. Velocity storage in the vestibulo-ocular reflex arc (VOR) *Exp Brain Res* 1979;35:229–248.
27. Waespe W, Cohen B, Raphan T. Role of the flocculus and paraflocculus in optokinetic nystagmus and visual-vestibular interactions: effects of lesions. *Exp Brain Res* 1983;50:9–33.
28. Raphan T, Cohen B. Velocity storage and the ocular response to multidimensional vestibular stimuli. In: Berthoz A, Melvill Jones G, eds. *Adaptive mechanisms in gaze control: facts and theories.* Amsterdam: Elsevier, 1985;123–143.
29. Waespe W. Cohen B, Raphan T. Dynamic modifications of the vestibulo-ocular reflex in the nodulus and uvula. *Science* 1985;228:199–202.
30. Lisberger S, Fuchs AF. Role of primate flocculus during rapid behavioral modification of vestibulo-ocular reflex. I. Purkinje cell activity during visually guided horizontal smooth-pursuit eye movements and passive head rotation. *J Neurophysiol* 1978;45:733–763.
31. Waespe W, Henn V. Visual-vestibular interaction in the flocculus of the alert monkey. II. Purkinje cell activity. *Exp Brain Res* 1981;43:349–360.
32. Waespe, W, Rudinger D, Wolfensberger M. Purkinje cell activity in the flocculus of vestibular neurectomized and normal monkeys during optokinetic nystagmus and smooth pursuit eye movements. *Exp Brain Res* 1985;60:243–262.
33. Zee DS, Yamazaki A, Butler PH, Gucer G. Effects of ablation of flocculus and paraflocculus on eye movements in primate. *J Neurophysiol* 1981;46:878–899.
34. Waespe W, Henn V. Neuronal activity in the vestibular nuclei of the alert monkey during vestibular and optokinetic stimulation. *Exp Brain Res* 1977;27:523–538.
35. Waespe W, Henn V. Vestibular nuclei activity during optokinetic after-nystagmus (OKAN) in the alert monkey. *Exp Brain Res* 1977;30:323–330.
36. Uemura T, Cohen B. Effects of vestibular nuclei lesions on vestibulo-ocular reflexes and posture in monkeys. *Acta Otolaryngol [Suppl] (Stockh)* 1973;315:1–71.
37. Collewijn H. Impairment of optokinetic (after-)nystagmus by labyrinthectomy in the rabbit. *Exp Neurol* 1976;52:146–156.
38. Zee DS, Yee RD, Robinson DA. Optokinetic response in labyrinthine-defective human beings. *Brain Res* 1976;113:423–428.
39. Cohen B, Suzuki JI, Raphan T. Role of the otolith organs in generation of horizontal nystagmus; effects of selective labyrinthine lesions. *Brain Res* 1983;276:159–164.
40. DeJong JMBV, Cohen B, Matsuo V, Uemura T. Midsagittal pontomedullary brainstem section: effects on ocular adduction and nystagmus. *Exp Neurol* 1980;68:420–442.
41. Blair SM, Gavin M. Brainstem commissures and control of time constant of vestibular nystagmus. *Acta Otolaryngol (Stockh)* 1981;91:1–8.
42. Collewijn H. Latency and gain of the rabbit's optokinetic reactions to small movements. *Brain Res* 1972;36:59–70.
43. Precht W, Cazin L, Blanks R, Lannou J. Anatomy and physiology of the optokinetic pathways to the vestibular nuclei in the rat. In: Roucoux A, Crommelinck M, eds. *Physiological and pathological aspects of eye movements.* The Hague: Dr. Junk, 1982;153–172.
44. Evinger C, Fuchs AF. Saccadic, smooth pursuit, and optokinetic eye movements of the trained cat. *J Physiol (Lond)* 1978;285:209–229.
45. Hoffmann KP. Visual inputs relevant for the optokinetic nystagmus in mammals. In: Freund H-J, Buttner U, Cohen B, Noth J, eds. *The oculomotor and skeletalmotor systems: differences and similarties.* Progress in Brain Research, vol 64. Amsterdam: Elsevier, 1986;75–84.
46. Ter Braak JW. Untersuchungen ueber optokinetischen Nystagmus. *Arch Neerl Physiol* 1936;21:309–376.
47. Raphan T, Cohen B. Multidimensional organization of the vestibulo-ocular reflex. In: Keller

EL, Zee DS, eds. *Adaptive processes in visual and oculomotor systems.* Advances in the Biosciences, vol 57. Oxford/New York: Pergamon Press, 1986;285–292.
48. Raphan T, Cohen B. Three dimensional structure of velocity storage and its functional significance. *Ann NY Acad Sci* 1988;545:239–247.
49. Huerta MF, Weber JT, Rothstein LR, Harting JK. Subcortical connections of area 17 in the tree shrew: an autoradiographic analysis. *Brain Res* 1985;340:163–170.
50. Newsome WT, Wurtz RH, Dursteler M, Mikami A. Deficits in visual motion processing following ibotenic acid lesion of the middle temporal visual area of the macaque monkey. *J Neurosci* 1985;5:825–840.
51. Dursteler M, Wurtz RH, et al. Effects of lesions of MT and MST on optokinetic nystagmus in monkeys. *J Neurophysiol (in press).*
52. Cohen B, Buettner-Ennever JA. Projections from the superior colliculus to a region of the central mesencephalic reticular formation (cMRF) associated with horizontal eye movements. *Exp Brain Res* 1984;57:167–176.
53. Cohen B, Waitzman D, Buttner-Ennever JA, Matsuo V. Horizontal saccades and the central mesencephalic reticular formation. In: Freund H-J, Buttner U, Cohen B, Noth J, eds. *The oculomotor and skeletalmotor systems: differences and similarities.* Progress in Brain Research, vol 64. Amsterdam: Elsevier, 1986;243–256.
54. Zee DS, Tusa RJ, Butler PH, Herman SJ, Gucer C. Effects of occipital lobectomy upon eye movements in primates. *J Neurophysiol* 1987;58:883–901.
55. Magnin M, Courjon JH, Flandrin JM. Possible visual pathways to the cat vestibular nuclei involving the nucleus prepositus hypoglossi. *Exp Brain Res* 1983;51:198–203.
56. May JG, Keller EL, Suzuki DA. Smooth pursuit eye movement deficits with chemical lesions in the dorsolateral pontine nucleus of the monkey. *J Neurophysiol* 1988;59:952–977.
57. Ferrier D. *The functions of the brain.* New York: GP Putnam, 1876.
58. Wagman IH. Eye movements induced by electric stimulation of cerebrum in monkeys and their relationship to bodily movements. In: Bender MB, ed. *The oculomotor system.* New York: Hoeber Medical Division, Harper and Row, 1964;18–39.
59. Lachmann J, Bergmann F, Monnier M. Central nystagmus elicited by stimulation of the meso-diencephalon in the rabbit. *Am J Physiol* 1958;193:328–334.
60. Bergmann F, Chaimovitz J, Gutman J, Zelig S. Optokinetic nystagmus and its interaction with central nystagmus. *J Physiol (Lond)* 1963;168:318–331.
61. Cohen B, Henn V, Raphan T, Dennett D. Velocity storage, nystagmus and visual-vestibular interactions in human. In: Cohen B, eds. *Vestibular and oculomotor physiology. Ann NY Acad Sci* 1981;374:421–433.
62. Lafortune S, Ireland DJ, Jell RM, Duval L. Human optokinetic afternystagmus. Charging characteristics and stimulus exposure time dependence in the two-component model. *Acta Otolaryngol (Stockh)* 1986;101:353–360.
63. Komatsuzaki A, Alpert J, Harris HE, Cohen B. Effect of mesencephalic reticular formation lesions on optokinetic nystagmus. *Exp Neurol* 1972;34:522–534.
64. Bender MB, Shanzer S. Oculomotor pathways defined by electric stimulation and lesions in the brainstem of monkeys. In: Bender MB, ed. *The oculomotor system.* New York: Hoeber Medical Division, Harper and Row, 1964;81–140.
65. Pasik P, Pasik T, Bender MB. The pretectal syndrome in monkeys. I. Disturbances of gaze and body posture. *Brain* 1969;92:521–534.
66. Christoff N. A clinicopathological study of vertical eye movements. *Arch Neurol* 1974;31:1–8.
67. Bender MB. Brain control of conjugate horizontal and vertical eye movements. A survey of the structural and functional correlates. *Brain* 1980;103:23–69.

Vision and the Brain,
edited by B. Cohen and I. Bodis-Wollner.
Raven Press, Ltd., New York © 1990.

Developing a Functional Anatomy of the Human Visual System with Positron Emission Tomography

Marcus E. Raichle

Mallinckrodt Institute of Radiology, Department of Neurology and Neurological Surgery, McDonnell Center for Studies of Higher Brain Function, The Washington University Medical Center, St. Louis, Missouri 63110

Emission tomography is a technique that produces an image of the distribution of a previously administered radionuclide in any desired section of the body. Positron emission tomography (PET) uses the unique properties of the annihilation radiation that is generated when positrons are absorbed in matter (1) to provide an image that is a highly accurate representation of the spatial distribution of the radionuclide at a selected plane through the tissue. Such an image is effectively equivalent to a quantitative tissue autoradiogram obtained with laboratory animals, but PET has the added advantage that it is noninvasive, hence studies are possible in living animals, including humans. PET has been used in humans to measure brain blood flow, blood volume, metabolism of glucose and oxygen, acid-base balance, receptor pharmacology, and transmitter metabolism (for an introduction to this literature, see [2]). In this chapter, I focus on the measurement of brain blood flow.

Interest in the relationship between brain blood flow and local functional activity has spanned nearly a century. The initial interest crystallized when Roy and Sherrington (3) published their seminal paper in 1890 in which they put forth the suggestion that there exists an "automatic mechanism" that provides for a local variation of the blood supply in accordance with local variations of the functional activity of the brain. Although the experiments of Roy and Sherrington were imperfect in many ways by today's standards, their hypothesis has compelled investigators to pursue the envisioned relationships in order to better understand the function of the brain.

Even before the development of modern tracer methodology in the middle of this century, several early experiments indicated the correctness of the hypothesis of Roy and Sherrington (3) and gave us our first *in vivo* observations of the visual system of humans. In 1928 Fulton (4) studied a patient of Dr. Harvey Cushing at the Peter Brent Brigham Hospital in Boston. The patient was operated on for an arteriovenous malformation of the occipital lobe that proved to be unresectable, and he was left with a craniotomy defect over which a bruit associated with the malformation was easily heard with a stethoscope. The patient reported that the noise in the back of his head intensified whenever he used his eyes. Fulton pursued this observation and was able to confirm that the audible bruit over the occipital lobe increased during visual stimulation and that no other stimulus had an effect on it. Within 10 years, two additional experiments (5,6), both involving studies of the visual system in laboratory animals, confirmed the hypothesis of Roy and Sherrington that functional activity in the visual system as well as elsewhere in the brain is associated with local changes in brain blood flow. The subsequent development of radiotracer techniques for the measurement of local brain blood flow and metabolism in laboratory animals and in humans led to confirmation of these pioneering observations (see [7] for review of this literature).

In this chapter I outline a strategy employing PET measurements of local brain blood flow that we have developed to do highly accurate functional mapping of the human brain and present data that we have obtained on the human visual system in support of the hypothesis that PET is useful in developing a detailed functional anatomy of the human brain.

THE DEVELOPMENT OF A PET STRATEGY

The facts that PET can measure local brain blood flow in humans and local blood flow is closely linked to changes in functional activity should make PET an ideal technique for functional mapping of the human brain. However, a number of important questions must be answered before using PET in this way. Thus, why do we measure blood flow instead of metabolism? How can responses measured with PET be related objectively to brain anatomy? How accurately can responses measured with PET be localized given the low spatial resolution of PET? How can low-level responses be distinguished from noise? Finally, how do we know which responses are significant? I would like to address each of these questions briefly and then outline the actual strategy that we employ.

Blood Flow or Metabolism: What Should Be Measured?

Conventional wisdom suggests that functionally induced changes in neuronal activity are accompanied by changes in oxygen consumption and glucose utilization supported by an increase in blood flow to supply needed oxygen and replenish depleted glucose stores. Thus, any one of the three could be used to develop a functional anatomy with PET. In fact, all three have been used by different investigators working with PET (7). However, recent work from our laboratory has produced the somewhat surprising finding that local increases in functional activity are accompanied by parallel increases in blood flow and glucose consumption but only minimal increases in oxygen consumption (8,9). Thus, the measurement of oxygen consumption can be eliminated as sensitive marker of changes in neuronal activity during increases in functional activity.

Although glucose consumption parallels blood flow during changes in functional activity, its measurement with PET is hampered by the fact that measurement of brain glucose consumption, using the deoxyglucose method developed by Sokoloff and colleagues (10) and the tracer ^{18}F-fluorodeoxyglucose (11), requires 45 min to complete and is difficult to repeat even once in a single setting (the feasibility of a single repeat study in one setting has been increased somewhat by the use of ^{11}C-deoxyglucose [12]). Because of the long measurement time (i.e., 45 min) the measurement of glucose utilization is vulnerable to fatigue on the part of the subject as well as adaptive changes in the brain during such a prolonged period of time. Experience in our laboratory (*unpublished data*) confirms the existence of both of these problems.

In comparison with the lack of sensitivity of oxygen consumption to changes in functional activity and the rather slow and cumbersome nature of the measurement of glucose metabolism (11), measurement of local blood flow with PET following the intravenous bolus injection of ^{15}O-water (13–16) using an adaptation of the classic Kety tissue autoradiographic technique is fast (40 sec for a single measurement), sensitive, and easily repeatable (as many as 10 measurements in a single setting) due to the short half-life of the radionuclide (^{15}O, half-life 2 min) used to label the tracer ^{15}O-water and the short measurement time. Although actual quantitation of blood flow in units of ml/(min × 100 g) requires timed sampling of arterial blood during the measurement, which we have done safely from the radial artery in nearly 1,500 subjects, responses to functional activation can be estimated accurately from the regional radioactive counts obtained in the PET image because of the near-linear relationship between radioactive counts and the computed blood flow using this method (14). It should be noted that other methods of measuring blood flow with PET (17) do not exhibit this linear relationship between blood flow and radioactive counts in the tissue.

Anatomical Localization

Determining the relationship between physiology and anatomy is one of the objectives of most functional studies with PET. Although physiological images of the brain often contain some anatomical information, correspondence between physiology and anatomy cannot be assumed. Despite this fact, some investigators have based their judgments about anatomical localization on the appearance of the physiological PET image of blood flow or glucose uptake. This practice is not satisfactory. Localization schemes based on scanning in planes parallel to a standard cranial reference plane (e.g., the orbitomeatal line) with subsequent regional comparisons with a tomographic atlas of the brain have been widely used. Yet this approach is both subjective and inaccurate due to the well-described variability in the relationship of the brain to standard reference planes (see [7] for a review of the literature). Some investigators have attempted to circumvent these difficulties by also making a structural image for each subject in closely matched anatomical planes using either X-ray computed tomography or magnetic resonance proton images. Although this approach is attractive in many respects potentially permitting accurate anatomical localization in each subject, its shortcomings must be appreciated. First and most important, accurate regional comparisons of the PET images of different subjects are not possible with a method that is based on the comparisons of each subject's PET image with his or her own structural image. Differences in subject positioning cannot be easily overcome. Second, localization depends on the presence of gross anatomical boundaries evident on the structural image. A lack of such demarcation between different cortical regions makes localization within the cerebral cortex difficult.

In order to overcome these difficulties we have developed an anatomical localization procedure for physiological imaging that is based on the well-established principles of neurosurgical stereotaxy (18). This approach determines the anatomical location of a PET region of interest with the coordinate system of atlases for stereotaxic neurological surgery. Measurements made from a lateral skull radiograph and from a tomographic transmission scan form the basis of this method. The method is accurate, objective, and not dependent on visual inspection of either a physiological or structural tomographic image. Regions defined by this procedure can be easily compared among subjects in a study and among different subject populations within a laboratory. Comparisons of data from different laboratories are also possible when this procedure is used.

Response Localization versus Spatial Resolution

Spatial resolution has always been a concern to investigators contemplating the use of PET for physiological studies. Operationally, the spatial resolution of PET is based on the spatial distribution of measured radioactivity produced by a single point source of radioactivity. This spatial distribution of radioactivity is a blurred representation of the original point source of radioactivity with the highest counting rate at its center. The resolution of a PET system is defined as the width of this distribution of radioactivity at one-half of the maximum counting rate, the so-called full width at half maximum, usually abbreviated FWHM. One very important consequence of this definition of resolution is that when two point sources of radioactivity occur simultaneously in the field of view of a PET device, they cannot be distinguished as two separate sources if they are closer than a distance of 1 FWHM. Further, accurate quantitation of radioactivity in a particular region of the brain requires that the region be approximately twice the FWHM in all dimensions. PET devices currently operational have spatial resolutions, defined as the FWHM, in the range of 10 to 20 mm. The ultimate resolution of PET defined in this way has not been clearly established but will be limited by factors such as the distance traveled in tissue by the positron before annihilation (usually approximately 2 to 3 mm), slight deviation of the paths of the two annihilation photons from colinearity, and the statistical quality of the data. It is realistic to anticipate that reconstruction of some PET images to a resolution of 5 to 6 mm will be possible, although this is still less than optimal for functional mapping.

Functional studies with PET allow an additional, very important perspective on the issue of spatial resolution. By functional studies I mean studies in which some type of activation paradigm is employed to produce a change in local blood flow from a resting or control state. Under such circumstances the data can be used to determine whether areas separated by significantly less than 1 FWHM are differentially activated by specific alterations in the stimulus condition (19,20). This expectation is based on signal detection theory, which has also been used to explain the phenomenon of hyperacuity in vision perception. Experimental strategy rather than the inherent spatial resolution of the tomograph defines the operational resolution of such a study. To implement such a strategy we obtain paired images of blood flow measured with ^{15}O-water, one in a control state and one during a desired type of functional activity different from the control state. These two images are obtained from the same subject in the same experimental setting. By first linearly scaling the images to a laboratory standard we eliminate global changes in blood flow between measurements and permit direct subtraction of the activated state from the control state. Physiologic responses then appear as foci of change with clearly discernible maximums and minimums from which the actual location can be determined using computer-based search routines designed to determine the actual center-of-mass of such responses (21). Using this strategy we have been able to demonstrate response localization that exceeds the spatial resolution of a PET device (in our case PETT VI with a reconstructed image resolution of 18 mm [22]) by almost an order of magnitude (19,20).

Detection of Low-Level Responses

Blood flow responses obtained during functional activities such as opening and closing the hand, viewing flashing lights, or having a large, electric vibrator placed in the hand or elsewhere on the body (19,20,23) are robust (typically 20%–40% above control) and easily seen with the naked eye. However, responses related to higher level processing in the brain including internal mental operations (25) are of considerably lower magnitude (typically 2%–5% above control) and therefore are not easily distinguished from background noise in the image. In order to circumvent this problem we adopted a strategy of image averaging (21) that, like electrical signal averaging, suppresses noise and enhances the signal. The signal in our case is the local blood flow response, which represents a local change in the physiologic activity of the brain. This type of image averaging is based on data obtained from the subtraction of two blood flow images in a single subject obtained in a resting and an activated state (see previous section). Such a subtraction image contains the blood flow responses to functional activation plus noise due to the statistical quality of the data. A very important feature of these data is that all of the "responses," whether reflecting noise or true changes in local neuronal activity, can be localized in a standard stereotaxic space because of the system of anatomical localization we employ (see anatomical localization section). As a result, we can add responses from individual subjects to a standard stereotaxically defined space after appropriate anatomical scaling to account for differences in brain dimensions between each individual and the standard brain (in our case we use the HD6 brain in the stereotaxic atlas of Talairach et al. [25]), to obtain an image of average responses. In so doing it can be clearly demonstrated, as anticipated, that there is a dramatic improvement in the signal-to-noise ratio (26). It should be noted that in producing these average images of blood flow responses, the data from individual subjects are linearly interpolated in all three spatial dimensions to create data sets in which the volume elements (i.e., voxels) have uniform dimensions (i.e., $2 \times 2 \times 2$ mm). The details of these data manipulations and the computer search routines designed to locate and quantitate the blood flow responses are presented elsewhere (21,26).

Statistical Analysis

One of the great difficulties in working with PET data of the type previously described or its counterpart, tissue autoradiographic data of cerebral metabolism obtained from laboratory animals (10), is to determine which of the many changes observed are actually statistically significant. In a typical study, using the strategies outlined earlier for image averaging, our computer search routines frequently identify several hundred responses to a particular type of functional activity. If one uses these responses to make comparisons between a control and activated state (e.g., using a paired t-test) and assumes that the blood flow data are normally distributed about the means of these two groups, there is an obvious risk of encountering statistically significant differences between a resting and a stimulated state because of chance alone. In order to circumvent this problem we adopted a strategy based on a distribution analysis of the averaged blood flow change images (see detection of low-level responses section) using outlier detection by the gamma-2 statistic (26). Such a strategy permits an objective means of determining the presence of significance responses to functional activation in the population of all responses (i.e., signal plus noise) present in the averaged images.

In summary, our strategy for the functional mapping of neuronal activity in the human brain with PET is composed of a number of important elements. These include the deliberate selection of blood flow as the most accurate and flexible signal of changes in neuronal activity that can be detected with PET. Linearly scaled images of blood flow in a control state are subtracted from images obtained during functional activation in each subject (i.e., paired image subtraction). These subtraction images form the basis of a data set that is composed of responses averaged across many individual subjects (i.e., stereotaxic intersubject averaging) that is objectively searched using computer-based algorithms that determine with an accuracy of 1 to 2 mm the location of the responses (i.e., response localization) as well as the magnitude of the changes. Finally, we use statistical procedures based on distribution analysis of these responses to objectively determine the presence of statistically significant responses.

A final caveat in the analysis of PET data of this type needs to be mentioned. When a response has been localized, it is important to remember what is likely to be responsible for the observed change in blood flow. As has been elegantly demonstrated by Schwartz and colleagues (27), blood flow and metabolic changes occurring during functional activation occur in cell processes rather than cell bodies. The cell bodies can often be located some distance from the site of the observed change in blood flow or metabolism. Thus, the observation that changes in blood flow have occurred in a particular region of the brain should immediately stimulate a review of the connectivity of this region with other regions of the brain.

OBSERVATIONS ON THE HUMAN VISUAL SYSTEM WITH PET

Since the introduction of PET in the early 1970s, the visual system has been a popular area for investigation, in part, because it responds so vigorously to a variety of stimuli ranging from simple-patterned flashes to complex patterns including outdoor scenes (for a general review of this literature see [7]). In the remainder of this chapter I would like to review some of the studies we performed with visual stimuli using the techniques previously outlined.

Elementary Stimulus Variables

Elementary stimulus variables such as the repetition rate of a visual stimulus are very important in determining the blood flow response during a particular activation paradigm. This is due to the temporal resolution of measurements of blood flow that represent values averaged over the time of the measurement (i.e., 40 sec). Unless neuronally induced changes in blood flow occupy a sufficient portion of the measurement time, the average blood flow change measured during a period of activation will not differ significantly from the control.

Pursuing this issue experimentally we examined the response of primary visual cortex to patterned-flash stimuli varying in frequency from 1 to 61 Hz (28). In every subject striate cortex blood flow varied systematically with stimulus rate. Between 0 and 7.8 Hz blood flow increased as a linear function of the stimulus repetition rate (Fig. 1). Assuming a uniform response to each stimulus repetition, increases in stimulus rate will directly affect the mean neuronal synaptic activity integrated over the scanning interval and directly affect measurements of blood flow. Our results agree with this expectation. In order to exclude the possibility that our results were due to changes in stimulus luminance, we repeated the study using a reversing checkerboard (29). The results were the same (Fig. 1), confirming our hypothesis that blood flow responses were due to the frequency of the stimulus.

Patterned-flash stimulation beyond the range of 7.8 to 61 Hz produced a decline in blood flow (Fig. 1). This result is in keeping with the response characteristics of the visual pathways as a function of stimulus frequency, which have been described for both photic and electrical stimuli (see [28] for a review of this literature).

This rather simple experiment underscores the importance of properly selecting such elementary stimulus variables as stimulus presentation rate when studying the responses in a particular neuronal system. Response amplitudes can obviously be maximized by proper selection of such variables as rate of stimulus presentation. Conversely, the absence of a response can occur due to the selection of too high or too low a repetition rate and not to the nature of the activation condition itself.

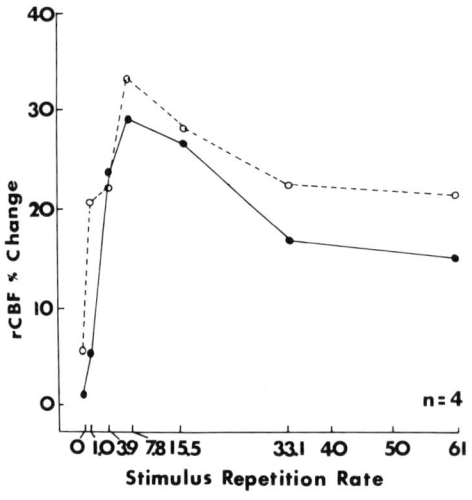

FIG. 1. Local blood flow response measured in the human striate cortex with PET as a function of stimulus repetition rate. Note that for both the reversing checkerboard (○) and the patterned flash (●), the blood flow response peaked at 7.8 Hz and declined thereafter, supporting the hypothesis that the observed response was a function of the stimulus rate and not the stimulus luminance. (Adapted from ref. 29.)

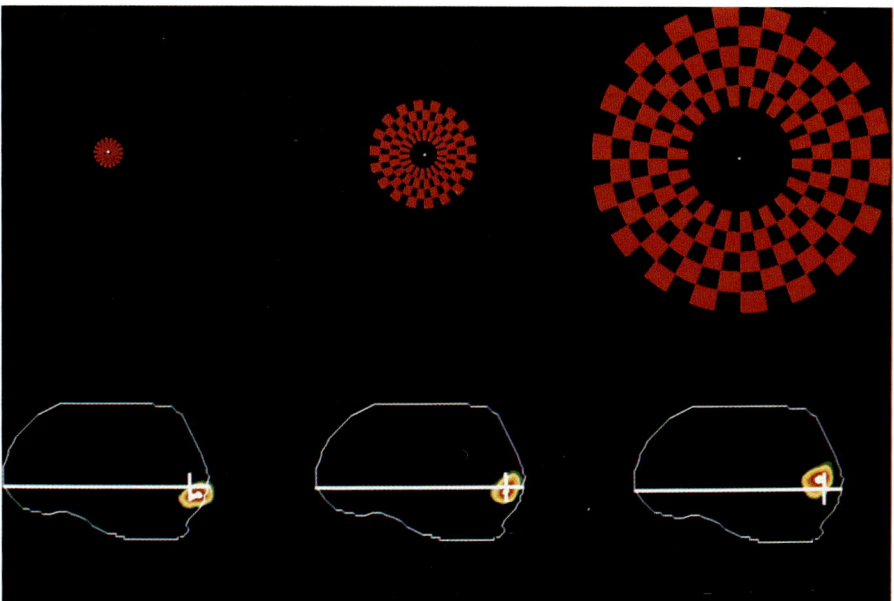

FIG. 2. Local blood flow responses in human striate cortex measured with PET during stimulation of the retina with a reversing annular checkerboard alternating colors at 10 Hz. The checkerboard was presented at three different eccentricities (**top**), whereas the subjects fixed gaze on a small fixation point. Blood flow responses were obtained for each individual in each condition by subtraction of a control state image (viewing the fixation point) from the stimulated state. The summed responses for seven individuals during the three different stimulus presentations are shown at the bottom. The brain boundary was obtained from a summed control state midsagittal image of blood flow. The horizontal line passes through the anterior and posterior commissures of the brain. The vertical lines are 2 cm in length and transect the bicommissural line 6.2 cm posterior to its center. Note the movement of the blood flow response as the stimulus moves from the center to the periphery of the retina. The exact locations of these responses are shown in Fig. 3.

Retinotopic Organization of Visual Cortex

In an attempt to extend to humans the detailed knowledge of visual cortex that has been accumulating for nonhuman species (30,31) and to demonstrate the feasibility of doing high resolution response localization with PET using the strategy previously outlined (see development of a PET strategy section), we mapped the retinotopic organization of the human visual cortex on the medial wall of the occipital lobe using PET measurements of blood flow (19,20).

The visual stimuli consisted of checkerboard annuli with a central fixation point. The macular annulus extended radially from 0.1 to 1.5°. The perimacular annulus extended radially from 1.5 to 5.5° and the peripheral stimulus extended radially from 5.5 to 15.5°. Radial check size increased with eccentricity from 0.5 to 2.0° to emulate the magnification factor of striate cortex. Checks were red on black and alternated colors at 10 Hz to maximize the induced blood flow response as predicted from our earlier experimental work (28,29; see elementary stimulus variables section). Upper and lower hemifield stimulation was achieved with a hemiannulus positioned on either side of the horizontal meridian and extending radially from 5.5 to 15.5°.

The general arrangement of retinal projections to striate cortex are well understood (see [20] for review); that is, central retina projects caudally, in the vicinity of the occipital pole, whereas peripheral retina projects rostrally; superior retina projects above the calcarine fissure and inferior retina projects beneath the fissure. Our results (Figs. 2 and 3) agree completely with this arrangement. Whereas earlier studies of retinal projections to striate cortex in humans depended on the vagaries of missile injuries and strokes (32,33), our results were obtained safely in normal subjects. The success of this initial PET study of the organization of primary visual cortex clearly demonstrates the feasibility of detailed neurophysiological experimentation in normal human subjects with PET.

In this study it should be noted that activated brain areas were located with a precision surpassing the spatial resolution of the imaging system employed. Cortical regions separated by as little as 3 mm were distinguished using images with a resolution of 18 mm (FWHM; see response localization versus spatial resolution section). This study provides strong evidence that the PET method we developed for functional mapping of the human brain performs as expected (see development of a PET strategy section).

Cortical Responses During Voluntary Saccades

During the early development of our strategy for mapping functional activity in the human brain with PET we studied voluntary saccades to determine the cortical areas active during this type of eye movement (34). The results of

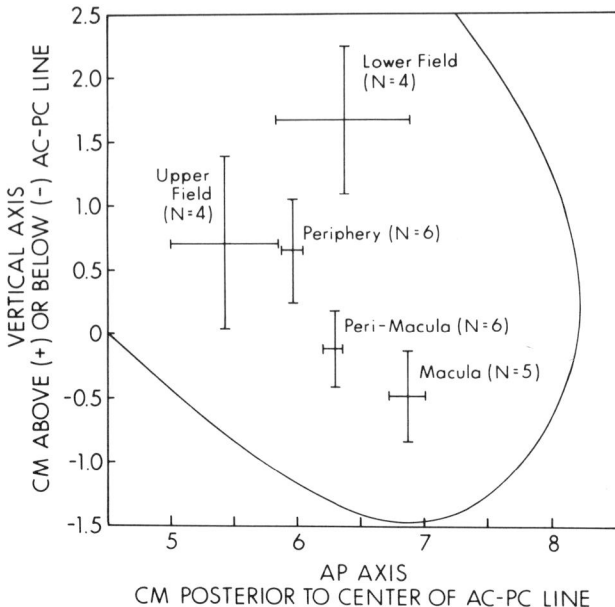

FIG. 3. Midsagittal stereotaxic plot of the retinotopic organization of the human striate cortex made from the data shown in Fig. 2 as well as stimulations of the upper and lower visual fields using a hemiannular checkerboard (Fig. 2) divided along the horizontal plane. The horizontal axis represents distance posterior to the center of the line running through the anterior commissure (AC) and the posterior commissure (PC). The vertical axis represents distance above the AC-PC line. Distances relate to the HD6 brain of the Talairach atlas of human anatomy (25). The error bars and ±1 SD. The curved line represents an outline of the occipital pole of the brain. (From ref. 20.)

this study, based on a data analysis strategy quite primitive by our current standards as outlined in this chapter, were not entirely surprising. Increased blood flow was observed in the supplementary motor area, bilaterally in an area of frontal cortex that we termed frontal eye fields (FEF) and, in the targeted conditions (see below), in primary visual cortex. The subsequent development of the full strategy for data analysis of this type (see the development of a PET strategy section) prompted us to reevaluate these data (*unpublished*) and define in greater detail the role of the FEF in the generation of voluntary saccadic eye movements. I would like to comment briefly on the new analysis of our data on the FEF.

We were prompted to reexamine our data on the FEF during voluntary saccades because we believed that it might provide support for the hypothesis that FEF may keep track of visuospatial information over time (35), especially when the subject is required to keep visuospatial information in mind in the absence of the target. Support for this hypothesis already comes from the observations that FEF lesions impair delayed eye movements in monkeys to visual targets that are no longer present (36) and impair the generation of goal-directed saccades in patients (37,38). Our data are appropriate to address this question because of two of the conditions employed: auditorily cued, targeted saccades and auditorily cued, nontargeted saccades. The hypothesis was that the FEF would be more active during the auditorily cued, nontargeted condition in which the subject was required to keep target information in mind in the absence of the target.

For these experiments, subjects were fitted with a pair of plastic, light-proof goggles, each containing a 1.5-cm long, vertical target line consisting of five 0.2-cm diameter, round monochromatic (6400 A) light-emitting diodes (modified from the Grass S10VS goggles). The distance between the two target lines was 90° of arc. Black felt covers were placed over the apertures of the tomograph to assure that no ambient room light reach the subjects. In the first condition the target lights were illuminated bilaterally throughout the measurement of blood flow. A metronome, audible to the subject, struck every 500 msec. Saccades were generated in time to the metronome alternating between the targets. In the second condition no target lights were illuminated. The subjects were instructed to saccade alternately right and left to the points occupied by the targets during the targeted conditions. Saccades were cued by the metronome as in the first condition.

The results of this new analysis of our data support the hypothesis that the FEF are involved in keeping target information (i.e., visuospatial information) in mind during the execution of voluntary saccades in the absence of a target. Blood flow was increased significantly in the FEF bilaterally only during voluntary saccades in the dark. In a more general sense these results support the hypothesis that areas in prefrontal cortex access and hold "on line" sources of representational information for as long as necessary to guide a particular response (39). Finally, this study supports the notion that PET can be used effectively to examine issues of high-level information processing in the human brain. The final experiment to be presented, in the next section, further supports that contention.

Extrastriate Responses to Visually Presented Words

We recently examined the visual responses to passively presented words as part of a larger project designed to study the cortical anatomy of single-word processing (25). In this project we used four behavioral conditions in each subject to form a three-level subtractive hierarchy in which each task state was intended to add a small number of mental operations to those of its subordinate (control) state. In the first-level comparison that I will discuss briefly in this chapter, the visual presentation of single words without a lexical task was compared with visual fixation without word presentation. Words were presented for 150 msec at the rate of once per second on a television screen during the 40-sec measurement of blood flow. No motor output or volitional lexical processing was required in this task; rather, simple sensory input and involuntary word-form processing were targeted by this subtraction.

The areas of cortex identified as active during the passive viewing of words appear to support two different computational levels, one of passive sensory processing in primary visual cortex and a second level of modality-specific word-form processing in extrastriate areas. The main cortical activations were in striate cortex bilaterally and three inferior, lateral-prestriate areas, one on the left and two on the right, extending as far anterior as the temporo-occipital boundary on the right. The primary striate responses were similar to those produced by simple sensory stimuli such as the checkerboard annuli used in our retinotopy experiments (Figs. 2 and 3). The regions in prestriate cortex, however, have so far only been activated by the presentation of visual words. Thus, these regions may represent a network that codes for visual word form. In this regard it is important to note that lesions near the left prestriate region sometimes cause pure alexia, i.e., the inability to read words without other language deficits (40), suggesting that it may be the component of such a network most concerned with visual word form whereas the regions on the right may contribute to the analysis of the more primitive features of the stimulus. Experiments are currently underway to explore these issues further.

This experiment demonstrates the capacity of PET to explore higher level processing in the normal human brain. As expected, response magnitudes were considerably less in this study (2%–5%) than those observed during the presentation of simple visual stimuli (20%–40%) (Fig. 2) and yet they were objectively detected and accurately localized using the strategy developed in our laboratory. Such studies support the idea that PET will be useful in developing a detailed functional anatomy of the normal human brain.

ACKNOWLEDGMENTS

The research reviewed in this chapter was supported by the McDonnell Center for Studies of Higher Brain Function at Washington University, The John D. and Catherine T. MacArthur Foundation and NIH grants HL 13851, NS 14834, AG 03991, and NS 06833.

REFERENCES

1. Raichle ME. Positron emission tomography. *Annu Rev Neurosci* 1983;6:249–268.
2. Raichle ME. Neuroimaging. *Trends Neurosci* 1986;9:525–529.
3. Roy CS, Sherrington CS. On the regulation of the blood supply of the brain. *J Physiol (Lond)* 1890;11:85–109.
4. Fulton JF. Observations upon the vascularity of the human occipital lobe during visual activity. *Brain* 1928;51:310–320.
5. Schmidt CF, Hendrix JP. The action of chemical substances on cerebral blood vessels. *Res Publ Assoc Res Nerv Ment Dis* 1937;18:229–276.

6. Serota HM, Gerard RW. Localized thermal changes in the cat's brain. *J Neurophysiol* 1938;1:115–124.
7. Raichle ME. Circulatory and metabolic correlates of brain function in normal humans. In: Mountcastle VB, Plum F, eds. *Handbook of physiology. The nervous system* sec 1, vol V, pt 2. Bethesda: American Physiological Society, 1987;643–674.
8. Fox PT, Raichle ME. Focal physiological uncoupling of cerebral blood flow and oxidative metabolism during somatosensory stimulation in human subjects. *Proc Natl Acad Sci USA* 1986;83:1140–1144.
9. Fox PT, Raichle ME, Mintun MA, Dense C. Nonoxidative glucose consumption during focal physiologic neural activity. *Science (in press)*.
10. Sokoloff L, Reivich M, Kennedy C, et al. The ^{14}C-deoxyglucose method for the measurement of local glucose utilization: theory, procedure and normal values in the conscious and anesthetized albino rat. *J Neurochem* 1977;28:897–916.
11. Rcivich M, Alavi A, Wolf A, et al. Glucose metabolic rate kinetic model parameters determination in humans: the lumped constants and rate constants for ^{18}F-fluorodeoxyglucose and ^{11}C-deoxyglucose. *J Cereb Blood Flow Metab* 1985;5:179–182.
12. Reivich M, Alavi A, Wolf A, et al. Use of 2-deoxy-D [1]^{11}glucose for the determination of local cerebral glucose metabolism in humans: variation within and between subjects. *J Cereb Blood Flow Metab* 1982;2:307–319.
13. Herscovitch P, Markham J, Raichle ME. Brain blood flow measured with intravenous $H_2^{15}O$. I. Theory and error analysis. *J Nucl Med* 1983;24:782–789.
14. Raichle ME, Martin WRW, Herscovitch P, Mintun M, Markham J. Brain blood flow measured with $H_2^{15}O$. II. Implementation and validation. *J Nucl Med* 1983;24:790–798.
15. Videen TO, Perlmutter JS, Herscovitch P, Raichle ME. Brain blood volume, flow and oxygen utilization measured with O-15 radiotracers and positron emission tomography: revised metabolic computations. *J Cereb Blood Flow Metab* 1987;7:513–516.
16. Herscovitch P, Raichle ME, Kilbourn MR, Welch MJ. Positron emission tomographic measurement of cerebral blood flow and permeability-surface area product of water using ^{15}O-water and ^{11}C-butanol. *J Cereb Blood Flow Metab* 1987;7:527–542.
17. Herscovitch P, Raichle ME. Effect of tissue heterogeneity on the measurement of cerebral blood flow with equilibrium $C^{15}O_2$ inhalation technique. 1983;4:407–415.
18. Fox PT, Perlmutter J, Raichle ME. A stereotactic method of anatomical localization for positron emission tomography. *J Computer Assist Tomog* 1985;9:141–153.
19. Fox PT, Mintun MA, Raichle ME, Meizen FM, Allman JM, Van Essen DC. Mapping human visual cortex with positron emission tomography. *Nature* 1986;323:806–809.
20. Fox PT, Meizen FM, Allman JM, Van Essen DC, Raichle ME. Retinotopic organization of the human visual cortex mapped with positron emission tomography. *J Neurosci* 1987;7:913–922.
21. Mintun MA, Fox PT, Raichle ME. A highly accurate method of localizing regions of neuronal activation in the human brain with positron emission tomography. *J Cereb Blood Flow Metab (in press)*.
22. Yamamoto M, Ficke DC, Ter-Pogossian MM. Performance study of PETT VI, a positron computed tomograph with 288 cesium fluoride detectors. *IEEE Trans Nucl Sci* 1982;29:529–533.
23. Fox PT, Burton H, Raichle ME. Mapping of somatic sensory cortex with positron emission tomography. *J Neurosurg* 1987;67:34–43.
24. Petersen SE, Fox PT, Posner MI, Mintun MA, Raichle ME. Positron emission tomographic studies of the cortical anatomy of single word processing. *Nature* 1988;331:585–589.
25. Talairach J, Sxikla G, Tournoux P, et al. *Atlas d'anatomie stereotaxique du telencephale*. Paris: Masson, 1967.
26. Fox PT, Mintun MA, Reiman EM, Raichle ME. Enhanced detection of focal brain responses using intersubject averaging and distribution analysis of subtracted PET images. *J Cereb Blood Flow Metab (in press)*.
27. Schwartz WJ, Smith CB, Davidsen L, et al. Metabolic mapping of functional activity in the hypothalamo-neurohypophysial system of the rat. *Science* 1979;205:723–725.
28. Fox PT, Raichle ME. Stimulus rate dependence of regional cerebral blood flow in human striate cortex demonstrated by positron emission tomography. *J Neurophysiol* 1984;51:1109–1120.

29. Fox PT, Raichle ME. Stimulus rate determines regional brain blood flow in striate cortex. *Ann Neurol* 1985;17:303–305.
30. Allman JM, Kaas JH. The organization of the second visual area (v-II) in the owl monkey: a se order transformation of the visual hemifield. *Brain Res* 1974;76:247–265.
31. Van Essen DC, Newsome WT, Maunsell JHR. The visual field representation in striate cortex of the macaque monkey: asymmetries, anistropies, and individual variability. *Vision Res* 1984;24:429–448.
32. Holmes G, Lister WT. Disturbances of vision in cerebral lesions with special reference to the cortical representation of the macula. *Brain* 1916;39:34–73.
33. McAuley DL, Ross-Russell RW. Correlation of CAT scan and visual field defects in vascular lesions of the posterior visual pathways. *J Neurol Neurosurg Psychiatry* 1979;42:298–311.
34. Fox PT, Fox JM, Raichle ME, Burde RM. The role of cerebral cortex in the generation of voluntary saccades: a positron emission tomographic study. *J Neurophysiol* 1985;54:348–369.
35. Bruce CJ, Goldberg ME. Primate frontal eye fields. I. Single neurons discharging before saccades. *J Neurophysiol* 1985;53:603–635.
36. Deng S-Y, Segraves MA, Ungerleider LG, Mishkin M, Goldberg ME. Unilateral frontal eye field lesions degrade saccadic performance in the rhesus monkey. *Soc Neurosci Abstr* 1984;10:59.
37. Gross CG, Bruce CJ, Desimone R, Fleming J, Gatass R. Cortical visual areas of the temporal lobe. In: Woolsey CN, ed. *Cortical sensory organization. Multiple visual areas*. Clifton, NJ: Humana, 1982;187–216.
38. Gross CG, Weiskrantz L. Some changes in behavior produced by lateral frontal lesions in the macaque. In: Warren JM, Akert K, eds. *The frontal granular cortex and behavior*. New York: McGraw-Hill, 1964;74–101.
39. Goldman-Rakic PS. Circuitry of primate prefrontal cortex and regulation of behavior by representation memory. In: Mountcastle VB, Plum F, eds. *Handbook of physiology. The nervous system*, sec 1, vol V, pt 1. Bethesda: The American Physiological Society, 1987; 373–417.
40. Damasio AR, Damasio H. The anatomic basis of pure alexia. *Neurology* 1983;33:1573–1583.

Vision and the Brain,
edited by B. Cohen and I. Bodis-Wollner.
Raven Press, Ltd., New York © 1990.

Neuromagnetic Localization of Neuronal Activity in Visual and Extravisual Cortex

Lloyd Kaufman and Samuel J. Williamson

Neuromagnetism Laboratory, Departments of Psychology and Physics, New York University, New York, New York 10003

Extensive investigations on infrahuman species for more than 25 years, have led to major advances in understanding the functional anatomy of visual systems. However, for obvious reasons, direct extrapolation to humans from work on other species is somewhat risky. The methods of neuromagnetism permit us to test the generality of the principles of functional organization of visual systems across species, including humans, as well as to define unique attributes of the human visual system by noninvasive means. These methods have the advantage that they reveal functionally disparate regions of the visual cortex. In this chapter we summarize the evidence that precise three-dimensional localization of sources of neuronal activity is indeed possible and that it extends from the primary visual projection areas to the extravisual areas of the human brain. We present the hypothesis that the activity of small populations of cells measured magnetically has some of the specialized characteristics of single-cell responses, and, moreover, this activity is closely related to human psychphysical data.

Since the first observation of the visually evoked magnetic field (1), our understanding of the origin of these fields and the techniques for measuring them have advanced dramatically. It is now clear that extracranial magnetic fields measured perpendicular to the scalp are due to *intracellular* current flowing within the active neurons of the brain (for an introduction to these concepts, see [2]). Because tissue of the head is transparent to such "neuromagnetic" fields, they emerge without distortion, and mapping the extracranial field pattern provides a means for locating its source in three dimensions with considerable precision. In addition, the strength of the source can be determined, which, in turn, can be translated in an estimation of the number of neurons involved in the average response. It should be noted that the intracellular current is accompanied by a *volume current* flowing within the conducting medium of the head, but this current does not contribute significantly to conventional field measurements over occipital and parietal areas of the scalp. The reason is that for an ideal head that can be modeled as a sphere or concentric spherical shells of various conductivities, the volume current makes no contribution at all to the extracranial field normal to the head. In the case of real heads (which are nonspherical), the volume current makes such a small contribution that it is generally inconsequential (3–5).

The underlying source of the visually evoked neuromagnetic field is the intracellular flow of current within dendrites of functionally open-field neurons. As in the electroencephalograph (EEG), candidate sources are the apical dendrites of pyramidal cells, since these have an open-field structural configuration, and, when active at the same time, their magnetic fields summate to produce a field that can be detected outside the human scalp. We have estimated that relatively small populations of neurons contribute to the neuromagnetic field related to sensory stimulation, e.g., typically 10,000 neurons can give rise to the event-related neuromagnetic field (6).

NEUROMAGNETIC METHODS

To record changes in the brain's magnetic field related to visual stimulation, one or more sensors are placed near the scalp to record temporal variations in the magnetic field that are time-locked to the presentation of the stimulus. Despite the fact that the amplitudes of the field variations are extremely weak relative to the field of the earth and of other sources of magnetic fields in the environment, in many cases, and with proper precautions, such measurements can be carried out in a normal laboratory environment. However, to achieve maximum sensitivity, especially at frequencies below a few hertz, a magnetically shielded room provides important advantages. Figure 1 illustrates the arrangement of magnetic sensors in our laboratory at New York University. The subject either lies on a bed, sits in a chair, or sits in a "kneeling" chair, as illustrated, while magnetic fields at various locations over the scalp are recorded. The subject's head rests on a vacuum "cast," which helps to keep it still. The signals of interest are very weak, typically 100 femtotesla (100 × 10^{-15} fT) or less, approximately 10^{-9} of the earth's steady field.

The principle behind the magnetic sensors in Fig. 1 is shown in Fig. 2. The only instrument with sufficient sensitivity for brain studies is the *S*uperconducting *Qu*antum *I*nterference *D*evice (SQUID), which must be cooled to low temperatures to exhibit its superconducting properties. Conventionally this is achieved by immersing the device in a bath of liquid helium (4.2 K or −266.8°C) maintained in a vacuum-insulated vessel called a dewar (named for Sir James Dewar who was the first to liquify hydrogen and used his cryogenic vessel for lectures to the public in the late 19th century). The conventional SQUID is not suitable for detecting biomagnetic fields directly. Instead, the field is sensed by a detection coil of superconducting wire, and this wire forms a closed circuit when connected to a second, much smaller coil placed near the SQUID. This closed superconducting circuit has the important property that

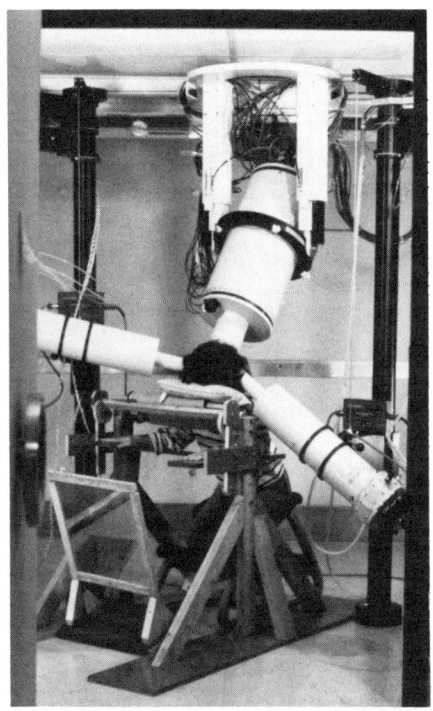

FIG. 1. Magnetic sensors placed near the head of a subject in the magnetically shielded room at the Neuromagnetism Laboratory of New York University. The overhead gantry supports a five-channel system, and independent gantries extending from the side walls of the room each support a single channel system. The subject rests in a kneeling chair to view a visual display projected from outside the room.

when a field is applied to the detection coil, a current flows around the circuit to keep the net magnetic flux within the circuit unchanged. The portion of the flux produced in the smaller coil is sensed by the SQUID, and its response is monitored by room temperature electronics. The voltage output of the electronics is strictly proportional to the field applied to the detection coil, and the system is capable of recording fields in the bandwidth from dc to several kilohertz. One reason for not using the SQUID to detect directly the field of interest is that with the superconducting circuit the detection coil can have a variety of geometries, depending on the particular application. The one shown in Fig. 2 is called a second-order gradiometer and is particularly effective in rejecting noise from remote sources such as electric elevators, subways, and metal doors being opened and closed. The output of the SQUID electronics goes through computer-controlled amplifiers and bandpass filters and continues to a computer for analysis and storage. A detailed explanation of biomagnetic instruments and their applications has been given by Romani et al. (7).

In Fig. 1 the dewar suspended from the ceiling contains an array of five SQUID sensors, so that simultaneous measurements are possible at five locations over the scalp separated by approximately 2 cm from each other. Each of the other two smaller dewars contains a single sensor. The reason the dewars

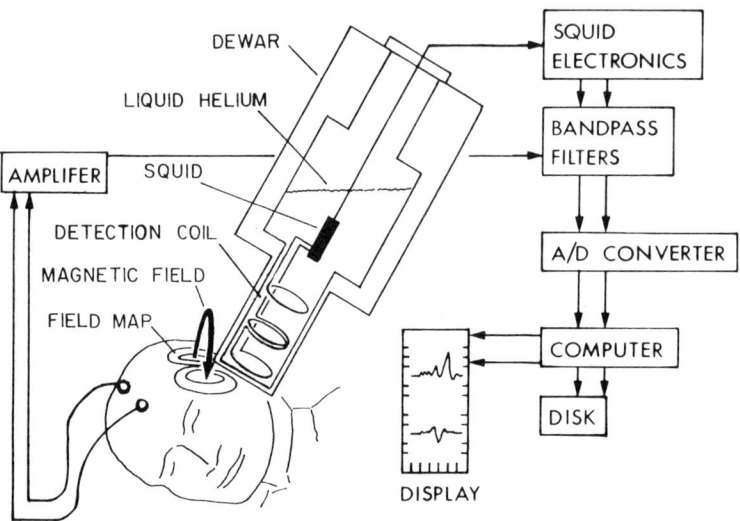

FIG. 2. Arrangement for recording MEG and EEG simultaneously. The superconducting detection coil and SQUID are mounted in a dewar containing a bath of liquid helium. The outside of the dewar is well insulated from the bath by a vacuum insulated space. The detected magnetic and electric signals are filtered and sent to a computer for processing.

can be tipped at such large angles from the vertical is that they do not require liquid helium for operation: They rely on a refrigerator that achieves liquid helium temperatures with a multistage process whereby cooling is achieved when helium gas is allowed to expand (8). Such sensors can be tipped in any direction, including upside-down, for sensing neuromagnetic fields.

RETINOTOPIC SEQUENCE

An illustration of the neuromagnetic precision obtained in localizing neuronal activity in visual cortex is the earliest noninvasive determination of a portion of the retinotopic sequence in a human subject. As Fig. 2 indicates, a small region of neuronal activity produces a field that emerges from the scalp in one region and enters at another. The source, if modeled by an equivalent current dipole (or short element of current), lies directly under the center of the pattern. Its depth is determined by the distance between the two points of maximum radial field (*field extrema*) in comparison with the radius of the head. This relationship is valid as long as the curvature of the inner surface of the skull above the source is well approximated by a spherical model. The model can be generalized to include a variation of conductivity with radial position, without any effect on the analysis. The procedures for analyzing neuromagnetic data have been recently reviewed by Williamson and Kaufman (6). In situations in which neuronal activity extends over larger areas, with dimensions of several centimeters, these same methods provide an accurate estimate for the center of mass of activity (9).

The retinotopic sequence was explored by presenting a sine-wave grating in a portion of the right visual field, with the contrast of the grating reversing at 13 Hz. The luminance of the display was 50 cd/m^2, and the contrast 33%. The magnetic response was detected in synchrony with the 13 Hz reversal rate, and the amplitude and phase lag of the field component at the frequency were determined. This is called a steady-state paradigm because the neuronal response to one stimulus has not worn away before the next stimulus is presented. Earlier neuromagnetic studies showed that the field pattern of evoked neuronal activity lies over the occipital area contralateral to the visual field in which the stimulus is presented (10), as expected for neuronal activity in the contralateral visual cortex. The grating was bounded by either a semicircle or semi-annulus in the right visual field, as depicted at the top of Fig. 3. Figure 3 (bottom) shows the pattern of strongest evoked field, indicated at each measurement position by the length of the vector displayed there (11). The orientation of each vector indicates the phase lag, so these vectors alternatively can

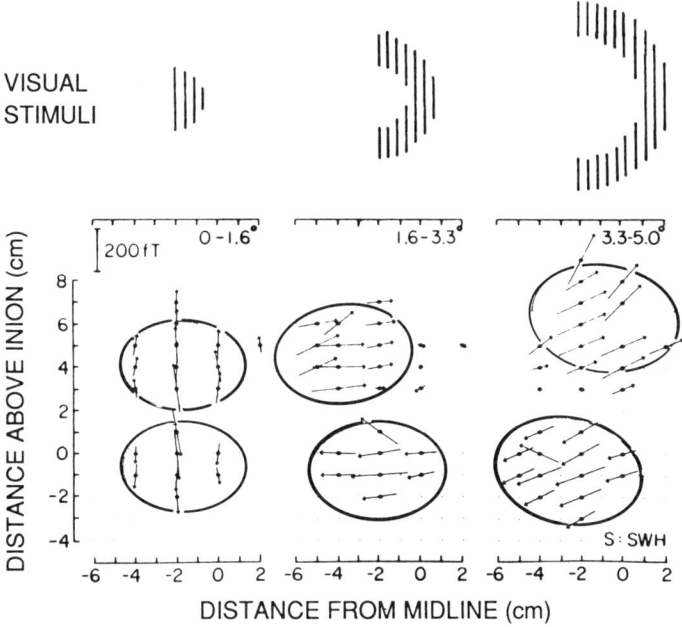

FIG. 3. Top: Depiction of contrast reversal gratings presented in various portions of the right visual field. **Bottom:** Corresponding steady-state evoked fields over the occipital area of the subject's scalp. *Ellipses* denote the regions of the field extrema where responses are substantially above the noise level, for stimuli presented within the indicated angular ranges of the visual field. Each *arrow* is a phasor centered at a measurement position, with the phase lag indicated by the angle measured counterclockwise from the right.

be called phasors. Two regions of strong field, of opposite direction lie to the left of the midline as expected for activity in the left hemisphere. The equivalent current dipole accounting for the field pattern is oriented perpendicular to the line joining the two field extrema. Thus, the dipole lies approximately perpendicular to the midline for each of the depicted stimulus patterns. This is expected if the primary contribution to the field is from neurons oriented perpendicular to the surface of the cortex in the upper and lower segments of the longitudinal fissure. The orientation of the current dipole implies that the fields from neurons in the roof and floor of the calcarine fissure are largely self-canceling, as may be predicted from the cruciform model for cortex. The center of the source actually lies closer to the midline than the center of the field pattern shown in the figure because it lies on the radius that projects out from the center of the head through the midpoint of the pattern on the scalp. Figure 3 shows that as the eccentricity of the stimulus is increased, the two field extrema move apart, indicating the source lies deeper within the longitudinal fissure.

The corresponding positions of deduced neuronal activity are shown in sagittal view in Fig. 4: There is a systematic increase in depth with increasing peripheral presentation. The dashed outline is a typical boundary for visual cortex obtained from an atlas, and it need not represent the boundary for this particular subject. Our interest in the retinotopic sequence is not merely to display this correspondence between visual space and cortical position, which in this case is already well-known, but ultimately to determine whether there is an exact mathematical description for the correspondence. We are motivated by the discovery of a tonotopic sequence across human auditory cortex by

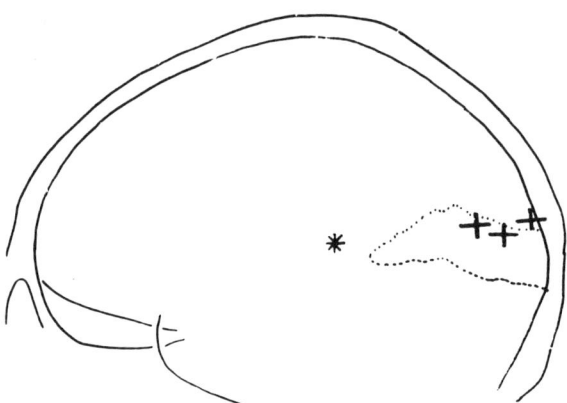

FIG. 4. Sagittal view of the deduced positions of the current dipoles that account for the field extrema in Fig. 3. *Asterisk* indicates the center of curvature for the occipital region of the subject's scalp, used as the center of the sphere that modeled the head. *Broken line* is a representative outline of visual cortex, although not obtained for this particular subject.

neuromagnetic techniques (12), a sequence that is accurately described by the cumulative distance across cortex from one place of activity to the next varying as the logarithm of the frequency. It is generally agreed that the retinotopic projection of striate cortex is roughly described by the distance d of evoked activity from the cortical apex varying as the logarithm of the angular position z of the stimulus in the visual field. Schwartz (13) predicted a specific form for this projection: $d = A\ln(z + \alpha)$, which appears to well describe projections across animals studied by autoradiography (13), although there has been some controversy (14,15). It is of considerable interest that this form of logarithmic conformal transformation preserves certain features of the image (e.g., angles) that may provide computational advantages for information processing in cortex. The data in Fig. 4 are not sufficiently precise to afford a rigorous test of such an expression; however, our present magnetic sensing system is three times as sensitive as was the system used to obtain the original recordings described earlier. In addition, the present system allows for far greater accuracy in determining the locations of the detection coils with respect to the scalp, thus permitting a commensurate improvement in source localization. Therefore, a replication of this study in which the data would benefit from the improved sensitivity and accuracy of positioning is now justifiable.

CONTRAST THRESHOLD

Neuromagnetic localization provides an opportunity to study the functional characteristics of populations of neurons within circumscribed locations in visual cortex. For instance, Okada et al. (16) studied the effects of different spatial frequency, temporal frequency of contrast reversal, and luminance contrast on the strength of the neuromagnetic response to sinusoidal gratings presented to one-half of the visual field. The stimuli were presented on an oscilloscope screen subtending a visual angle of $9° \times 19°$. Magnetic response strengths peaked between 3 and 5 c/deg, as normally observed in psychophysical contrast sensitivity functions (17,18) and for the evoked scalp potential (19). The spatial frequency for peak response decreased with increasing temporal frequency, shifting from near 3 c/deg to 1 c/deg as temporal frequency was increased from 3.5 Hz to 11.5 Hz, as observed in psychophysical (17,18) and in visually evoked potential (19) experiments. The effect on these curves of decreasing contrast was explored for a contrast reversal rate of 13 Hz. The overall trends were also similar to those of the evoked potential (19). This suggests that the same neuronal population was giving rise to both electric and magnetic signals, as may be expected for sources lying close to the skull with a predominantly tangential orientation. To test this, electrodes were applied to the occipital area of the scalp, and the magnetic and electric amplitudes as a function of spatial frequency were compared directly. A linear relationship was found between voltage and field amplitudes, but the proportionality factor varied significantly with spatial frequency. This variation indicates that the responding neuronal populations varied with spatial frequency. The observed differences could be explained by changes in either the direction of dominant intracellular current, position of neuronal activity, or extent of cortex that is active. Which factor is most important could not be determined in this study. However, this does not detract from the principle that was established, namely, that macroscopic magnetic and electric measurements carried out simultaneously reveal the presence of spatial-frequency selective populations within visual cortex. This is consistent with the known functional architecture of monkey striate cortex (20).

THRESHOLD RELATIONSHIPS

Variation in the strengths of the fields evoked by sensory stimuli correspond to psychophysically determined thresholds for the same stimuli. Thus, Okada et al. (16) extrapolated the strength of the evoked neuromagnetic field back to the noise level on the basis of response magnitude to several different contrast levels. This was done for patterns of several different spatial frequencies. It was found that these extrapolated values displayed a variation with spatial frequency that was in excellent correspondence with psychophysically determined contrast thresholds for these same patterns. One subject's contrast sensitivity function (the reciprocal of the threshold values) was essentially identical to the function inferred from the neuromagnetic data, whereas for another subject the psychophysical sensitivity was a factor of two higher than the inferred sensitivity. Nevertheless, this result is in essential agreement with those obtained by Campbell and Kulikowski (21) and Campbell and Maffei (22) and using a steady-state evoked potential measure. Okada et al. attributed the difference to the possibility that the subjects employed different criteria in using the method of adjustment to determine thresholds.

A remarkable example of the complementary relationship between magnetic and electric recordings was found (16) by comparing the phase lags of electrical and magnetic responses to stimuli of different spatial frequencies and different contrast reversal rates (temporal frequencies). For one thing, the phase lags of the two responses agreed for low spatial frequencies, indicating from the signs of potential and field that the electrical currents of the two flow in opposite directions. This is consistent with the fact that the (extracellular) current associated with the evoked potential flows opposite to the (intracellular) current associated with the evoked field. (One caveat to be kept in mind, however, is that this conclusion is predicated on the assumption that the observed fields and potentials arise from a common source.) Second, with stimulus spatial frequencies higher than approximately 6 c/deg, the visually evoked potential phase lags became larger than the visually evoked field phase lags, implying that the neuronal populations responsible for the two measures differ. This indicates that one of these measures was affected by a second population of neurons that is not as well represented in the signal detected by the other. Although neither the visually evoked field nor the visually evoked potential would have revealed the presence of activity from at least two different populations of neurons, both measures make this inference possible. Of course, the identification of these two populations has yet to be ascertained.

RELATIONSHIP BETWEEN LATENCY AND REACTION TIME

It is well established that differential sensitivity to classes of stimuli may be reflected in behavioral reaction time (RT) to the same types of stimuli, even when they are at suprathreshold levels. However, measures of RT have a usefulness that extends beyond the assessment of differential sensitivity. Since RT measures are widely used in cognitive science as well as in studies of sensory processes, it is of some importance to consider the levels of the nervous system at which changes in neuronal response latency contribute to changes in RT.

The latency with which the magnetic field occurs after a stimulus with which it is in step can be determined from the measured phase lag of the response and the period between successive stimuli. Figure 5 shows that the corresponding "apparent" latencies increase monotonically with increasing spatial frequency of the grating (23).

These latencies may be compared with the values of simple RTs to the appearance of a grating, as reported by Breitmeyer (24): RT increases with spatial frequency. A close qualitative agreement is obtained between the two if a value of 115 msec is subtracted from the RTs, for the two trends from Breitmeyer's two subjects then overlap the range of evoked field measurements. Okada (*unpublished data*) has shown that the neuromagnetic latency also increases with decrease in luminance or contrast, and RTs of the same subjects show similar increases. The results of Okada et al. (16) at low contrast agree with the relationship between simple RT and contrast reported by Harwerth and Levi (25) for evoked potential measurements.

These agreements between the latency of activity in visual cortex and RT suggest that the neuromagnetic signal occurring with a particular apparent latency reflects a degree of sensory processing related to the spatial frequency and other stimulus parameters. It is plausible to infer that neuronal effects of stimuli of low spatial frequency and high contrast are transmitted to visual cortex along faster pathways, and that early cortical processing following the arrival of these signals also occurs more rapidly. By the same token, high spatial frequencies and patterns of low contrast are processed more slowly. The difference in this processing time within the visual system fully accounts for the variations in RT, thus suggesting that the motor reaction as well as its

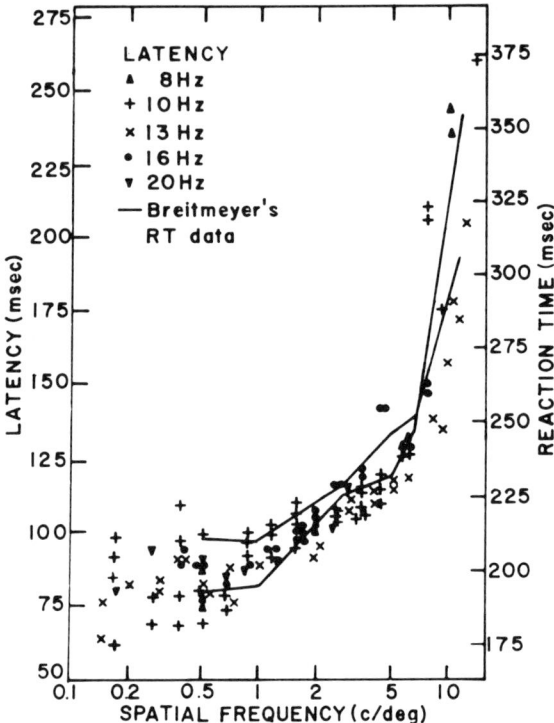

FIG. 5. Increase in latency of the steady-state response of a subject evoked by contrast reversing gratings of various spatial frequencies, presented in the central visual field for the indicated spatial frequencies. Symbols indicate the latencies computed from the observed phase lags at the indicated reversal rates. Breaks in each of the two *solid lines* indicate reaction times reported by Breitmeyer (24) for two subjects responding to the appearance of gratings. (From ref. 23.)

immediate antecedents are essentially independent of the properties of the sensory input. It remains to be seen whether the neuronal populations in primary sensory cortex or earlier in the visual system also reflect the increases in RT that accompany more complicated tasks, e.g., as in the choice RT paradigm, or whether other neural centers are involved. This would permit us to realize the goals expressed by Donders (26), who hoped to use the RT method in illuminating decision processes. Thus far this goal has been approached using exclusively behavioral methods (27).

PARALLEL PROCESSING CHANNELS

Breitmeyer (24) proposed one theory as to why the RT to high spatial frequency patterns is longer than that for patterns of low spatial frequency. He suggested that the longer RT for high spatial frequencies is related to the fact that neuronal signals associated with such patterns are conveyed via the so-called X cells of the visual system (28,29), and these units are presumed to be related to pattern vision. Sometimes these cells are associated with the sustained cells that have been observed in the lateral geniculate nucleus of cat (30). These cells are most sensitive to patterns of high spatial frequency and low temporal frequency. By contrast, the Y cells of the visual system are known to be most strongly affected by patterns of low spatial frequency and high temporal frequency. These are called transient cells because they respond to stimulus onset and offset, which is a response at twice the fundamental frequency of stimulation by a pattern that is periodically turned on and off. On the other hand, X cells respond in a sustained manner at the frequency of stimulation and are presumed to be involved in the detection of motion by the visual system (31,32). Breitmeyer (24) proposed that the transient channels do respond more rapidly than do the sustained channels. Since the transient channels are more strongly affected by patterns of low spatial frequency, he proposed that their activity accounts for the relatively short RT. Also, as the spatial frequency of the pattern becomes higher, this implies an increasing contribution of the slower responding sustained channels.

One implication of this explanation is that Y cells (transient channels) should play a stronger role in the overall response for high rates of reversal of the contrast of grating patterns than for low rates. Now, as intimated above, the apparent latency of a steady-state response may be defined by the slope of the line relating the phase lag of the response to stimulus reversal rate (33). This definition of the so-called apparent latency provides results that are equivalent with those in Fig. 5 for low reversal rates, as illustrated on the left in Fig. 6. The greater slope for the lines below 20 Hz corresponding to higher spatial frequency indicate longer apparent latency, in agreement with the data of Fig. 5.

A remarkable feature in Fig. 6 is the change in phase trends when the contrast reversal rate exceeds approximately 20 Hz (34,35). All of the trends for the high spatial frequencies increase less rapidly, and their slopes virtually coincide with the slope displayed at lower rates by responses to the lowest spatial frequency. In other words, at high reversal rates the apparent latency becomes independent of spatial frequency and takes the low value seen at lower rates for the lowest spatial frequency. This is consistent with the two-channel model if the response at high reversal rates is indeed dominated by the Y cells or their counterpart, the transient or movement channels. This is, to our knowledge, the first physiological evidence in humans for the parallel channel model of visual information processing.

ACTIVITY IN AN EXTRAVISUAL AREA

Neurons in medial temporal cortex (MT) of rhesus macaque are now known to be selectively sensitive to motion and not to orientation of visual patterns

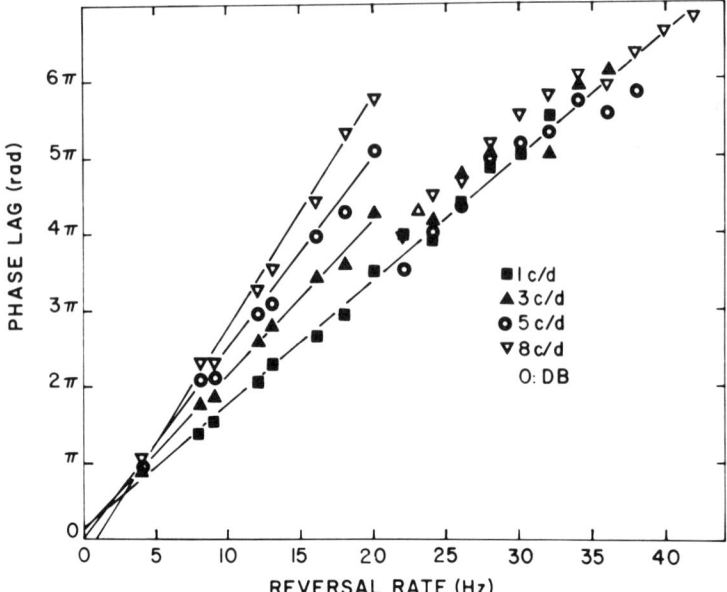

FIG. 6. Increase of the phase lag of steady-state responses with contrast reversal rate for various spatial frequencies. The spatial frequency dependence of the slopes at low reversal rates is lost at rates above approximately 20 Hz. For convenience in comparing slopes, 2π has been subtracted from phase lags for 5 c/deg and 8 c/deg above 20 Hz. (From ref. 34.)

(36,37). This raises the question of the identification of the homologous area of the human brain. Motivated by this question we sought to develop a stimulus that would permit the detection of neuronal activity in response to motion. Realizing that a smoothly moving pattern does not provide a temporal reference for detecting fields that are time locked to a specific stimulus event, we sought to detect responses to *changes* in velocity of a pattern instead. What was found was another region of neuronal activity that previously had not been known to respond to visual stimulation: a region of neuronal activity within the central cortex, in or near the rolandic fissure.

A vertically oriented grating of 1.5 c/deg spatial frequency for one subject (3 c/deg for a second subject) was drifted horizontally across an oscilloscope, and its speed was sinusoidally modulated at 7 Hz. The modulation produced a velocity contrast of 50% expressed by the modulation amplitude as a percentage of the mean velocity. With the subject fixated on the center of the screen, the grating drifted unidirectionally and its speed changed repetitively from slow to fast.

Neuromagnetic responses were observed over a wide area of the scalp by Lounasmaa et al. (38), as illustrated in the sagittal view in Fig. 7. An area of strong field having a common phase lag appears over the lower occipital region, at the lower left of the figure, with a weaker region of apparently

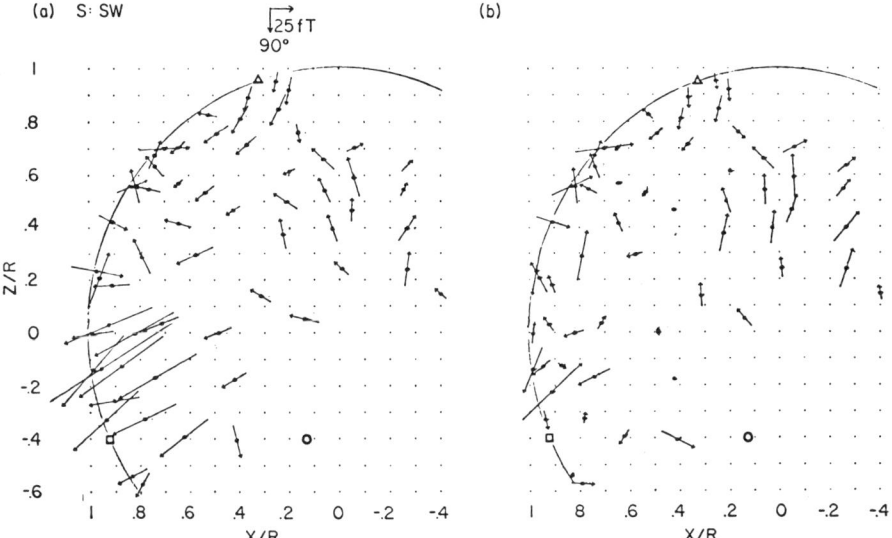

FIG. 7. Sagittal projection of steady-state responses observed over the right hemisphere for a moving grating whose speed is sinusoidally modulated. **a:** Phasors representing the evoked field pattern, with lengths showing strong responses in the occipital region and additional weaker activity in the central region but of a different phase lag. **b:** Residual field pattern when neuronal activity in visual cortex is modeled by a current dipole in each hemisphere and the dipole fields are subtracted from the data. Only a few phasors remain strong in the occipital area, but these are attributed to noise. The only consistent phase lags are found in the central area. *Solid line* shows the outline of sphere of radius $R = 10$ cm used to model the head. △, vertex; ○, ear canal; □, inion.

random phase appearing just above. In separate studies with half-field presentations this lower and upper area can be identified as the regions of inward and outward field from activity in visual cortex of the right hemisphere; and a similar pattern of two oppositely directed field areas is found over the left hemisphere. The occipital sources appear to be tipped so that the strong field patterns (of opposite field direction) over the upper occipital area largely superimpose, thus accounting for the weak magnetic field there for full visual field presentation.

When the occipital sources in left and right hemispheres are modeled by equivalent current dipoles, and their field patterns are subtracted from the measured fields, only nonoccipital sources should be represented by the neuromagnetic data. This result is illustrated in Fig. 8. An interesting feature in this plot of the residual field is the presence of two regions over the rolandic fissure whose phase lags differ by 180°, one area lying near the border of the diagram just posterior to the vertex (phasors pointing nearly downward), and the other to the lower right of it (phasors pointing nearly upward). This phase difference of 180° indicates that one area represents magnetic field emerging from the scalp and the other represents field entering the scalp. A similar

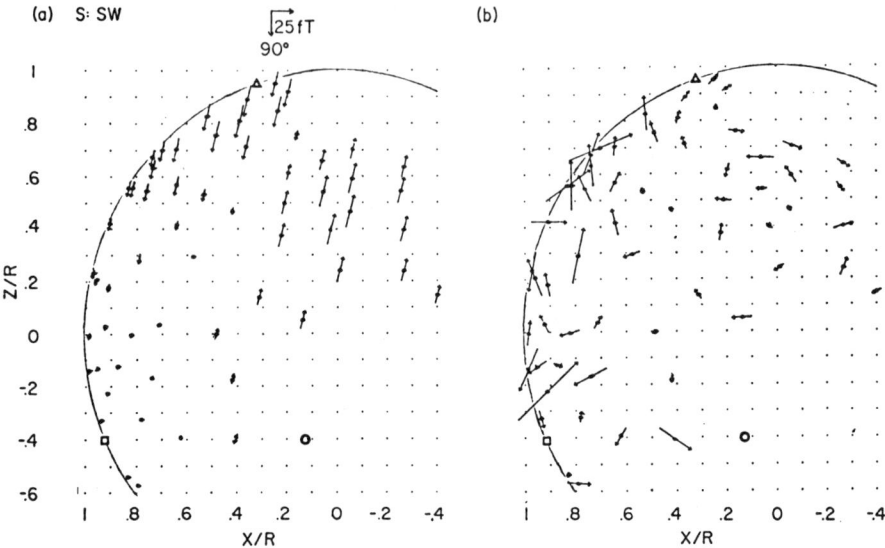

FIG. 8. a: Phasors representing the field pattern from a current dipole modeling the hypothesized source near the rolandic fissure. **b:** Residual field pattern when this dipole pattern is subtracted from the field pattern of Fig. 7b, showing no systematic phase lag for residual phasors in the central region. The amplitude of these residual phasors is at the noise level. △, vertex; ○, ear canal; □, inion.

pattern is found over the left hemisphere as well (not shown), except the field directions are reversed. Thus, each source in the left and right central areas may be modeled by an equivalent current dipole lying under the midpoint of each pattern, pointing approximately in the direction of the heavy arrow as illustrated in Fig. 8. When the predicted field pattern is subtracted from the data of Fig. 7, the resulting residual field pattern is without any regions of appreciable amplitude and consistent phase, implying that no additional sources contribute to it. Thus, within the precision of the measurements, the field pattern is explained by two bilaterally placed sources in visual cortex and two bilaterally placed sources in the central area.

The central source in the right hemisphere lies within or close to the rolandic fissure, which is well established on the subject characterized in Figs. 7 and 8. The source in this subject's right hemisphere lies 2 cm lower along the rolandic fissure than the projection area for motor and somatosensory response for voluntary ballistic flexure of the left index finger (39). Its orientation is perpendicular to the fissure, and its depth is 3 cm beneath the scalp, thus placing it within the fissure. To our knowledge, this is the first identification of visually related activity in this area. Although the somatosensory representation of some facial areas and related motor regions lie in this approximate area, we are unaware of any reports of evidence of eye muscle control here. Furthermore, it is not possible for subjects to move their eyes precisely in step with a pattern changing speed at rates within the range of 7 to 12 Hz where responses were observed, which would be required if coherent activity of motor cortex were responsible for the observed field pattern. Indeed, an increasing feature of the central magnetic fields is that activity appears whether the stimulus is presented in right or left halves of the visual field. Such bilateral responses distinguish neuronal activity due to visual stimulation in the central region from activity in visual cortex.

Thus, neuromagnetic measurements made it possible to detect a new region of activity in an extravisual area that had not been identified previously by microelectrode studies on primates. Activity is evoked by changes in the velocity of the stimulus, which would seem to imply that the population is involved in a tracking function. There is preliminary evidence that the latency of this activity is comparatively long (approximately 200 msec), and we have speculated elsewhere that this neuronal activity may follow processing in visual cortex for comparison purposes (38), such as determining whether an image moving across the retina is due to movement of the object or of the eye. Thus, the proximity of the visually active region to motor cortex suggests that it may be the site to which reafferent signals are distributed for comparison purposes.

CONCLUSIONS

Although this chapter is not a complete survey of the study of visual processes using neuromagnetic methods, it is quite representative. In fact, given the precision of results obtained using these methods in other modalities, it is somewhat surprising that more has not been accomplished during the past dozen years. This is attributable to several factors. Previously it has been difficult to provide visual stimulation without producing magnetic artifacts. Also it was difficult to keep a subject in a fixed position while measuring the field over a broad region at the back. Exploring the field over other regions of the head was particularly difficult because that required placing subjects on their sides, in order to investigate the temporal cortex, while also appropriately adjusting the position of the visual display. These problems have been alleviated by a variety of modern devices such as video projectors that can be used to project images into magnetically shielded rooms, vertatile gantries that ease the task of positioning the dewar over the head, CryoSQUID sensors that can be oriented in any direction, and innovative dewars in which the sensors themselves are canted with respect to the dewar's axis (40). These advances in instrumentation promise to markedly enhance the productivity of neuromagnetic studies of the human visual system and encourage more researchers to become involved.

ACKNOWLEDGMENTS

We are grateful for support from the Air Force Office of Scientific Research through grant F49620-86-C-0131.

REFERENCES

1. Brenner D, Williamson SJ, Kaufman L. Visually evoked magnetic fields of the human brain. *Science* 1985;190:480–482.
2. Williamson SJ, Romani GL, Kaufman L, Modena I, eds. *Biomagnetism: an interdisciplinary approach.* New York: Plenum Press.
3. Hämäläinen M, Sarvas J. Feasibility of the homogeneous head model in the interpretation of neuromagnetic data. *Phys Med Biol* 1987;32:91–97.
4. Meijs JWH, Peters MJ. The EEG and MEG, using a model of eccentric spheres to describe the head. *IEEE Trans Biomed Eng* 1987;BME-34:913–920.
5. Barth DS, Beatty J, Broffman J, Sutherling W. Magnetic localization of a dipolar current source implanted in a sphere and a human cranium. *Electroencephalogr Clin Neurophysiol* 1985;63:260–273.
6. Williamson SJ, Kaufman L. Analysis of neuromagnetic signals. In: Gevins A, Rémond A, eds. *Handbook of electroencephalography and clinical neurophysiology, revised vol 1.* Amsterdam: Elsevier, 1987;405–448.
7. Romani GL, Williamson SJ, Kaufman L. Biomagnetic instrumentation. *Rev Sci Instrum* 1982;53:1815–1845.
8. Buchanan DS, Paulson D, Williamson SJ. Instrumentation for clinical applications of neuromagnetism. In: Fast RW, ed. *Advances in cryogenic engineering, vol 33,* New York: Plenum Press, 1987;97–106.
9. Okada Y. Discrimination of localized and extended current dipole sources and localized single and multiple sources. In: Weinberg H, Stroink G, Katila T, eds. *Biomagnetism: applications and theory.* New York: Pergamon Press, 1985;266–272.
10. Brenner D, Okada Y, Maclin E, Williamson SJ, Kaufman L. Evoked magnetic fields reveal different visual areas in human cortex. In: Erné SN, Hahlbohm HD, Lübbig H, eds. *Biomagnetism.* Berlin: Walter de Gruyter, 1981;431–444.
11. Maclin E, Okada Y, Kaufman L, Williamson SJ. Retinotopic map on the visual cortex for eccentrically placed patterns: first noninvasive measurements. *Il Nuovo Cimento* 1983;2D:410–419.
12. Romani GL, Williamson SJ, Kaufman L. Tonotopic organization of the human auditory cortex. *Science* 1982;216:1339–1340.
13. Schwartz EL. A quantitative model of the functional architecture of human striate cortex with application to visual illusion and cortical texture analysis. *Biol Cybern* 1980;37:63–76.
14. Schwartz EL. On the mathematical structure of the visuotopic mapping of macaque striate cortex. *Science* 1985;227:1065–1066.
15. Tootell RBH, Silverman MS, Switkes E, De Valois RL. Deoxyglucose analysis of retinotopic organization in primate striate cortex. *Science* 1982;218:902–904; also, *Science* 1985;227:1066.
16. Okada Y, Kaufman L, Brenner D, Williamson SJ. Modulation transfer functions of the human visual system revealed by magnetic field measurements. *Vision Res* 1982;22:319–333.
17. Robson JG. Spatial and temporal contrast-sensitivity functions of the visual system. *J Opt Soc Am* 1966;56:1141–1147.
18. Kelly DH. Frequency doubling in visual responses. *J Opt Soc Am* 1966; 56:1628–1633.
19. Regan D. Assessment of visual acuity by evoked potential recording: ambiguity caused by temporal dependence of spatial frequency selectivity. *Vision Res* 1978;18:439–443.
20. Hubel D, Weisel TN. Receptive fields and functional architecture of monkey striate cortex. *J Physiol (Lond)* 1968;195:215–243.
21. Campbell FW, Kulikowski JJ. The visual evoked potential as a function of contrast of a grating pattern. *J Physiol (Lond)* 1972;222:345–356.

22. Campbell FW, Maffei L. Electrophysiological evidence for the existence of orientation and size detectors in the human visual system. *J Physiol (Lond)* 1970;207:534–652.
23. Williamson SJ, Kaufman L, Brenner D. Latency of the neuromagnetic response of the human visual cortex. *Vision Res* 1978;18:107–110.
24. Breitmeyer B. Simple reaction time as a measure of the temporal response properties of transient and sustained channels. *Vision Res* 1975;15:1411–1412.
25. Harwerth RS, Levi DM. Reaction time as a measure of suprathreshold grating detection. *Vision Res* 1978;18:1579–1586.
26. Woodworth RS. *Experimental psychology.* New York: Henry Holt, 1938.
27. Posner MJ. *Chronometric explorations of mind.* Hillsdale NJ: Erlbaum, 1978.
28. Enroth-Cugell C, Robson JG. The contrast sensitivity of retinal ganglion cells of the cat. *J Physiol (Lond)* 1966;187:517–552.
29. Cleland BG, Dubin MW, Levick WR. Sustained and transient neurones in the cat's retina and lateral geniculate nucleus. *J Physiol (Lond)* 1971;217:473–496.
30. Hochstein S, Shapley RM. Linear and nonlinear spatial subunits in Y cat retinal ganglion cells. *J Physiol (Lond)* 1976;262:265–284.
31. Kulikowski JJ, Tolhurst DL. Psychophysical evidence for sustained and transient detectors in human vision. *J Physiol (Lond)* 1973;232:149–162.
32. Tolhurst DL. Sustained and transient channels in human vision. *Vision Res* 1975;15:1151–1155.
33. Regan D. *Evoked potentials in psychology, sensory physiology, and clinical medicine.* London: Chapman and Hall, 1972.
34. Williamson SJ, Kaufman L, Brenner D. Evoked neuromagnetic fields of the human brain. *J Appl Phys* 1979;50:2418–2421.
35. Kaufman L, Williamson SJ. The evoked magnetic field of the human brain. *Ann NY Acad Sci* 1980;340:45–65.
36. Zeki S. Functional specialization of a visual area in the posterior bank of the superior temporal sulcus of the rhesus monkey. *J Physiol (Lond)* 1974;236:549–573.
37. Van Essen DC. Visual areas of the mammalian cerebral cortex. *Annu Rev Neurosci* 1979;2:227–263.
38. Lounasmaa OV, Williamson SJ, Kaufman L, Tanenbaum R. Visually evoked responses from non-occipital areas of human cortex. In: Weinberg G, Stroink G, Katila T, eds. *Biomagnetism: applications and theory.* New York: Pergamon, 1985;348–353.
39. Okada Y, Williamson SJ, Kaufman L. Magnetic field of the human sensorimotor cortex. *Int J Neurosci* 1982;17:33–38.
40. Knuutila J, Ahlfors S, Ahonen A, Hämäläinen M, Ilmomiemi R, Kajola MJ. Large-area low-noise seven-channel dc SQUID magnetometer for brain research. *Rev Sci Instrum* 1987;58:2145–2156.

The Pattern Electroretinogram in Animals and Humans: Physiological and Clinical Applications

L. Maffei and A. Fiorentini

Istituto di Neurofisiologia del CNR, 56100 Pisa, Italy

THE FLASH ELECTRORETINOGRAM AND THE PATTERN ELECTRORETINOGRAM IN ANIMALS FOLLOWING SECTION OF THE OPTIC NERVE

The pattern electroretinogram (PERG), although it may appear a recently discovered diagnostic tool, has a rather long history. The first report of an electroretinographic potential that was not evoked by a light flash but by a pattern temporally modulated in color contrast was made by Riggs et al. (1). This small retinal potential remained a sort of curiosity because it was not realized at that time that it could have substantially different bioelectrical sources from the classic electroretinogram (ERG).

A new insight was indirectly suggested by the fruitful development of the recording of visual evoked potentials (VEP) in response to patterned stimuli.

The pattern VEP, different from those evoked by uniform light, were correlated with visual functions. It soon became clear that different neural sources contribute to the potentials evoked by patterned and unpatterned stimuli. This view was supported by the electrophysiological properties of cortical neurones that are known to be rather insensitive to homogeneous light stimuli.

By analogy, it appeared likely that also at a retinal level homogeneous and patterned stimuli could excite preferentially different classes of neurons.

This was proved by a simple experiment in the cat and monkey. One optic nerve was transected intracranially to cause retrograde degeneration of ganglion cells. The steady-state PERG (in response to sinusoidal gratings phase reversed at several hertz) was found to deteriorate and eventually to disappear in parallel with the time course of ganglion cell degeneration (2,3). The flash ERG remained unaltered (Fig. 1). Histological examination using light and electron microscopy showed that the cells in retinal layers distal to the ganglion cells were morphologically normal (4).

The degeneration of ganglion cells progresses for a few weeks in the monkey (5) and for 2 to 3 months in the cat (6). During this period the deteriora-

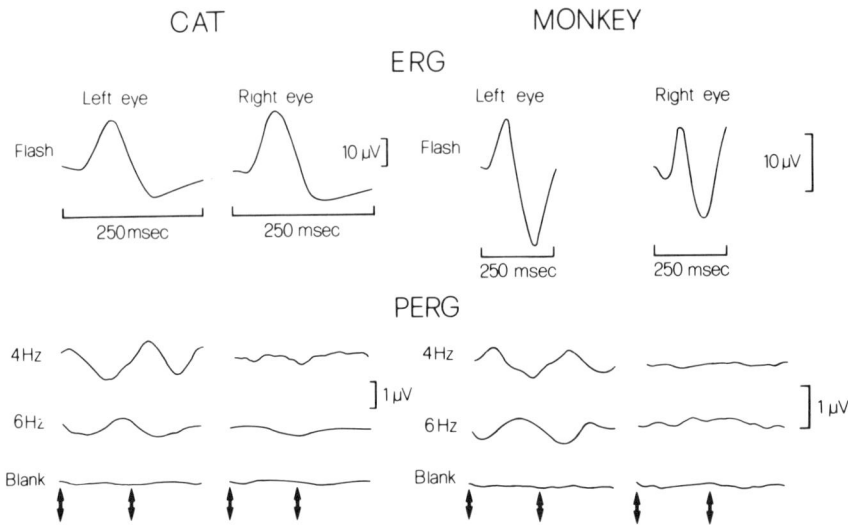

FIG. 1. Examples of electroretinographic records obtained from both eyes of a cat **(left)** and a macaque pigtail monkey **(right)**, in which the right optic nerve had been transected intracranially 9 months (cat) or 26 months (monkey) before recording session. **Top:** ERG response to 50-msec flashes of homogeneous light (averaged over 20 stimuli). **Bottom:** PERG responses to sinusoidal gratings reversed in phase at 4 and 6 Hz and averaged over 800 stimulus periods. The *double arrows* indicate stimulus reversals. Stimulus spatial frequency: 0.5 c/deg (cat), 1.5 c/deg (monkey). Stimulus contrast: 80% (cat); 60% (monkey). Mean luminance: 7 cd/m^2 (cat); 100 cd/m^2 (monkey). Artificial pupil: 3 mm. (From unpublished data obtained in collaboration with S. Bisti and C. Trimarchi.)

tion of the PERG also progresses. Initially, at least in the cat, the responses to low spatial frequencies are mainly depressed.

This raised the question whether the deterioration of the PERG was correlated with the degeneration of a particular class of ganglion cells. The approach was to correlate the time course of ganglion cell degeneration in the cat with the progressive alteration in the PERG recorded at various times after optic nerve section. It was found that the first observable alteration of the PERG, which occurs in the low spatial frequency range, is correlated with the degeneration of the mid-sized ganglion cells (most probably β neurones) (4).

Recent experiments on the rhesus monkey in which ganglion cell degeneration was induced by localized burns of the retinal fiber layer confirm the rapid loss of PERG responses to gratings of medium spatial frequency following the lesion (7).

The conclusion is that ganglion cell degeneration prevents the PERG recording. This should not be taken as evidence that this potential directly originates in the ganglion cell layer. The degeneration of the ganglion cells could affect the function of other retinal neurons indirectly, such as bipolar cells, which do not appear to be altered morphologically (4). The spatial frequency tuning of the PERG, with a marked low-frequency attenuation at least in humans and monkeys, suggests that the retinal cells involved in PERG generation have receptive fields with concentric antagonistic organization.

As is known, this organization favors the cell's responsiveness to patterns of suitable size and contrast, whereas the dc component (uniform luminance) tends to be filtered out.

Experimental findings obtained in animals with optic nerve section do not permit one to localize the electrical sources of the PERG precisely. Despite this uncertainty about the precise origin of the PERG, the important point is that the degeneration of the ganglion cells affects only the PERG.

Below we review other experimental evidence that complements findings after ganglion cell degeneration pointing to the existence of at least partially different retinal sources for the PERG and the flash ERG.

OTHER METHODS TO DISTINGUISH THE FLASH ERG FROM THE PERG

Increase of Intraocular Pressure

Another method to dissociate the sources of the flash ERG from those of the PERG is to induce retinal ischemia by increasing the intraocular pressure in the cat's eye. This is also an attempt to mimic the situation of acute glaucoma in humans. This experiment (8) was performed by injecting physiological saline solution into the posterior chamber of the eye, thus increasing the intraocular pressure to the point at which the mass response to a flickering light recorded from the lateral geniculate nucleus (LGN) just vanishes. Under these conditions, there is no ERG response either to light flashes or to pattern reversal. When the injection is discontinued after 15 to 20 min, the responses to light flashes and to contrast-reversal gratings recover, the former after only a few minutes, the latter more slowly.

If the increased intraocular pressure is maintained for at least 30 min, the dissociation between the responses to light flashes and phase-reversed gratings is more apparent and long-lasting. Similar findings have been recently obtained by Siliprandi et al. (9).

Experimental glaucoma has also been induced in the monkey (10), and the PERG has been found to be reduced in amplitude by an amount related to the increase in intraocular pressure. The uniform field ERG was unaffected.

Interfering with Spike Activity of Retinal Cells Affects the PERG, Not the Flash ERG

In the cat, antidromic activation of the optic nerve by stimulation with a train of electrical impulses causes a depression of the PERG but leaves the flash ERG unaltered (8). This shows that interfering with spike activity in the ganglion cell axons selectively affects the PERG. Further support of this point has been obtained recently by Bisti et al. (*unpublished data*). It has been found that injection of a solution of tetrodotoxin (TTX) to block the retinal spike input to the LGN has the effect of depressing dramatically the PERG, leaving the flash ERG unchanged.

Flash ERG and PERG Following Block of the Retinal Artery in the Cat

The b wave of the flash ERG is known to be impaired by retinal ischemia. This effect is, however, to a large extent, reversible. The b wave recovers after restoration of retinal circulation. The effects of a temporary block of the retinal artery on the PERG are much more severe (8).

Intraretinal Recording of PERG

Intraretinal recordings have provided another basis for distinguishing the PERG from the flash ERG.

Sieving and Steinberg (11) recorded intraretinally in the cat and found that the amplitude of the PERG generated by a square-wave grating phase-reversed at 8 Hz has its maximum amplitude in the proximal layers of the retina, whereas the amplitude of the luminance ERG is highest more distally. They conclude that the generators contributing to the PERG are located proximal to the inner nuclear layer and are different from the generators of the flash ERG. Similar results were obtained by Baker et al. (12) from intraretinal recording in the monkey.

Properties of the PERG in Humans

In humans, as in cats and monkeys, the PERG in response to a grating phase-reversed at a sufficiently high temporal frequency (6–8 Hz or 12–16 reversals/sec) has an approximately sinusoidal waveform corresponding to the second harmonic of the stimulus frequency. The second harmonic is largest at 8 Hz, and there is a secondary peak at approximately 2 Hz where the waveform is much more complex (13).

The PERG shows a spatial frequency tuning, with the maximum at approximately 2 to 4 c/deg and attenuation at both lower and higher spatial frequencies. The attenuation at low spatial frequencies suggests that the PERG has neural sources with center-surround antagonistic organization. Vaegan and Arden (14) recently showed that the amplitude of the PERG in response to various types of patterns is correlated with the amplitude of the fundamental Fourier component of the pattern and not with the local luminance or peak-to-peak luminance change. This property is not consistent with an interpretation of the PERG resulting from local responses to luminance modulation (15).

The human PERG shows a dramatic increase in amplitude when the mean luminance increases in the photopic range. At illuminances below 1 troland, the PERG is very small even with a large stimulus field, suggesting the predominant contribution to the PERG of photopic mechanisms (16,17).

THE PERG AS A DIAGNOSTIC TOOL IN THE CLINICAL PRACTICE

The PERG is widely used at present in the clinic since, different from the flash ERG, it is a sensitive indicator of optic nerve pathology and ganglion cell dysfunction. A number of cases have been reported in which the PERG is severely depressed or totally absent, whereas the flash ERG is normal. These include cases of retinal ischemia, glaucoma, and optic neuritis.

Similar to findings in the animal (see previously), a temporary block of the retinal artery has profound effects on the PERG. We reported a case of retinal ischemia caused by a block of the retinal artery in which the flash ERG was normal although the PERG was completely abolished (18).

Another pathological state that compromises the PERG, but not the flash ERG, is increased intraocular pressure. In glaucoma, which is known to affect predominantly the ganglion cells (19), impairment of PERG responses is particularly evident at medium spatial frequencies (20). To some degree this impairment seems to correlate with the amount of intraocular pressure elevation (21).

A reduction in PERG amplitude has also been reported in many cases of patients with retrobulbar optic neuritis, in which the flash ERG was normal (16). In the early acute phase of neuritis, the PERG may remain normal, whereas the VEP are depressed. Subsequently, however, the PERG response becomes abnormal, suggesting a progressive dysfunction of retinal ganglion cells.

Maculopathies may also profoundly affect the amplitude of the PERG. As suggested by Celesia and Kaufman (22), this might be due to the predominant contribution to the PERG of the macular region where the density of ganglion cells is highest.

PERG IN PATIENTS WITH TRAUMATIC LESIONS OF THE OPTIC NERVE

The dissociation between the luminance ERG and the PERG produced by transection of the optic nerve in animals is reproduced in humans with lesions of the optic nerve fibers. There has been a number of reports of such patients with partial or complete interruption of the optic fibers. ERG responses were recorded from their eyes a long time after the lesion, and their retinae were therefore likely to have undergone ganglion cell degeneration. In some of these cases, a complete suppression of PERG (with spared ERG to flash) was reported (23,24). In other cases, however, the PERG was reported to be present, although somewhat reduced in amplitude (25–27).

Obviously, in patients with accidental traumatic lesions, the anatomical control of the lesion is not available, and therefore it is difficult to have precise information on the proportion of nerve fibers severed. This could be one of the reasons for the diversity of results reported for the various cases.

Recently, two patients with unilateral surgical transection of the optic nerve were studied, one by us. The latter was a 10-year-old girl operated on 36 months before testing. The operated eye was totally blind and no VEP response was present. The flicker ERG was normal, but the PERG, in response to sinusoidal gratings of 2 and 5 c/deg, 50% contrast, phase-reversed at 8 Hz, did not exceed the noise level in amplitude.

A report of the second case was published recently (28). The results of PERG recorded in the normal and affected eye are reproduced in Fig. 2. The stimulus consisted of checkerboards of very high contrast (99%) that reversed in phase 10 times per second (5 Hz). For very large checks the responses of the two eyes were equally large and did not change in amplitude when the retinal image was defocused. The authors rightly point out that these are not

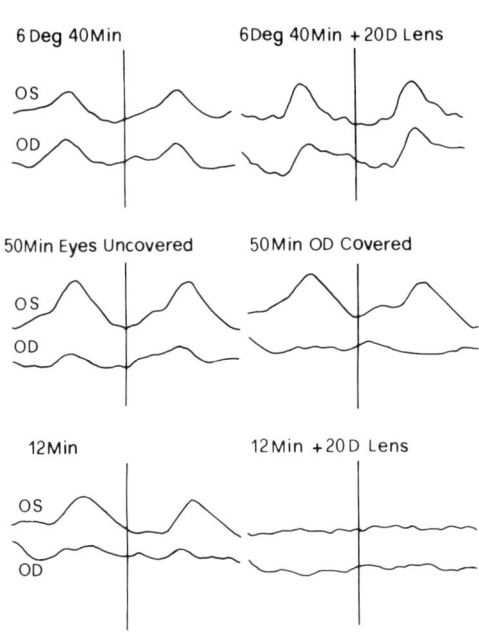

FIG. 2. PERGs in a human patient after resection of the right optic nerve. Vertical lines mark reversal. Positive at the active electrode on the cornea is indicated by an upward deflection. **Top:** PERGs produced by 6-deg/40-min checks with normal viewing **(left)** and with +20 diopter lens in front of the eyes **(right)**. **Middle:** PERG produced by 50-min checks in the left and right eyes (top and bottom traces). **Left:** both eyes uncovered; **right:** right eye covered. **Bottom:** PERGs produced by 12-min checks with normal viewing **(left)** and with +20 diopter lens in front of the eyes **(right)**. (Replotted from ref. 28.)

pattern responses. For checks smaller than 5 deg/side, the responses of the affected eye dropped dramatically, approaching noise level.

In Fig. 2 (middle), the responses to 50-min checks are reported. A PERG of small amplitude is present in the records from the affected eye. Unfortunately, the control with defocused images is lacking. This small response could still be a local luminance response (Fig. 2, top), in view of the check size that is still large and of high contrast. A single 50-min check covers a large portion of the human fovea. At the bottom of Fig. 2 are the responses of the two eyes to 12-min checks. The authors conclude that a small response is present in the affected eye. On inspection of the records, we would tend to conclude the opposite. This is an example of the degree of uncertainty in the interpretation of this type of record from patients, particularly when no quantitative analysis of the data is available.

REFERENCES

1. Riggs LA, Johnson EP, Schick AML. Electrical responses of the human eye to moving stimulus patterns. *Science* 1964;144:567.
2. Maffei L, Fiorentini A. Electroretinographic responses to alternating gratings before and after section of the optic nerve. *Science* 1981;211:953–955.
3. Maffei L, Fiorentini A, Bisti S, Holländer H. Pattern ERG in the monkey after section of the optic nerve. *Exp Brain Res* 1985;59:423–425.
4. Holländer H, Bisti S, Maffei L, Hebel R. Electroretinographic responses and retrograde changes of retinal morphology after intracranial optic nerve section. A quantitative analysis in the cat. *Exp Brain Res* 1984;55:483–493.
5. Radius LR, Anderson DR. Retinal ganglion cell degeneration in experimental optic atrophy. *Am J Ophthalmol* 1978;86:673–679.
6. Stone J. The number and distribution of ganglion cells in the cat's retina. *J Comp Neurol* 1978;180:753–771.
7. Dawson WW, Stratton RD, Hope GM, Parmer R, Engel HM, Kessler MJ. Tissue responses of the monkey retina: tuning and dependence on inner layer integrity. *Invest Ophthalmol Vis Sci* 1986;27:734–745.
8. Maffei L, Fiorentini A. Electroretinographic responses to alternating gratings in the cat. *Exp Brain Res* 1982;48:327–334.
9. Siliprandi R, Cannella R, Carmignoto G. Pressure effects on pattern electroretinogram in the cat. *Soc Neurosci Abst* 1986;12:638.
10. Marx SM, Podos SM, Bodis-Wollner I, et al. Flash and pattern electroretinograms in normal and laser-induced glaucomatous primate eyes. *Invest Ophthalmol Vis Sci* 1986;27:378–386.
11. Sieving PA, Steinberg H. Proximal retinal contribution to the intraretinal 8-Hz pattern ERG of cat. *J Neurophysiol* 1987;57:104–120.
12. Baker CL, Hess RF, Zrenner E, Olsen BT. Current source density analysis of linear and non linear components of the primate ERG. *J Neurophysiol* (*in press*).
13. Baker CL, Hess RF. Linear and non-linear components of the human electroretinogram. *J Neurophysiol* 1984;51:952–967.
14. Vaegan Arden GB. Effect of pattern luminance profile on the pattern ERG in man and pigeon. *Vision Res* 1987;27:883–892.
15. Riemslag FCC, Ringo JL, Speckreijse H, Verduyn-Lunel H. The luminance origin of the pattern electroretinogram in man. *J Physiol* (*Lond*) 1985;363:191–209.
16. Maffei L, Fiorentini A. Generator sources of the pattern ERG in man and animals. In: Cracco RQ, Bodis-Wollner I, eds. *Evoked potentials,* Frontiers of Clinical Neuroscience, vol 3. New York: Alan R. Liss, 1986;101–116.

17. Hess RP, Baker CL, Zrenner E, Schwarzer J. Differences between electroretinograms of cat and primate. *J Neurophysiol* 1986;56:747–768.
18. Fiorentini A, Maffei L. Pirchio M, Spinelli D, Porciatti V. The ERG in response to alternating gratings in patients with diseases of the peripheral visual pathway. *Invest Ophthalmol Vis Sci* 1981;21:490–493.
19. Quigley HA, Addicks EM, Green WR, Marimenal AE. Optic nerve damage in human glaucoma. II. The site of injury and susceptibility to damage. *Arch Ophthalmol* 1981;99:635–649.
20. Porciatti V, Falsini B, Brunori S, Colotto A, Moretti G. Pattern electroretinogram as a function of spatial frequency in ocular hypertension and early glaucoma. *Doc Ophthalmol Proc Ser* 1987;65:349–355.
21. Papst M, Bopp N, Schnandigel OE. The pattern evoked electroretinogram associated with elevated intraocular pressure. *Graefes Arch Clin Exp Ophthalmol* 1984;222:34–17.
22. Celesia GG, Kaufman D. Pattern ERGs and visual evoked potentials in maculopathies and optic nerve diseases. *Invest Ophthalmol Vis Sci* 1985;26:726–735.
23. Groneberg A, Teping C. Topodiagnostik von Sehstoerungen durch Abteilung retinaler and kortikaler Antworten auf Umkehr-Kontrastmuster. *Ber Dtsch Ophthalmol Ges* 1980;77:409–415.
24. Dawson WW, Maida TM, Rubin ML. Human pattern-evoked retinal responses are altered by optic atrophy. *Invest Ophthalmol Vis Sci* 1982;22:796–803.
25. Sherman J. Simultaneous pattern-reversal electroretinograms and visual evoked potentials in diseases of the macula and optic nerve. In: Bodis-Wollner I, ed. *Evoked potentials*, Annals of the New York Academy of Sciences, vol 388. New York: Alan R. Liss, 1982;214–226.
26. Sherman J. ERG and VEP as supplemental aids in the differential diagnosis of retinal versus optic nerve disease. In: Cracco RG, Bodis-Wollner I, eds. *Evoked potentials*. Frontiers of Clinical Neuroscience, vol 3. New York: Alan R. Liss, 1986;343–353.
27. Caruso RC, Higgins KE. Origin of the pattern electroretinogram: evidence provided by the hemianopic retina. *Invest Ophthalmol Vis Sci* 1987;28 (suppl):62.
28. Harrison JM, O'Connor PS, Young RSL, Kinkaid M, Bentley R. The pattern ERG in man following surgical resection of the optic nerve. *Invest Ophthalmol Vis Sci* 1987;28:492–496.

Vision and the Brain,
edited by B. Cohen and I. Bodis-Wollner.
Raven Press, Ltd., New York © 1990.

The Visual System in Parkinson's Disease

Ivan Bodis-Wollner

*Department of Neurology, Mount Sinai School of Medicine,
New York, New York 10029*

Scattered studies in the clinical-neurophysiological literature have suggested vague sensory defects in patients affected by Parkinson's disease (PD). Such observations were generally attributed to impaired cognition. A primary sensory defect as a possible explanation would have run contrary to the accepted notion that PD is an exclusive motor system disorder with specific neuropathological changes affecting the basal ganglia, predominantly dopaminergic neurons and their circuits in the striatonigral pathway. It was surprising, therefore, when Bodis-Wollner and Yahr in 1978 (1) reported that a large number of patients suffering from PD have abnormal visual evoked potentials (VEP) and suggested that this result represents dopaminergic synaptic deficiency in the visual pathway. Initially, there was little support for this idea. By now, considerable support based on psychophysical and electrophysiological measurements exists attesting to visual dysfunction in a significant number of patients affected by PD. Animal studies using pharmacological manipulations have indicated an important role for dopamine (DA) in the retina, as we will discuss later. In addition, pathological and pathophysiological data obtained in monkeys suffering from a parkinsonian syndrome induced by 1-methyl-4-phenyl 1,2,3,6-tetrahydropyridine (MPTP), a neurotoxin specific for dopaminergic neurons, strengthens the notion that PD is a clinical syndrome based on specific but distributed lesions of various dopaminergic systems of the human CNS, including the visual pathway. As previously mentioned, studies of visual dysfunction in PD were instrumental in refocusing attention on the specific neurophysiopathology of this disease. In this chapter our studies, published elsewhere in greater detail, are summarized, as well as those of other investigators. Studies of visual dysfunction in PD patients and in monkeys with dopaminergic deficiency have challenging implications for visual physiology.

CONTRAST SENSITIVITY IN PD

It was shown nearly 20 years ago (2) that the use of contrast sensitivity (CS) can uncover hidden visual defects. CS quantifies the contrast needed to detect coarse targets, not only the smallest target size the observer can identify (Fig. 1). Usually sinusoidal gratings are used as targets for the test. It was shown

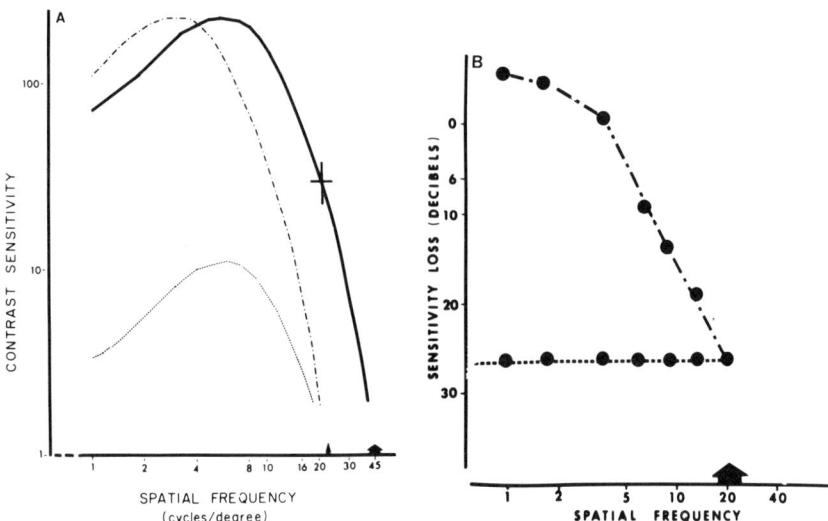

FIG. 1. A: The normal CS curve (*solid line*) is based on data from 10 observers. The inverse of contrast threshold is called CS. This is plotted as a function of spatial frequency and drawn by eye. There is a 4-dB spread between individual observers. Both coordinates are plotted on logarithmic scales. The extrapolated high frequency leg of the curve defines the finest detectable grating pattern at 100% contrast, the so-called cut-off frequency. This is 45 cpd under the conditions of this investigation for normal observers with 6/6 Snellen acuity. In angular size, a single bar at this frequency subtends 40 sec of arc at the eye. The *broad arrow* shows this extrapolated frequency. A *thin arrow* is placed at half the normal cut-off frequency (22.5 cpd) to symbolize a twofold reduction in the normal acuity (6/12). Extrapolation of either of the two CS curves shown with *broken lines* meets the abscissa at this frequency. The *dashed-dotted line* curve results from the uniform displacement of the normal curve to the left along the spatial frequency axis, whereas the *dotted line* curve results from the uniform depression of the normal curve along the CS axis. **B:** In order to demonstrate reduction in contrast sensitivity for 6/12 visual acuity, a visuogram was constructed. For corresponding spatial frequencies, the ratio of the altered to normal contrast threshold is plotted. This ratio is expressed in decibels. *Dashed-dotted lines* show the visuogram to be expected if 6/12 acuity resulted from a displacement of the normal contrast sensitivity curve to the left, as shown in A. The visuogram corresponding to a displacement of the normal curve downward in A is shown with *short dashed lines*. (From ref. 4.)

that for a given twofold change in visual acuity, CS may be altered by as much as a factor of 20. A patient's ability to detect patterns of varying sizes may be impaired without much effect on the visual acuity. Since then, CS measurements have been found increasingly useful for clinical application in the assessment of foveal vision in patients with neurological and ophthalmological disorders (3). Studies of patients with various neurological disorders (4,5) have established that it is not possible to predict a patient's ability to detect coarse patterns on the basis of visual acuity (for review, see [3]). CS is usually established with sinusoidal gratings as test targets. These were originally introduced into animal and human physiological studies by Campbell, Robson, and colleagues (6–8), whose work has established that the normal human CS function reflects both optical and neural attenuation. As opposed to a purely passive optical filter, the human CS curve shows a low spatial frequency decline. Low frequency CS attenuation is also observed at many levels of the visual system, including retinal ganglion cells, and its occurrence is attributed to the organization of center and surround mechanisms of the receptive field (7). Pattern electroretinogram (PERG) measurements in humans also reveal a low spatial frequency decline (9,10). It has been established that the PERG reflects ganglion cell activity in primates (11). It is therefore likely that the low spatial frequency decline of the human CS curve also reflects the retinal input to the cortex of neurons with center-surround organization. Analogous to the spatial CS curve is the flicker sensitivity function. Detectability of sinusoidal flicker is plotted against temporal frequency, and the resulting curve of the human temporal transfer function is named after de Lange (12). The de Lange curve also shows low (temporal) frequency attenuation, analogous to the spatial curve. Finally, Robson (13) explored the detectability of various spatial frequencies at different rates of flicker. Studies by Robson and by Kelly (14) revealed that the normal human spatiotemporal CS is a function with a single peak. When presented as a three-dimensional surface plot, it shows low and high frequency attenuation in both spatial and temporal frequencies.

During the past decade, using sinusoidal gratings as stimuli, we studied CS and evoked potentials (summarized in the second part of this chapter) of patients affected by PD. Kupersmith et al. (15) reported abnormal CS in patients with PD using printed grating targets. Regan and Neima (16) studied vision in PD using low-contrast Snellen optotypes and reported that patients have defects for relatively large letters. Following an inquiry as to whether we had found spatial CS losses in PD (D. Regan, 1984, *personal communication*), we reevaluated our own data and performed additional studies measuring flicker sensitivity and in particular spatiotemporal CS (17). In general, visual abnormalities that may be considered specific for this disease could be summarized graphically as a specifically distorted shape of the spatiotemporal CS function: the peak is flattened and low frequency attenuation is less apparent compared with normals. As we shall discuss, these and converging data from other investigators suggest that dopaminergic deficiency in PD affects the visual system, and DA is probably one of the crucial retinal neurotransmitters of receptive field organization in human vision.

Spatiotemporal CS

Methods

A total of 41 patients with PD (82 eyes) were tested. Flicker sensitivity (spatial frequency = 0 cpd [cycles/degree]) measurements were made at 1, 2, 4, 8, and 16 Hz. In addition, spatial CS was compared for 1 and 8 Hz over the spatial frequencies 0.5, 1, 2, 4, 6, 8, 12, and in some at 16 cpd. Sinusoidal modulation was employed. Stimuli were generated on cathode-ray tubes (CRT). The screen of the CRT was always surrounded by a homogeneously illuminated field with a hue similar to that of the stimulus screen (its mean luminance was 0.2 log units lower than the screen). Monocular testing with natural pupils was always employed. The nontested eye was patched with gauze, which transmitted light but blurred spatial detail. Viewing distance was always 1.44 m from the visual display.

CS was assessed monocularly using the method of constant stimuli (MCS) (4). Spatial contrast threshold was also determined with the MCS.

The input to the CRT from the z axis was increased in successive steps of half a log unit until the observer indicated that flicker or pattern, depending on the test, was visible. We then assumed that the threshold occurred within this range of half a log unit (or 10 dB). For all threshold measurements, we will refer to z axis attenuation in terms of decibels, in which 20 dB corresponds to 1 log unit (18). Once the 10 dB range was determined for a given temporal frequency, flicker stimuli that differed from each other by 2 dB (or 0.1 log unit) were presented to the observer. Following each presentation of the flicker, the observer was asked to indicate whether he or she detected the flicker. From these responses, the probability of detection was derived. We accepted 50% probability as the detection threshold. False negative and false positive responses were determined by random presentation of high and zero contrast stimuli (4). Patients were excluded from the study when they responded positively to zero contrast stimuli or negatively to high contrast stimuli on at least 6 of 20 presentations of a given stimulus condition.

In addition, we compared the threshold obtained by the MCS with the threshold obtained with a two-alternative temporal forced choice (2 AFC) technique in each eye of 16 of these patients with PD. It is thought that the 2-AFC procedure produces a less biased threshold measurement in which decision criteria play a lesser role. The MCS was much easier to employ with the patients of this study. Many patients could not follow the instructions for the 2-AFC procedure.

The critical fusion frequency (CFF) was also determined in each eye of these 41 patients with PD using the same stimulus display. The CFF was determined by first decreasing and then increasing the temporal frequency of the 100% modulated flicker. After six passes each way, the mean value was defined as the CFF.

Sensitivity Gain in Spatiotemporal Contrast Vision in PD

In normal observers, sensitivity decreases for low spatial frequencies with low rates of temporal modulation, and an increase in CS occurs when the rate of temporal modulation is increased (13). Our normal data, shown in Fig. 2, are consistent with those previously reported in the literature. In Fig. 2, we

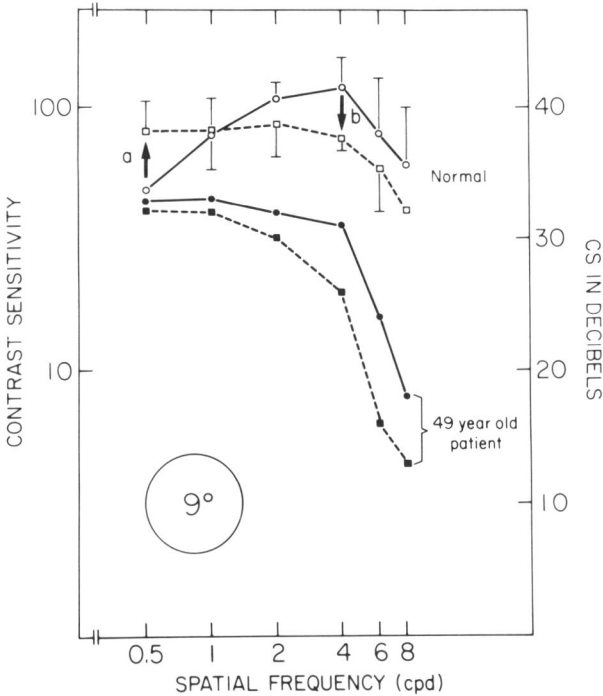

FIG. 2. Spatiotemporal CS to a 9° field is shown for five spatial frequencies that were on/off modulated using temporal frequencies of 1 Hz (*solid lines*) or 8 Hz (*broken lines*). CS (1/contrast threshold) is shown on the left vertical axis and CS is measured in decibels (dB) on the right vertical axis. The mean normal curves are represented by *open symbols*. The 1- and 8-Hz functions of a 49-year-old PD patient are represented by *solid symbols*. The 1-Hz functions are represented by *circles* and the 8-Hz functions by *squares*. Sensitivity gain is labeled a (*upward vertical arrow*) and refers to the increase from 1 to 8 Hz (see text). Notice that age does not determine the parkinsonian type of CS defects illustrated in this figure, as explained in the text. (From ref. 17.)

also present data from a patient with PD. Note that CS is attenuated in the 49-year-old patient, an age similar to the average of our normal controls. The peak is attenuated, and there is no low frequency decline in the patient. If we take the ratio of CS at the peak of the function to CS to the 0.5-cpd grating, the results indicate that there is a weakening of low frequency attenuation. Alternatively, the results could be viewed as a shift of the entire CS curve, down and to the left, as will be discussed later.

Figure 2 shows that differences between 1 versus 8 Hz CS at low spatial frequencies are not pronounced in PD. In normal observers, we refer to the increase of CS, which occurs to the 0.5-cpd grating when the rate of temporal modulation is increased from 1 to 8 Hz, as the "sensitivity gain" (represented as "a" in the figure). We found the average sensitivity gain to be +4.8 dB with an SD of 2.1 dB. We compared the sensitivity gain of the 17 PD eyes with the norm, and responses that were 2 SDs below the normal mean were counted as abnormal. Eight of the 17 eyes (or 6/11 patients with PD) were abnormal. Five of these abnormal eyes had *negative* sensitivity scores, indicating that CS for 1 Hz modulation was actually *higher* than CS for 8 Hz modulation.

The 1 and 8 Hz CS values to the different spatial frequencies in each patient were compared with the norm, and responses that fell 2 SDs below the normal mean for a given spatiotemporal condition were counted as abnormal. The breakdown of abnormal spatiotemporal CS in the patients with PD shows that the abnormality rates were significantly different for comparisons between 1 versus 8 Hz CS for the 0.5-cpd grating and for the 1-cpd grating (McNemar's test, $p < 0.05$). However, comparisons between spatial frequencies of 2 cpd and above failed to reach statistical significance. Thus, the greatest number of abnormal responses occurred with 8-Hz modulation of the low spatial frequency gratings, a result also suggested by our examination of sensitivity gain at 0.5 cpd.

To assess CS to 0.5 cpd and 8 Hz in more detail, we measured this response in a total of 25 additional patients with PD (50 eyes). Pearson's correlation coefficient was then calculated from these data with patient age as the x variable and the CS value as the y variable. Neither the correlation coefficient for the right eye nor that for the left reached statistical significance. CS did not vary significantly with increasing age in these patients with PD.

Spatiotemporal CS: The Effect of DA

All our data were obtained in patients receiving DA precursor therapy on a regular basis. To evaluate the presumed effect of DA on pattern vision, we examined 13 patients with the "on-off" syndrome. A significant portion of PD patients on long-term DA precursor therapy develop the on-off syndrome. This is characterized by sudden "switches" between relatively intact motor status to a rigid tremorous state with slowed movements. Clinical pharmacological studies have established that these changes correlate with switches in dopaminergic efficiency at the synapse. A patient in the on state has good DA synaptic function, whereas in the off state there is reduced responsiveness (19). Clear differences in spatiotemporal CS were observed in on versus off stages in six patients. These six (of the 13) patients showed sufficient segregation in time of on and off stages and a stability of their psychophysical responses during each stage. Stability was judged by the slope of the psychometric function obtained for each threshold measurement and by repeating selected spatial frequencies at the end of each session.

Subjects were tested at 0.5, 1, 2, 4, 6, and 8 cpd using 1- and 8-Hz on/off modulation. A total of 17 eyes was tested: both eyes were examined in six of these 11 patients; in the other five patients, only one eye was tested. We report data from all 17 eyes in all conditions except for the 6-cpd grating presented at 1 and 8 Hz, in which only 10 of the 17 eyes (7 of the 11 patients) were examined.

In this study, a special circuit Joyce Electronics CRT was used to present the vertical sinusoidal gratings. Mean luminance of the display was 100 cd/m. The field size was 9° of visual angle. By employing a larger field size, we were able to present spatial frequencies as low as 0.5 cpd. Contrast thresholds were assessed for the spatiotemporal conditions, as previously described, using the MCS.

In normal observers, the spatiotemporal surface is a function with a single peak at approximately 4 cpd. In general, the spatiotemporal surfaces of these PD patients tended to show less height than that of the normal surface (i.e., there is a generalized reduction in sensitivity). However, our results clearly show the importance of considering visual sensitivity separately in on and off states. We found that not only the height but, most important, the shape of the spatiotemporal surface changes between on and off states. Spatiotemporal surfaces were derived for six patients (one eye only in five patients, both eyes in the sixth patient). Of the seven patient eyes, five showed an *increase* in CS to 0.5 cpd at 1 Hz in the off versus the on condition, whereas CS in the other two eyes did not change. At 4 cpd and 1 Hz, five eyes showed an increase and two eyes showed a minor (-1 dB) decrease in the on condition. At 4 cpd and 1 Hz, five eyes showed an increase near the peak of the spatiotemporal surface and two eyes did not change when in the on state compared with the off state. Thus, for most patients CS is higher at the lower spatial frequency in the off condition, and CS is higher at the peak of the spatial frequency function in the on condition—in the same eye of a patient with PD. Spatiotemporal surfaces of one patient with PD were shown in Fig. 3. The spatiotemporal surface in the on state shows a peak as well as a relative attenuation to combinations of low spatial frequencies and low temporal frequencies. The spatiotemporal surface in the off state resembles a plateau and does not present a discernible peak. As mentioned before, it is thought that on and off states represent high versus low dopaminergic activity in patients with PD who are undergoing treatment (19,20). Therefore, by obtaining a difference in the CS function between the on and off states, one may infer the effect of DA in the visual system. Figure 3 also shows the on versus off sensitivity "difference." On the difference surface, notice that (a) there is a valley rather than a peak and (b) the edges dip slightly *below* the surface. An almost identical surface was obtained in four of the seven eyes. This difference surface leads us to suggest that the effect of DA at low spatial and temporal frequencies is to decrease CS and that the effect of DA at the peak of the spatiotemporal surface (and beyond) is to enhance CS. Thus, these data suggest that DA is involved in low frequency attenuation and medium and high frequency amplification (i.e., tuning) of human spatiotemporal contrast vision.

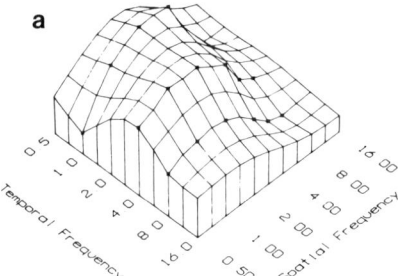
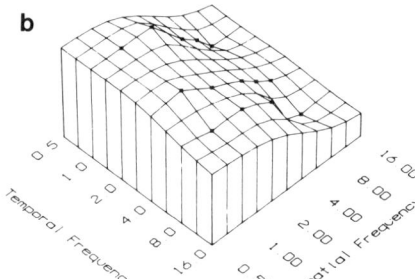
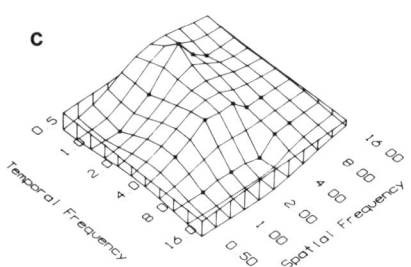

FIG. 3. Spatiotemporal CS to a 9° field is shown for six spatial frequencies and six temporal frequencies in a three-dimensional surface plot for PD patient 2 who shows the on-off syndrome. PD patient 2 is a 46-year-old man, with an age near that of the mean of the normal observers. Snellen visual acuity was 20/20 and 20/30. **a** represents the three-dimensional surface measured when this patient was in the on phase, and **b,** the surface measured when this patient was in the off phase. Since this patient serves as his own control by providing data during both on and off periods. **c** shows the difference three-dimensional surface resulting when the off-phase responses are subtracted from the on-phase responses. The shape of the difference surface suggests that DA enhances sensitivity at the peak of the spatiotemporal surface and attenuates sensitivity at the lower spatial frequencies (see text). (From ref. 17.)

VEP STUDIES IN PD

Measuring electroencephalogram (EEG) changes that are time locked to a visual stimulus are called VEP and provide a clinical diagnostic tool in the evaluation of patients suspected of suffering from demyelinating diseases or definite optic neuropathy. However, in 1978, we (1) described that patients affected by PD, hitherto not thought to have any visual defects, also have abnormal (delayed) VEP. In these studies the VEP delay occurred in more than half of the treated advanced patients. Pattern spatial frequency was 2.3 cpd and was modulated at 1-Hz counterphase. After several years of scepticism, however, there recently have been other studies describing VEP and also psychophysically measured alterations in the vision of PD patients. As summarized elsewhere (21), those studies that show visual changes in PD employ spatial frequencies above 2 cpd. In fact, diagnostic yield is highest for spatial frequencies for which a normal human observer is most sensitive: at the peak of the CS curve (22–24). Several studies show the effect of L-dopa therapy on pattern VEP latency (24–26a).

The Effect of Temporal Frequency on the VEP in PD

To evaluate the effect of varying the temporal frequency of stimulation, steady-state pattern VEP were studied in 16 patients and in an age-matched control group of 18 observers. In comparison with transient presentation, steady-state stimuli are delivered at a faster rate so that the response to one stimulus partially overlaps the response to the next stimulus. A steady-state response is analyzed by fast Fourier transform (FFT) in terms of the amplitude and phase (relative to the stimulus phase) of its harmonic components. If the stimulus is modulated at a frequency of FHz, then a response frequency of FHz is called the *first harmonic* or *fundamental*, whereas a response at twice the modulation frequency (2 FHz) is called the *second harmonic* response. In the case of counterphase or pattern-shift modulation, some consider the reversal rate as the modulation frequency.

In this study, we compared "routine" transient (1 Hz) counterphase results with the results of steady-state on-off modulation. With on-off modulation, the resulting VEP contains both first and second harmonic components; with counterphase modulation, the response is dominated by second harmonic components. Using FFT, one obtains VEP "power," which is converted into amplitude (in microvolts). Our amplitude measures are expressed as peak (or trough) to base line (i.e., one half of the peak-to-trough measure). The phase is expressed in radians or is converted into trigonometric components (sine-cosine). A vector plot presents both the amplitude and the phase of any harmonic component of the response. The length of the vector represents the amplitude, and the angle of the vector represents the phase of the response. From our studies it is evident that if a steady-state response contains energy at more than the fundamental frequency, the different harmonics can have identical amplitudes but different relative phases; hence the vector in PD is abnormal.

For the following discussion, it is essential to distinguish modulation frequency (input) from response frequency (output). The VEP response (output) contains power at the input frequency and at harmonically related frequencies. By examining the VEP response at the first and second harmonic frequencies, we can gain information concerning sequential processing in the visual system. We have shown (26) that PD patients exhibit abnormalities when the modulation frequency (input) is near a 4- to 5-Hz frequency band rather than some other frequency. Such an abnormality might reflect a distortion arising, not in the visual system, but in the generation of electrocortical rhythms near 4 to 5 Hz. We can, however, demonstrate that the VEP abnormality is evident not only at the response frequency that corresponds to the 4-Hz input (the fundamental frequency), but also at the second harmonic frequency (8 Hz). However, using an 8-Hz input frequency, we find that the same patient may not show an abnormality of the response at 8 Hz. An abnormal response to a narrow range of input frequencies and their harmonics, but not to identical output frequencies arising from different inputs, suggests that the pathology in PD affects an early stage of visual signal processing. Early may be defined as being prior to or at the same site where the harmonics of the input frequency are generated.

Methodology

A Joyce Electronics CRT-type display unit subtending 9° at the eye was used to present the stimuli. The screen had an average luminance of 170 cd/m and was surrounded by an unpatterned field of approximately the same luminance. Patterns were vertical sinusoidal gratings of 55% contrast.

The EEG activity was recorded using a Z5-Z63 (midline) referential montage and both lateral occipital electrodes. Signal averaging was performed on-line with a Nicolet 1170, and Fourier analysis was performed with an LSI-11.

Results

We found that VEP delays in PD are related to the temporal frequency of modulation. Temporal modulation of the pattern at 4.19 Hz induced abnormal VEP with phase alterations of the first harmonic component in 70% and of the second harmonic in 75% of the PD patients. Only 35% of the patients showing abnormal VEP to 4.19-Hz modulation had delayed transient (1 Hz) VEP, and only 48% of them had abnormal responses to 8.41 Hz modulation. Steady-state VEP cannot be measured by applying the common peak latency criterion used for transient VEP; rather, time-domain measurements are substituted by frequency analysis (27). The phase of steady-state VEP can be converted into apparent latency with the following calculations: 1/360 multiplied by phase change/frequency range of stimulation. The product of this equation expresses latencies in seconds that can be converted into milliseconds. The observed phase alterations of steady-state VEP in PD could therefore be consistent with a latency alteration of the VEP in PD. However, the applicability of this method to a system that induces nonlinear changes of the input is problematic.

The data of PD patients nevertheless emphasize that VEP in PD depend on temporal frequency of the stimuli and that delays depend on both temporal and spatial factors.

The Effect of Contrast on the VEP in PD

We have shown that pattern contrast affects the steady-state VEP in normal observers (28). Using on-off temporal modulation of a 2.3-cpd grating, we found that the amplitude of both the first and second harmonic components of the response grow with increasing contrast. In addition, the phase of the response advances; that is, the response quickens as the level of contrast is increased. Given our present notion of DA's role in spatial tuning in the retina, we became interested in the effect of contrast on the VEP in PD.

Results

We studied eight untreated PD patients and six control observers. All visual acuities were 20/25 or better. A 4-cpd sinusoidal grating was modulated in the on-off mode at 4.19 Hz. Mean contrast was varied from 5% to 55%. VEP were recorded over midline and lateral channels and then Fourier analyzed in terms of amplitude and phase of the first and second harmonic frequency components.

In the normal observers, the amplitudes of both the first and second harmonic components of the VEP increased, and their phases advanced with increasing contrast; that is, high-contrast VEP responses were larger and faster. In PD, the amplitude function appeared flattened and even declined in some patients with levels of contrast above 14%; instead of a phase advance there was a plateau, and in some patients there was a phase lag with increasing contrast. If DA is involved in spatial tuning in the human retina, the present results suggest that its effect extends over a range of contrasts.

VISION OF THE MONKEY WITH SYSTEMIC OR RETINAL DOPAMINERGIC DEFICIENCY

Systemic Dopaminergic Deficiency: The Effect of MPTP

The pattern VEP (PVEP) and PERG were studied in five cynomolgus monkeys before and during the development of a parkinsonian syndrome induced by MPTP. The stimuli were vertical bars of four spatial frequencies (0.5, 1.2, 2.5, and 3.5 cpd) modulated at temporal rates of 1, 4, 6, and 8 Hz. Following MPTP administration, all monkeys developed parkinsonian signs accompanied by changes in the amplitude and latency of the PVEP and PERG. Sinemet (L-dopa with carbidopa) administration produced temporary recovery of both PVEP and PERG. Two of the monkeys were followed for a prolonged period: 30 to 40 days after MPTP, the parkinsonian signs showed partial recovery; the PVEP latency and amplitude to 2.5- and 3.5-cpd stimuli and the latency to 1.2 cpd showed improvement but remained abnormal. The latencies of PERGs were normal, but the amplitudes were significantly reduced when stimuli of 2.5 and 3.5 cpd were used. Both PVEP and PERG to 0.5-cpd stimuli returned to normal. No further modifications were seen in the recordings performed 6 months and 1 year later (29) (Figs. 4 and 5). Retinal

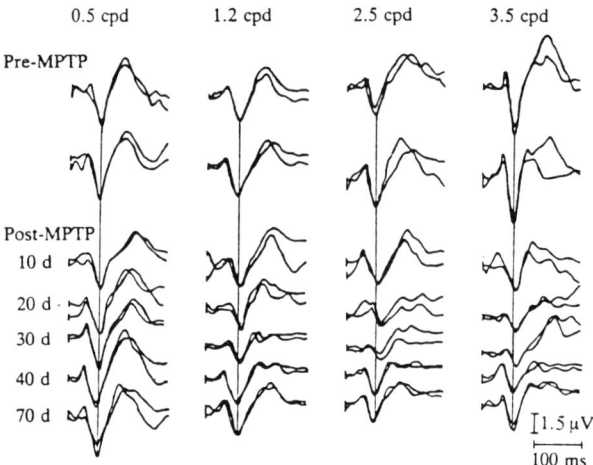

FIG. 4. PERGs recorded in monkey 3, before and after MPTP administration. The b wave is the major positivity (peak down) and the a wave the preceding negative peak (up). The latency and amplitude in the pre-MPTP recordings were replicable. The *vertical lines* indicate the normal latency of the b wave. In the recordings of days 10 to 30, a delay in the b-wave latency and a marked reduction in amplitude are evident, whereas from day 40, only an amplitude decrement was seen for the PERG obtained with 2.1- and 3.5-cpd stimuli. (From ref. 29.)

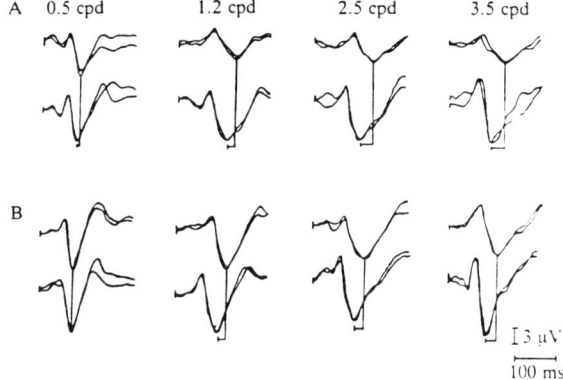

FIG. 5. Acute effect of the administration of Sinemet in monkey 3 showing the traces obtained for the four spatial frequencies tested. The experiment was performed 20 **(A)** and 40 days (B) after the last MPTP injection. Upper traces, pre-Sinemet; lower traces, post-Sinemet. Partial recovery of PVEP latency is evident at day 20 and full recovery at day 40, reaching the range of the pre-MPTP recordings. (From ref. 29.)

DA and dihydroxyphenylacetic acid contents were measured in four MPTP-treated monkeys and in three normal monkeys. DA and dihydroxyphenylacetic acid levels were significantly lower in the retinas of the MPTP-treated animals ($p < 0.001$), suggesting that DA has a specific function in the visual system of primates (30).

Following this study showing that systemically administered MPTP produced a chronic parkinsonian syndrome accompanied by retinal DA deficiency and spatial frequency-dependent abnormalities, we studied the effect of intravitreally administered 6-hydroxydopamine (6-OH-DA) on the PERG and PVEP of three aphakic monkeys (31). Because of the aphakic condition, several complexities of intravitreal injection of 6-OH-DA could be avoided. Nevertheless, following 6-OH-DA treatment, both the phase and amplitude of PERG and PVEP became abnormal. This abnormality was most pronounced for the higher spatial frequencies (2.5 and 3.5 cpd), whereas lower spatial frequency (0.5 and 1.2 cpd) were less impaired (Fig. 6). The effects of systemically administered MPTP on PERG and PVEP are similar to the effects of intravitreal injections of 6-OH-DA, suggesting that a retinal catecholaminergic system plays an important role in pattern vision of primates.

To examine the effect of dopaminergic blockade on signal processing in the primate retina, both light- and dark-adapted flash ERGs were measured in

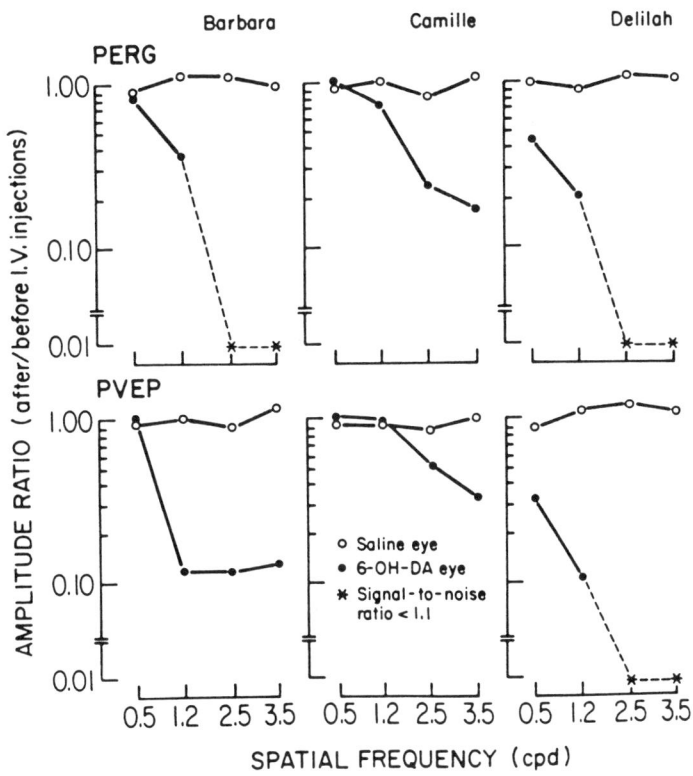

FIG. 6. The amplitude ratios (after/before the intravitreal injections) are illustrated as functions of spatial frequency for the three monkeys. The amplitude ratios of the saline eyes show little variability, whereas the responses from the 6-OH-DA-treated eyes are either reduced or absent for the higher spatial frequencies used (i.e., 2.5 and 3.5 cpd). (From ref. 31.)

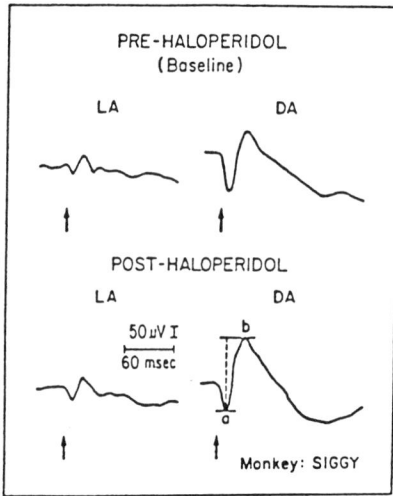

FIG. 7. Both light-adapted (LA) and dark-adapted (DA) flash ERG waveforms are shown for one monkey, Siggy. Positivity of the waveform is upward. In this figure, the LA flash ERGs were recorded after 5 min of light adaptation and the DA flash ERGs were recorded after 25 min of dark adaptation. The flash ERGs recorded prehaloperidol (i.e., baseline) are presented on the top row; flash ERGs recorded posthaloperidol are presented on the bottom row. The *vertical arrows* at the beginning of each waveform indicate when the flush stimulus was presented. Amplitude was measured from the peak of the a wave to the peak of the b wave, represented by the *vertical dashed line* on the flash ERG in the lower right corner. Amplitude and latency calibrations are indicated. (From ref. 32.)

five normal cynomolgus monkeys prior to and following the systemic administration of haloperidol, a blocker of DA receptors (32). The stimulus was delivered as a single flash of Intensity 16 (Grass PS2 Photo Stimulator, which is roughly 3 log units above the photopic threshold), which subtended 25.8° of visual angle. Base-line flash ERGs appeared similar to those recorded in the human. Flash ERG amplitude was measured from the trough of the a-wave to the peak of the b-wave. Following base-line recordings, haloperidol was administered (0.1 mg/kg, i.m.). Haloperidol caused a statistically significant increase in the amplitude of both light- and dark-adapted flash ERGs in all monkeys (Fig. 7). In conclusion, DA receptor blockade in the primate retina enhances both light- and dark-adapted flash ERGs, a result suggesting that DA is active in both the light and dark in response to flash stimulation.

These studies demonstrate that (a) spatial frequency-dependent electrophysiological abnormalities occur in the MPTP-treated monkey, a result previously found in humans with PD, (b) there is retinal dopaminergic deficiency in the parkinsonian monkey, and (c) DA has a specific function in neurotransmission in the visual system of primates.

DISCUSSION

The studies reviewed show that the CS defect in PD involves patterns that, for the normal observer, require the least contrast to detect. Most patients when properly refracted do not have any acuity changes. The parkinsonian visual defect is not, in an ordinary sense, a simple reduction in visual sensitivity, rather it appears to involve spatiotemporal interactions and demonstrates itself in the change of the shape of the spatiotemporal CS function. This change implies that spatial and temporal tuning functions are altered in the processing of visual signals in the CNS in PD. Tuning relies on the existence of spatial interactions with a finite time course and implies both subtractive and additive processes. Mammalian retinal ganglion cells show spatial tuning, albeit less narrowly than cortical neurons. Indeed, one of the prime candidate sites for altered spatiotemporal processing in PD is the retina itself.

The Evidence for Retinal Abnormality in PD

The pathognomic feature of PD is a loss of DA neurons of the substantia nigra and an abnormally low concentration of DA in the basal ganglia. In addition to the basal ganglia, low DA concentration has been demonstrated in other areas of the CNS; however, the retina has not been traditionally included in either morphological or neuropharmacological postmortem studies. A single neuropharmacological study did show, however, reduced DA content in the retina of PD patients (33). The bulk of evidence of retinal dysfunction in PD is therefore primarily electrophysiological: ERG studies reveal alteration of the ERG of PD patients in comparison to age-matched controls (34–40a). Not only is the ERG abnormal in PD, but in most patients the alterations can be corrected by L-dopa therapy. L-dopa, the precursor of DA crosses the blood-retina barrier, which is largely analogous to the blood-brain barrier. It is taken up by terminals of retinal DA neurons and converted *in situ* into the active neurotransmitter DA. There is little evidence of noradrenergic retinal neurotransmission and little doubt of a retinal DA-dependent dysfunction in PD. A specific effect of DA on spatiotemporal vision, as we have summarized, was proved in the human visual system but not in the retina. However, it was seen in monkeys with MPTP-induced parkinsonian syndrome—in these monkeys as we have seen, PERG alterations were pronounced at the peak spatial frequency and the abnormality responded to L-dopa. Intravitreal injection of 6-OH-DA induced similar changes. In these monkeys, postmortem examination did demonstrate reduced DA content, thus the evidence strongly favors the role of DA in spatial vision. However, a missing piece of evidence in both monkeys and humans is lack of morphological studies concerning specific damage to retinal DA neurons.

The Functional Significance of Retinal DA Deficiency

DA was among the first clearly demonstrated neurotransmitters of the retina (28). Recent evidence suggests a neuromodulatory role in several species (41). The retina of all vertebrates contains dopaminergic neurons, which differ in some characteristics (42), although some similarities are evident: in no species are dopaminergic neurons involved in straight-through processing (43). In cynomolgus monkeys, DA amacrines (more precisely tyrosine hydroxylase-labeled amacrines) receive their input from cone bipolars (44,45). Their output is not yet clearly defined. In humans, a morphological study revealed DA-containing interplexiform cells in the retina (46). Such neurons could be in the position to feed back signals from the proximal to the distal retina. In either case, whether DA neurons of the human retina are simple amacrines or interplexiforms, it is most certain that DA cells are not involved in a straight-through pathway from receptors toward the brain. They are involved either in a proximal lateral interconnecting system or, as the human morphological evidence implies, in a circuit feeding back signals from the proximal to the distal retina and hence providing indirect modification of straight-through signals. In lower vertebrates, in particular, in the turtle (47) and in fish (48,49), the evidence is strong for the disjunctive effect of DA on electrotonic coupling between one type of horizontal cells. It has been proposed, but not universally accepted, that horizontal-cell signals dominate the surround mechanism of ganglion cells. However, all studies agree that DA has an important effect in modulating receptive-field organization. This action is mediated by cyclic AMP-linked D_1, and functionally antagonistic D2 receptors (50). In addition, Mangel and Dowling (51) suggested that DA is crucial for receptive-field reorganization in the dark in all, including higher vertebrates. In monkeys, this is unlikely to be the sole function of DA: both the anatomical evidence concerning DA amacrine cells being in the cone pathway and the lack of differential effect of haloperidol on monkey light- or dark-adapted ERG, as we have shown (35–37,39,40) and the evidence of photopic ERG changes in PD (as many have shown) do suggest that DA's effect is not exclusive to the dark-adapted state in primates. However, it is true that at this point the precise physiological role of DA in the primate retina cannot be stated. On the whole, several of the ERG studies used broad-band or flash ERG stimuli, thus a specific effect of DA on spatiotemporal tuning of the retina has not been established in humans. Nevertheless, our suggestion, based on our studies and those reviewed, is that DA, either in a feedback or lateral interconnecting system is involved in receptive-field organization. As we have seen, changes in the spatial CS curve in DA deficiency in PD can be viewed as either a shift to the left and down or as a change from a normal band-pass function to a low-pass curve without tuning. Both have implications for center-surround mechanisms. The effect of DA agonist therapy in human volunteers (52) and our results in PD summarized in this chapter are perhaps slightly more compatible with a notion that DA enhances center-dominated responses. Whether this is achieved by suppressing surround antagonism or enhancing center summation is not clear. The distinction between these two supposed mechanisms of DA is not entirely trivial, however. One significance of a feedback circuit is that, in addition to negative feedback, it is able to provide tuning and hence amplification of input signals (53). In order to gain insight into the output properties of the negatively coupled feedback circuit with a finite time constant, it would be necessary to analyze its temporal properties. Such studies have not been performed in any species. The only hint concerning the temporal effects of DA is hidden in an observation by Teranishi et al. (49) that DA speeds up retinal response. This is not inconsistent with our studies, which show that lack of DA causes a temporal tuning defect. One of the most noticeable effects of DA deficiency in PD is at low spatial frequencies where sensitivity is enhanced by temporal modulation in normals but not in patients. Assuming that normally DA attenuates the surround of the final ganglion cell organization and hence *lack of DA* strengthens surround inhibition, the temporal frequency data become particularly challenging. They raise the need to study the effect of DA on temporal properties of "center" and surround mechanisms in the retina and beyond.

Studies Suggesting Additional Nonretinal DA-Dependent Visual Dysfunction in PD

Two studies (54–56) found evidence of orientation-dependent CS abnormalities in PD. What is the evidence of orientation bias in retinal ganglion cells? In monkeys there is none; however, in cats Levick and Thibos (57) found that cells have a bias according to their location in polar coordinates with the origo at the macula. In this case, small retinal or corresponding segmental nerve fiber lesions oriented toward the macula could cause orientation-dependent CS defects. Ophthalmoscopy in PD is generally nonrevealing to this supposed mechanism. Unless we assume that retinal ganglion cells have an orientation bias of at least 4:1 (preferred sensitivity/nonpreferred sensitivity), the human data could not be explained by retinal dysfunction without some additional hypothesis. Hence we must assume that these defects may be caused by cortical organization, the fact notwithstanding that there is no evidence for DA in visual cortical mechanisms. Studies using tilt illusion or alignment of vertical/horizontal lines have found neuropsychological evidence for orientation-specific deficits in spatial vision in PD (58). In addition, there are neuropsychological tests, in particular, the Benton line orientation test, that reveal body-centric defects in visual orientation in PD. The relationship of these various defects to each other and the neurophysiological mechanism underlying them merits further studies.

In summary then at this point several issues relating the role of dopaminergic mechanisms to the parkinsonian visual dysfunction are still unresolved. At the basic level, the role of D1 and D2 receptors in the primate retina is unknown. There is no morphological evidence in humans suffering from PD of a specific defect of normal catecholamine-containing neurons, although this has been shown in MPTP monkeys. There is clear, but not retinal, evidence of dysfunction of center-surround type organization in humans. It has been shown that DA content is reduced in the PD retina. There is direct evidence in monkeys suffering from a parkinsonian syndrome of retinal dysfunction of spatial processing demonstrated with the ERG. It has also been shown that MPTP-treated monkeys have reduced DA and homovanillic acid levels several months following the development of a chronic, stable parkinsonian syndrome. MPTP is toxic to retinal dopaminergic neurons (59). Unfortunately, MPTP monkeys, as remarkable as they are in clinically and neuropharmacologically resembling human PD, do not provide a perfect analogue of PD. All in all, however, there is significant evidence concerning the pathological importance of DA mechanisms of the primate retina. It remains to be seen whether direct retinal studies of feedback circuits will directly reveal the role of DA in spatiotemporal tuning. Such studies could lead to a more thorough understanding of the significance of DA-containing neurons in other local neuronal circuits of the CNS.

ACKNOWLEDGMENTS

This study was supported by National Institutes of Health grants EY01708, EY01867, and NS-11631.

REFERENCES

1. Bodis-Wollner I, Yahr M. Measurement of visual evoked potentials in Parkinson's disease. *Brain* 1978;101:661–671.
2. Bodis-Wollner I. Visual acuity and contrast sensitivity in patients with cerebral lesions. *Science* 1972;178:769–771.
3. Bodis-Wollner I, Camisa JM. Contrast sensitivity measurement in clinical diagnosis. In: Lessell S, Van Dalen JTW, eds. *Neuro-ophthalmology. A series of critical surveys of the international literature.* Amsterdam: Excerpta Medica, 1980;373–401.
4. Bodis-Wollner I, Diamond SP. The measurement of spatial contrast sensitivity in cases of blurred vision associated with cerebral lesions. *Brain* 1976;99:695–710.
5. Regan D, Silver R, Murray TJ. Visual acuity and contrast sensitivity in multiple sclerosis—hidden visual loss: an auxiliary diagnostic test. *Brain* 1977;100:563–579.
6. Campbell FW, Green DC. Optical and retinal factors affecting visual resolution. *J Physiol (Lond)* 1965;181:576–593.
7. Enroth-Cugell C, Robson JG. The contrast sensitivity of retinal ganglion cells of the cat. *J Physiol (Lond)* 1966;187:517–552.
8. Campbell FW, Robson JG. Application of Fourier analysis to the visibility of gratings. *J Physiol (Lond)* 1968;197:551–566.
9. Hess RF, Baker CL. Human pattern-evoked electroretinogram. *J Neurophysiol* 1984;51:939–951.
10. Korth M, Ilschner S. The spatial organization of retinal receptive fields in light and darkness as revealed by the pattern electroretinogram. *Doc Ophthalmol* 1985;63:143–149.
11. Maffei L, Fiorentini A, Bisti S, Hollander H. Pattern ERG in the monkey after section of the optic nerve. *Brain Res* 1985;59:423–425.
12. De Lange DH. Research into the dynamic nature of the human fovea-cortex systems with intermittent and modulated light. *J Opt Soc Am* 1958;48:777–789.
13. Robson JG. Spatial and temporal contrast-sensitivity functions of the visual system. *J Opt Soc Am* 1966;56:1141–1142.
14. Kelly DH. Flickering patterns and lateral inhibition. *J Opt Soc Am* 1969;59:1361–1370.
15. Kupersmith MJ, Shakin E, Siegel IM, Lieberman A. Visual system abnormalities in patients with Parkinson's disease. *Arch Neurol* 1982;39:284–286.

16. Regan D, Neima D. Low contrast letter charts in early diabetic retinopathy, ocular hypertension, glaucoma and Parkinson's disease. *Br J Ophthalmol* 1984;68:885–889.
17. Bodis-Wollner I, Marx MS, Mitra S, Bobak P, Mylin L, Yahr M. Visual dysfunction in Parkinson's disease. *Brain* 1987;110:1675–1698.
18. Wolkstein M, Atkin A, Bodis-Wollner I. Contrast sensitivity in retinal disease. *Ophthalmology* 1980;87:1140–1149.
19. Clough CG, Bergmann KJ, Yahr MD. Cholinergic and dopaminergic mechanisms in Parkinson's disease after long-term L-DOPA administration. *Adv Neurol* 1984;40:131–140.
20. Marsden CD, Parkes JD. 'On-off' effects in patients with Parkinson's disease on chronic levodopa therapy. *Lancet* 1976;i:292–296.
21. Bodis-Wollner I, Onofrj M. The visual system in Parkinson's disease. In: Yahr MD, Bergmann KJ, eds. *Advances in neurology.* New York: Raven Press, 1986;323–327.
22. Tartaglione A, Pizio N, Bo I, Spadavecchia L, Favale E. Spatial properties of pattern as determinants of visual evoked potential changes in Parkinson's syndrome. In: Morocutti C, Rizzo PA, eds. *Evoked potentials: neurophysiological and clinical aspects.* Amsterdam: Elsevier, 1985;321–327.
23. Piccolino M, Bodis-Wollner I, Demontis G. Sistema dopaminergico retinico e visione spaziale. *Neuroscienze* 1988;2:1–23.
24. Onofrj M, Ghilardi MF, Basciani M, Gambi D. Visual evoked potentials in Parkinson's disease and dopamine blockade reveal a stimulus-dependent dopamine function in humans. *J Neurol Neurosurg Psychiatry* 1986;49:1150–1159.
25. Bhaskar PA, Vanchilingam S, Bhaskar EA, Devaprabhu A, Ganesan RA. Effect of L-dopa on visual evoked potentials in patients with Parkinson's disease. *Neurology* 1988;36:1119–1121.
26. Bodis-Wollner I, Yahr M, Mylin L, Thornton J. Dopaminergic deficiency and delayed visual evoked potentials in humans. *Ann Neurol* 1982;11:478–483.
26a. Sollazzo D. Influence of L-dopa/carbidopa on pattern reversal VEP: behavioural difference in primary and secondary parkinsonism. *Electroencephalogr Clin Neurophysiol* 1984;47:305–307.
27. Marx M, Bodis-Wollner I, Bobak P., Harnois C, Mylin L, Yahr M. Temporal frequency-dependent VEP changes in Parkinson's disease. *Vision Res* 1986;26:185–193.
28. Ames A III, Pollen DA. Neurotransmission in the central nervous tissue: a study of isolated rabbit retina. *J Neurophysiol* 1969;32:424–442.
29. Ghilardi MF, Bodis-Wollner I, Onofrj M, Marx MS, Glover AA. Spatial frequency-dependent abnormalities of the pattern electroretinogram and visual evoked potentials in a parkinsonian monkey model. *Brain* 1988;111:131–149.
30. Ghilardi MF, Chung E, Bodis-Wollner I, Dvorzniak M, Glover A, Onofrj M. Systemic 1-methyl, 4-phenyl, 1-2-3-6-tetrahydropyridine (MPTP) administration decreases retinal dopamine content in primates. *Life Sci* 1988;43:255–262.
31. Ghilardi MF, et al. The effect of intraocular 6-OH-dopamine on retinal processing in primates. *Ann Neurol* 1989;25:357–364.
32. Bodis-Wollner I, Marx MS, Ghilardi MF. Systemic haloperidol administration increases the amplitude of the light- and dark-adapted flash ERG in the monkey. *Clin Vis Sci* 1989;4:19–26.
33. Di Paulo T, Harnois C, Daigle M. Assay of dopamine and its metabolites in human and rat retina. *Neurosci Lett* 1989;74:250–254.
34. Iudice A, Virgili P, Muratorio A. The electroretinogram in Parkinson's disease. *Psychol Psychiatr Behav* 1980;5:283–289.
35. Nightingale S, Mitchell KW, Howe JW. Visual evoked potentials and pattern electroretinograms in Parkinson's disease and control subjects. *J Neurol Neurosurg Psychiatry* 1986;49:1280–1287.
36. Ellis CJK, Allen TGJ, Marsden CD, Ikeda H. Electroretinographic abnormalities in idiopathic Parkinson's disease and the effect of levodopa administration. *Clin Vis Sci* 1987;347–355.
37. Gottlob I, Schneider E, Heider W, Skrandies W. Alteration of visual evoked potentials and electroretinograms in Parkinson's disease. *Electroencephalogr Clin Neurophysiol* 1987;66:349–357.
38. Stanzione P, Pierelli F, Peppe A, Rizzo PA, Morocutti C. Pattern visual evoked potentials and electroretinogram abnormalities in Parkinson's disease: effects of L-dopa therapy. *Clin Vis Sci* 1989;4:115–128.

39. Jaffe MJ, Bruno G, Campbell G, Lavine RA, Karson CN, Weinberger DR. Ganzfeld electroretinographic findings in Parkinsonism: untreated patients and the effects of levodopa intravenous infusion. *J Neurol Neurosurg Psychiatry* 1987;50:847–852.
40. Pierelli F, Stanzione P, Peppe A, et al. Electrophysiological (PERG, VEP) abnormalities in Parkinson disease are reversed by L-dopa. In: Bodis-Wollner I, Piccolino M, eds. *Dopaminergic mechanisms in vision.* New York: Alan R. Liss, 1988;253–265.
40a. Cavallacci G, Perossini M, Wirth A. The interest of electroretinography in parkinsonism. *Doc Ophthalmol Proc Ser* 1979;23:121–125.
41. Bodis-Wollner I, Piccolino M. *Dopaminergic mechanisms in vision.* New York: Alan R. Liss, 1988.
42. Oyster CW, Takahashi ES, Brecha NC. Morphology of retinal dopaminergic neurons. In: Bodis-Wollner I, Piccolino M, eds. *Dopaminergic mechanisms in vision,* New York: Alan R. Liss, 1988;19–30.
43. Nguyen-Legros J, Savy C. Dopamine innervation of the vertebrate retina: morphological studies. In: Bodis-Wollner I, Piccolino M, eds. *Dopaminergic mechanisms in vision,* New York: Alan R. Liss, 1988;1–18.
44. Hokoc S, Mariani A. Tyrosine hydroxylase immunoreactivity in the rhesus monkey retina reveals synapses from bipolar cells to dopaminergic amacrine cells. *J Neurosci* 1987;7: 2785–2793.
45. Mariani AP, Hokoc JN. Synaptic organization of dopaminergic amacrine cells in the rhesus monkey retina. In: Bodis-Wollner I, Piccolino M, eds. *Dopaminergic mechanisms in vision,* New York: Alan R. Liss, 1988;31–40.
46. Frederick JM, Rayborn ME, Laties AM, Lam DMK, Hollyfield JG. Dopaminergic neurons in the human retina. *J Comp Neurol* 1982;210:65–79.
47. Piccolino M, Weyton J, Geschenfeld HM. Decrease of gap function permeability induced by dopamine and cyclic AMP in horizontal cells of turtle retina. *J Neurosci* 1984;4:2477–2488.
48. Cohen JL, Dowling JE. The role of retinal interplexiform cell. Effect of 6-hydroxydopamine on the spatial properties of carp horizontal cells. *Brain Res* 1988;264:307–310.
49. Teranishi T, Negishi K, Kato S. Regulatory effect of dopamine on spatial properties of horizontal cells in carp retina. *J Neurosci* 1984;4:1271–1280.
50. Piccolino M, de Montis G, Witkowsky P, Bodis-Wollner I, Mirolli M. D1 and D2 dopamine receptors involved in the control of electrical transmission between retinal horizontal cells. In: Spano PF, Biggio G, Toffano G, Gessa GL, eds. *Central and peripheral dopamine receptors. Biochemistry and pharmacology.* Padova, Italy: Liviana Press, 1988;265–275.
51. Mangel SC, Dowling JE. Responsiveness and receptive field size of carp horizontal cells are reduced by prolonged darkness and dopamine. *Science* 1985;229:1107–1109.
52. Domenici L, Trimarchi C, Piccolino M, Fiorentini A, Maffei L. Dopaminergic drugs improve human visual contrast sensitivity. *Hum Neurobiol* 1988;4:195–197.
53. Ratliff F, Knight BW, Graham N. On tuning and amplification by lateral inhibition. *Proc Natl Acad Sci USA* 1969;62:733–740.
54. Regan D. Visual sensory loss in patients with Parkinson's disease. In: Bodis-Wollner I, Piccolino M, eds. *Dopaminergic mechanisms in vision,* New York: Alan R. Liss, 1988; 221–225.
55. Regan D, Maxner C. Orientation-selection visual loss in patients with Parkinson's disease. *Brain* 1987;110:415–432.
56. Bulens C, Meerwaldt JD, van der Wildt GJ, Keemink CK. Contrast sensitivity in Parkinson's disease. *Neurology* 1986;36:1121–1125.
57. Levick WR, Thibos LN. Orientation bias of cat retinal ganglion cells. *Nature* 1980;286:389–390.
58. Harris JP, Gelbtuch MH, Phillipson OT. Effects of haloperidol and nomifensine on the visual aftereffects of tilt and movement. *Psychopharmacology* 1986;89:177–182.
59. Hadjiconstantinou M, Qu Z, Mariani A, Neff NH. MPTP neurotoxicity and retinal dopaminergic neurons. In: Bodis-Wollner I, Piccolino M, eds. *Dopaminergic mechanisms in vision.* New York: Alan R. Liss, 1988;193–203.

ns or sets of channels. (1).

To What Extent Can Visual Deficits Caused by Multiple Sclerosis Be Understood in Terms of Parallel Processing?

D. Regan

Department of Ophthalmology, University of Toronto, Toronto, Ontario, Canada M2H 1E8

There is growing evidence that some abstract features of the retinal image are processed in parallel functional units called "sets of channels," each of which operates rather independently of any other (1). It has been argued that there is a set of channels for color, one for orientation, one for spatial frequency, one for changing size, one for stereoposition in depth, one for stereomotion in depth, and so on. Each set of channels contains subunits called channels. For example, there are three color channels in the fovea (2), approximately six spatial frequency channels from any retinal point (3–5), perhaps eight orientation channels (6), eight stereomotion channels (7), two or three stereoposition channels (8,9), three flicker channels (10–13), two changing-size channels (1), and so on.

This channeling concept offers the possibility of functionally "dissecting" the visual pathway into parallel elements by using psychophysical stimuli that selectively activate different channels or sets of channels. (1).

One problem with the simple channeling concept outlined is that this initial analysis of the retinal image is far too coarse to explain our fine discriminations between slightly different shapes, sizes, line orientations, velocities, etc. A second problem is that, in itself, channeling does not reconcile our ability to effortlessly unconfound simultaneous changes in orientation, size, contrast, etc. with the fact that neurons in primary visual cortex confound all these visual parameters. These two problems can be explained if we assume that, after the initial channel analysis, channel outputs are compared. At this second stage, the neural connectivity mediates opponent-orientation, opponent-size, opponent-velocity, and other opponent processes that enhance discriminations of shape (1,4,14–16), line separation (18), velocity (1,17), depth (8,9), and flicker frequency (11) and could also unconfound covarying visual dimensions (1,6,14). This concept offers the further possibility of dissecting the visual pathway into *sequential* functional stages by means of psychophysical tests of discrimination.

Although it would be unrealistic to expect a one-to-one relationship between the functional and structural organization of the visual pathway, we will see that relationships have been found that can be used to (a) link the patterns of sensory loss experienced by multiple sclerosis (MS) patients with the underlying pathophysiologies, and (b) advance our understanding of the mechanism(s) of MS.

Among the physiological streams and subdivisions that are known to exist in the visual systems of nonhuman primates are the following: separate pathways for light on and off (19); three retinal color mechanisms (2); the parvocellular and magnocellular streams (20); X- and Y-type neurons; orientation columns in primary cortex (21); cytochrome oxidase blobs and interblob regions; "far" versus "near" binocular neurons (22); motion-in-depth versus position-in-depth neurons (23).

Figure 1 compares psychophysical and physiological models of the neural processing and unconfounding of spatial and motion information.

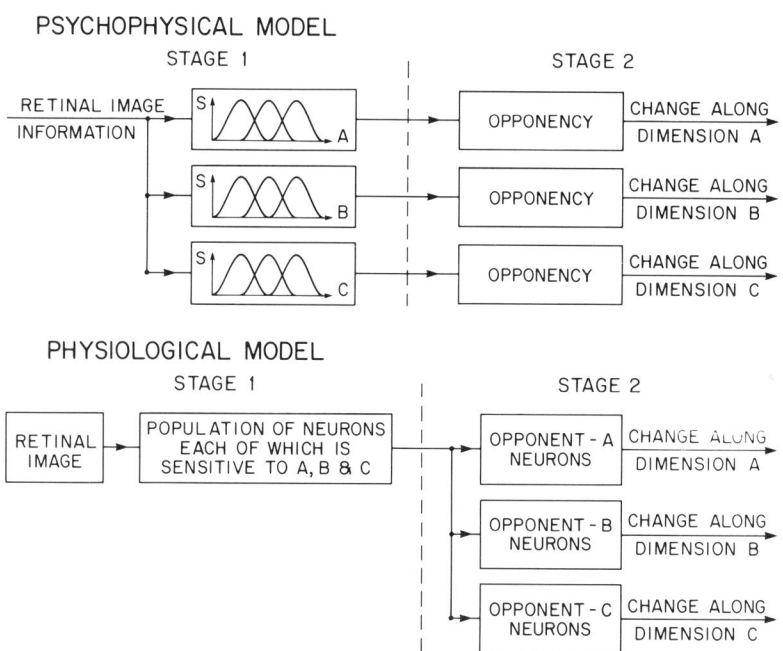

FIG. 1. Relation between psychophysical and physiological models of detection and discrimination. The upper half of the figure illustrates the psychophysical hypothesis that sensory information is processed along dimensions A, B, C, etc. by parallel sets of channels and that acute discriminations along the dimensions A, B, C, etc. are determined by the pattern of activity within a set of channels. The lower half of this figure illustrates the physiological hypothesis that retinal image information passes through a population of neurons in primary cortex, each of which is sensitive to dimensions A, B, C to varying extents and that changes along these dimensions are unconfounded by connectivity between these neurons. This connectivity also mediates acute discriminations along dimensions A, B, C, etc. (From ref. 45.)

ON/OFF MECHANISMS IN MS

Visual responses to light increment (on responses) and to light decrement (off responses) can be compared by means of the procedure set out in Fig. 2. The subject is presented with two light-emitting diodes (LEDs) L_1 and L_2 and instructed to fixate L_1 (Fig. 2A). When testing on responses, the rationale is as follows (24): the two lights increase in brightness (Fig. 2B), but unless neural signals from locations L_1 and L_2 travel at exactly the same speed from eye to brain the light increments will not be perceived as simultaneous when they are in fact physically simultaneous. If the perceptual delay from location L_2 is t sec longer than from location L_1, then the light increments will be seen as simultaneous when lamp L_2 increments t sec earlier than lamp L_2 rather than simultaneously. The value of t can be readily established by conventional psychophysical methods, and the variation of t over the visual field can be charted by successively measuring t for many different locations of lamp L_2 in the visual field, giving a so-called "delay field" (24). Variations of t over the visual field for a decrement of light intensity can be measured in a similar manner (Fig. 2C).

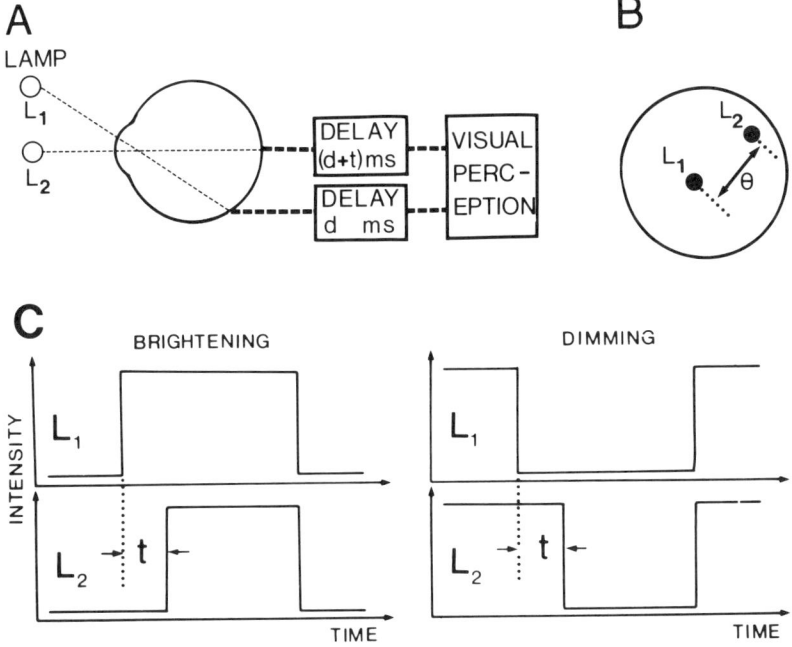

FIG. 2. A: Principle of the delay field test. The lamps appear to light simultaneously when lamp L_1 precedes lamp L_2 by delay t msec. **B:** The delay field tester as seen by the subject, showing lamps L_1 and L_2 and the matte white screen. **C:** Brightening and dimming stimuli. Intensity versus time plots for lamps L_1 and L_2. (From ref. 24.)

The visual fields of some patients include areas where the delay t is locally increased (24). This finding can be understood in terms of the slowing of neural conduction speed observed in partially demyelinated axons (25). A second parallel with experimental demyelination is that perceptual delay t sec increases when body temperature is elevated in some patients and decreases when the patient is cooled (26). But in our present context the more interesting point is that the on but not the off response may be delayed at one retinal site, whereas the off but not the on response is delayed at some other site (24). This observation can, perhaps, be understood in terms of the recent findings that the on and off pathways are neurochemically (19) and even anatomically (27) distinct at retinal and LGN level and possibly also at cortex.

TEMPORAL CHANNELS IN MS

It has been known for many years that the dynamic aspects of visual processing are abnormal in some patients with MS. For example, the ability to see high-frequency flicker may be lost (28,29). Again, the visual fields of some patients contain regions where a pair of flashes are seen as one flash even though control subjects see two flashes (30–33).

Two explanations for this degraded temporal resolution are (a) if neighboring axons suffered different degrees of demyelination so that signals were unevenly delayed, visual signals would be desynchronized (34); (b) evidence against this explanation was described by Regan (35) who alternatively suggested that reduced firing frequency caused by demyelination would degrade temporal resolution.

However, it may be an oversimplification to assume that the effect of MS on visual dynamics is merely to reduce the visual response to high flicker rates and to degrade temporal resolution. Both psychophysical and evoked potential evidence indicate that different flicker frequencies are processed in three parallel channels (10,11,13). Two lines of argument support the notion that MS can affect the balance of these different flicker channels: First, contrast sensitivity loss is greater at 2 Hz than at 16 Hz in some patients (37). Second, the ability of some patients to discriminate different flicker frequencies fails in a way that is consistent with selective damage to a single flicker channel (12).

SPATIAL FREQUENCY AND ORIENTATION CHANNELS IN MS

The idea that the spatial information in any small area of the retinal image is processed in multiple parallel channels, each selectively sensitive to a limited range of spatial frequencies and orientations, has been a major influence in human visual psychophysics during the past 20 years (3,5). It is widely assumed that the selectivity of these functional channels corresponds to the spatial frequency and orientation tuning of cortical neurons.

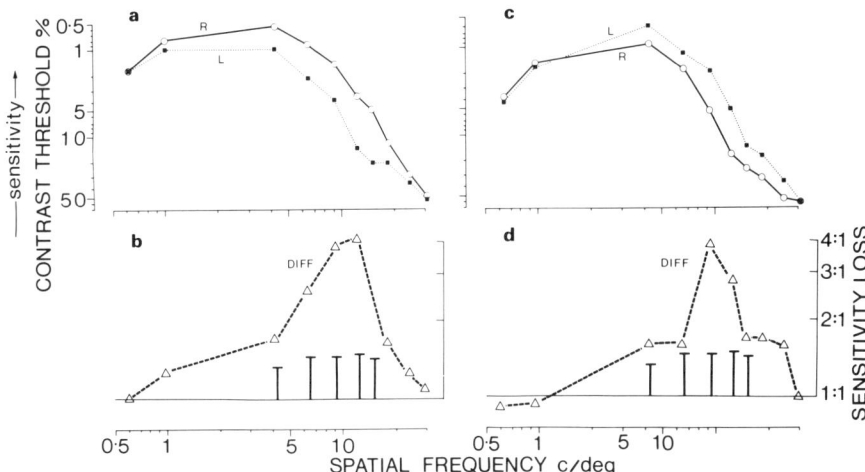

FIG. 3. Selective loss of contrast sensitivity over a range of intermediate spatial frequencies in two patients with MS. **a:** Contrast sensitivity curves for the left (L) and right (R) eyes of one patient. **b:** The sensitivity difference between the left and right eyes, showing a broad, intermediate-frequency loss that spared visual acuity. **c,d:** data for a second patient. (From ref. 37.)

This view of normal visual function provides a basis for understanding the finding that, although some patients with MS experience a loss of contrast sensitivity restricted to high spatial frequencies, other patients lose sensitivity over a broad range of intermediate spatial frequencies—most clearly shown as a difference between left and right eyes (Fig. 3). In these patients acuity may be spared. A third group of patients experiences contrast sensitivity loss at low spatial frequencies (and possibly intermediate frequencies also), high frequencies again spared (37–40). Indeed, in a longitudinal study comparing 16 patients with 15 controls for 12 months, substantial fluctuations of contrast sensitivity for low-frequency gratings occurred whereas visual acuity remained constant and in two instances heralded a subsequent relapse by several days. Changes in the large-check clinical visually evoked potential delay correlated more closely with psychophysical contrast sensitivity for low than for high spatial frequencies (Regan and Neima, *unpublished data*).

Figure 4A–C illustrates three patterns of contrast sensitivity loss observed in MS. (Mixed forms of loss are commonly seen also.)

The finding that contrast sensitivity loss is often tuned to orientation as well as to spatial frequency places the site of pathology at or central to primary visual cortex in those patients (40–42). The basis for this conclusion is that orientation-tuned neurons are not found peripheral to primary cortex in non-human primates. Further to this point, Fig. 5 illustrates that sensitivity to vertical and horizontal gratings can change independently of one another.

The idea that several channels serve each small area of the visual field (4,5) can explain why contrast sensitivity loss is often patchy, as illustrated in Fig. 6.

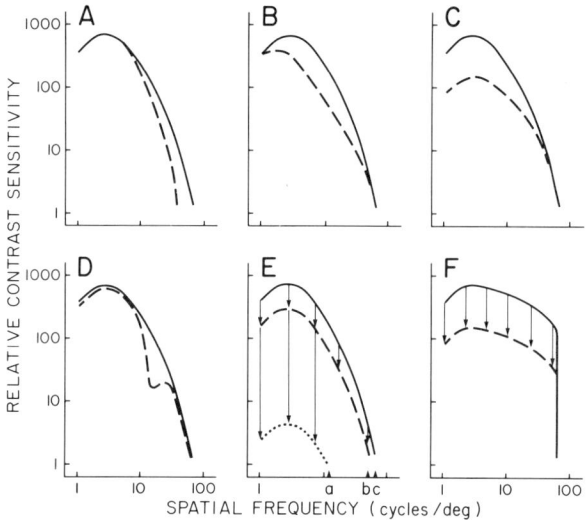

FIG. 4. Several kinds of abnormal contrast sensitivity curve. The continuous line is a normal curve. (From ref. 46.)

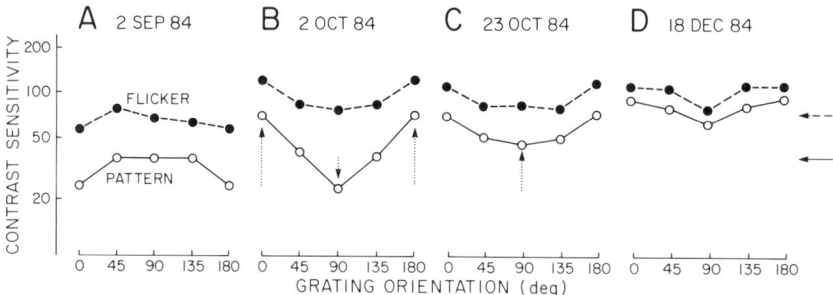

FIG. 5. Longitudinal changes in contrast sensitivity for a temperature-sensitive patient with MS. Orientation tuning for pattern was chiefly created by a selective improvement in sensitivity to horizontal gratings (0 deg, **A** and **B**), and then as the weather grew cooler, orientation tuning was abolished by a selective improvement of horizontal sensitivity (90 deg, **C**). The stimulus was a 2-c/deg grating, counterphase modulated at 8 Hz, and the patient was required to set thresholds for just-visible flicker and just-visible pattern. (From ref. 36.)

However, it is more difficult to explain why visual loss is often quite different at corresponding points in the left and right eyes (Fig. 6).

We should note here that an intermediate frequency loss of contrast sensitivity can be produced by monocular diplopia. The loss is orientation tuned and is seen either as a single sharp "notch" (Fig. 4D) or as a notch with one or more ripples (36,43). Figure 7 shows how the effect can be explained straightforwardly in terms of interference between the two diplopic images of a

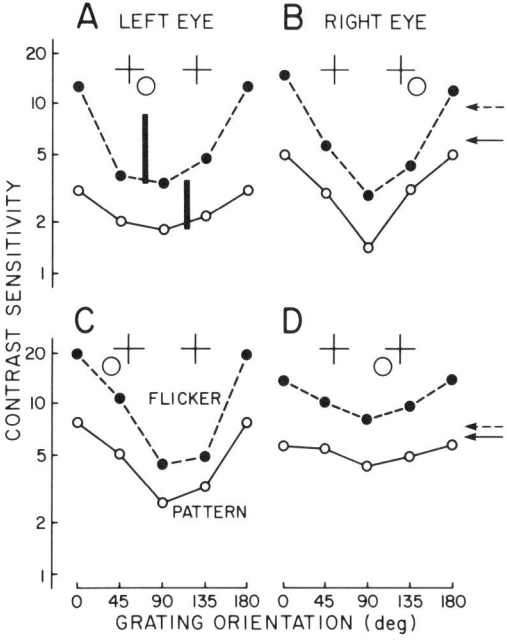

FIG. 6. Contrast sensitivity for pattern and for flicker sensations at 8 deg eccentricity at corresponding sites in the left and right eyes. Inserts indicate the stimulus location (○) relative to the fovea (+). The pattern of loss was quite different between different retinal sites in the same eye and between corresponding points in the left and right eyes. Technical details as in Fig. 5. (From ref. 36.)

repetitive grating target. If θ deg is the angle between the diplopic images, a notch in the contrast sensitivity curve occurs at $(\frac{1}{2} \theta)$ c/deg (perhaps with a second minimum at $(\frac{3}{2} \theta)$ c/deg and so on). A diplopic notch is easily distinguished from an intermediate frequency loss due to MS, because the MS defect is much broader (compare Fig. 4B and D). And, of course, diplopia is easily confirmed by asking the patient to describe the appearance of a narrow line stimulus. Monocular diplopia can be caused optically (43) or, in some individuals, can occur as a temporary condition following monocular occlusion (36).

The distinction between parvo- and magnocellular streams in the primate visual pathway described elsewhere is this volume may be related to the pattern of visual loss in some MS patients. This possibility is suggested by the observation that some patients experience the greatest sensitivity loss for low-contrast, low-frequency gratings modulated at high temporal rates: the magnocellular population has higher contrast sensitivity at low spatial frequencies, and many cells prefer higher temporal frequencies than cells in the parvocellular population (44).

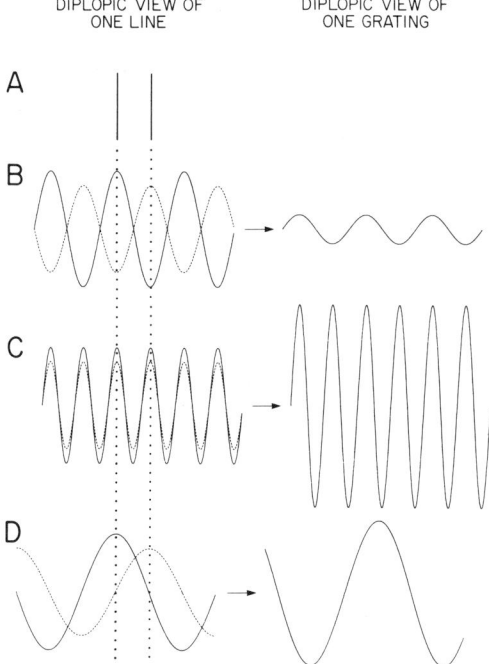

FIG. 7. Monocular diplopia can produce a sharp notch or even ripples in the contrast sensitivity curve. A single line is seen as two lines (**A**), and one grating as two gratings (**B–D**). Contrast sensitivity loss is greatest when the second grating image is shifted 0.5 cycles or 1.5 cycles, etc. (**B**), and is less for other shifts (**C,D**). (From ref. 45.)

RECOGNIZING AND SEEING

Some patients with MS may see an object quite clearly, yet see it incorrectly in a way that cannot be mimicked by a blurring lens or even easily imagined by normally sighted individuals. This is because the neurons that detect the presence of an object are not necessarily the same neurons that mediate the discrimination of one shape from another.

Figure 8 illustrates the basic idea. Panel C plots the firing rates of three neurons for stimulus gratings of different spatial frequencies. Consider a stimulus grating of frequency S_1 c/deg whose frequency is changed by a small amount to S_2 c/deg. The most strongly stimulated neuron (b in Fig. 8C) hardly changes its firing rate because S_1 and S_2 are both on the flat top of the Fig. 8C sensitivity curve. But the more weakly stimulated neurons a and b will change their firing rates. Note that the steep high-frequency slope of neuron a produces a greater effect than the shallow low-frequency slope of neuron b.

This hypothesis predicts that if neuron b is desensitized by adapting to a high-contrast grating of spatial frequency S_1 c/deg, the maximum contrast

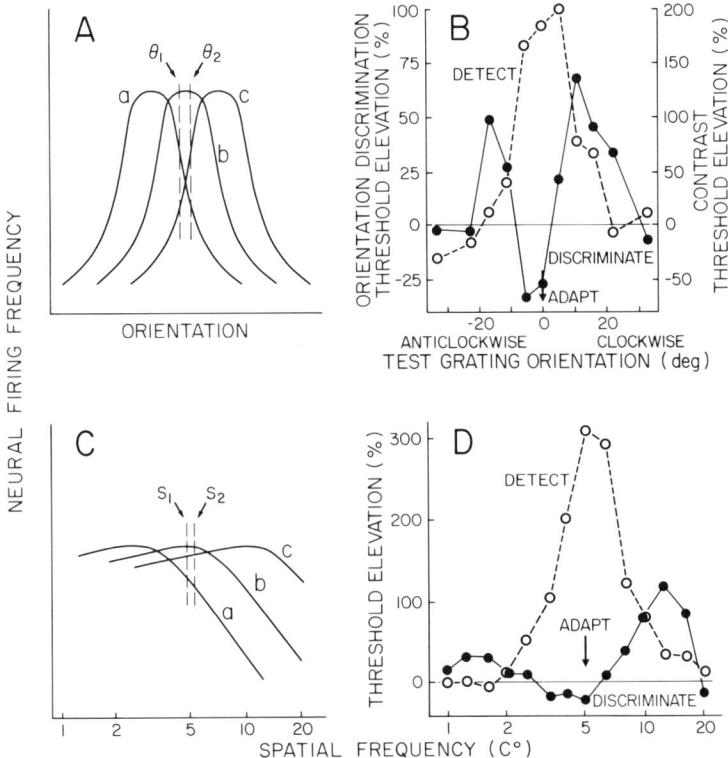

FIG. 8. The continuous lines in **A** and **C** represent tuning curves of three neurons that are driven from the same retinal location. **A:** When the orientation of a stimulus grating changes slightly from θ_1 to θ_2 (arrows), the response of the most active of the orientation-tuned neurons (b) changes negligibly, but there is a substantial change in the relative activations of neurons a and c. **B:** Postadaptation changes in orientation discrimination (solid line) and contrast detection (broken line) caused by inspecting a vertical grating (0 on abscissa). **C:** Test grating frequency changes from S_1 to S_2 c/deg. A small change in the spatial frequency of the test grating produces little change in the firing of the most excited neuron (b), but a considerable change in the balance of activity between neurons a and c, the greater contribution to this change in balance coming from a. **D:** Postadaptation changes in spatial-frequency discrimination (solid line) and contrast detection (broken line) caused by inspecting a sinewave grating of frequency 5 c/deg. (Modified from refs. 14 and 15.)

sensitivity loss will occur near S_1 c/deg, but the maximum loss of spatial frequency discrimination will occur, not at S_1 c/deg but at frequencies offset from S_1 (16). Figure 8D verifies this prediction in a normally sighted subject. After adapting to a 5-c/deg grating, the subject's spatial frequency discrimination was maximally degraded at approximately 12 and 2.5 c/deg rather than at 5 c/deg. The effect was asymmetric, in accord with the difference between the high- and low-frequency slopes in Fig. 8A (15).

Figure 9 illustrates a similar effect in an MS patient whose left eye showed contrast sensitivity loss for frequencies below approximately 8 c/deg whereas

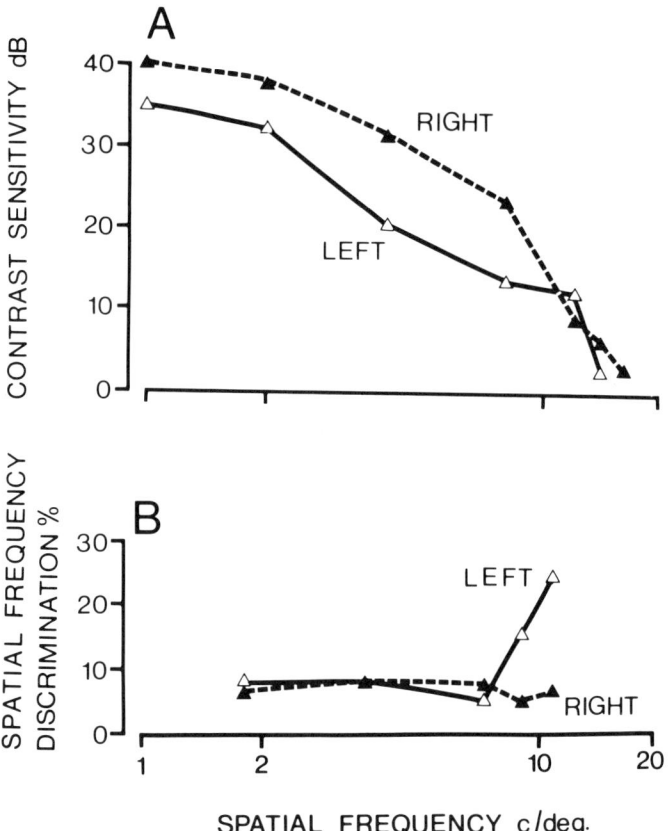

FIG. 9. A: Contrast sensitivity versus spatial frequency for the left and right eyes of a patient with MS. **B:** The just noticeable difference in spatial frequency between two successively presented gratings for the same patient. (From ref. 16.)

higher frequencies were spared (Fig. 8A). On the other hand, frequency discrimination in this left eye was normal below 8 c/deg where sensitivity was abnormal but was degraded above 8 c/deg where sensitivity was normal. Although this patient's sensitivity to high-frequency gratings was normal, she was unable to distinguish between high-frequency gratings whose bar widths differed by less than approximately 25%.

A similar argument holds for orientation discrimination (Fig. 8A and B). Desensitization of a channel tuned to orientation θ deg degrades orientation discrimination, not at θ deg but rather at orientations offset by approximately 10 to 20 deg on either side of θ (14).

If we assume that adequate spatial frequency discrimination and orientation discrimination are necessary for discriminating shapes then the visual losses previously described would be associated with impaired ability to recognize clearly visible objects.

CONCLUSIONS

A current hypothesis is that several abstract features of the retinal image are processed in parallel functional "set of channels" that operate rather independently of one another. MS is a demyelinating disease for which there is no effective treatment at the present time. Elucidation of the mechanism of MS may be requisite for the achievement of future rational therapy. This chapter describes an approach whose rationale is based on the channeling theory of visual processing and on empirical evidence that the disease can selectively affect individual visual channels. Such selective loss may be hidden to the Snellen and other clinical tests, and its detection may require a special test "tailored" to the affected channel. Comparing the pattern of loss among channels with emerging knowledge of the functional neuroanatomy and neurochemistry of neural streams promises insights into the mechanism(s) of the disease.

ACKNOWLEDGMENTS

Some of the experimental work outlined in this chapter was carried out in collaboration with S. Bartol, K. I. Beverley, R. Galvin, J. R. Heron, C. Maxner, B. A. Milner, T. J. Murray, D. Neima, R. Silver, and J. Whitlock. The author thanks J. Lord for assistance in preparing this chapter. This research was supported by the Medical Research Council of Canada, the National Eye Institute, and the E. A. Baker Foundation.

REFERENCES

1. Regan D. Visual information channeling in normal and disordered vision. *Psychol Rev* 1982;89:307–444.
2. Boynton RM. *Human color vision.* New York: Holt, Rinehart and Winston, 1979.
3. Braddick O, Atkinson J, Campbell FW. Channels in vision: basic aspects. In: Held R, Leibowitz HW, Teuber H-L, eds. *Handbook of sensory physiology,* vol 8. New York: Springer, 1978.
4. Wilson HR, Gelb DJ. Modified line-element theory for spatial-frequency and width discrimination. *J Opt Soc Am [A]* 1984;1:124–131.
5. Robson JG. Receptive fields: neural representation of the spatial and intensive attributes of the visual image. In: Carterette E, Friedman MP, eds. *Handbook of perception: Seeing,* vol 5. New York: Academic Press, 1975.
6. Regan D, Price P. Periodicity in orientation discrimination and the unconfounding of visual information. *Vision Res* 1986;26:1299–1302.
7. Beverley KI, Regan D. Evidence for the existence of neural mechanisms selectively sensitive to the direction of movement in space. *J Physiol (Lond)* 1973;235:17-29.
8. Richards W. Anomalous stereoscopic depth perception. *J Opt Soc Am* 1971;61:410–414.
9. Westheimer G. Cooperative neural processes involved in stereoscopic acuity. *Exp Brain Res* 1979;36:585–597.
10. Richards W. Quantifying sensory channels: generalizing colorimetry to orientation and texture, touch and tones. *Sensory Proc* 1979;3:207–217.
11. Hess RF, Plant G. Temporal frequency discrimination at and above threshold: evidence for a third temporal channel. *Vision Res* 1985;25:1493–1500.

12. Hess RF, Plant G. The psychophysical loss in optic neuritis: spatial and temporal aspects. In: Hess RF, Plant G, eds. *Optic neuritis.* Cambridge University Press, 1986.
13. Regan D. *Evoked potentials in sensory psychology and clinical medicine.* London: Chapman and Hall; New York: Wiley, 1972.
14. Regan D, Beverley KI. Postadaptation orientation discrimination. *J Opt Soc Am [A]* 1985; 2:147–155.
15. Regan D, Beverley KI. Spatial frequency discrimination and detection: comparison of postadaptation thresholds. *J Opt Soc Am* 1983;73:1684–1690.
16. Regan D, Bartol S, Murray TJ, Beverley KI. Spatial frequency discrimination in normal vision and in patients with multiple sclerosis. *Brain* 1982;105:735–754.
17. Beverley KI, Regan D. The relation between discrimination and sensitivity in the perception of movement in depth. *J Physiol (Lond)* 1975;249:387-398.
18. Morgan MJ, Regan D. Opponent model for line interval discrimination: interval and vernier performance compared. *Vision Res* 1987;27:107–118.
19. Schiller PH. The central visual system. *Vision Res* 1986;26:1351–1386.
20. Van Essen D. Functional organization of primate visual cortex. In: Peters A, Jones EG, eds. *Cerebral cortex,* vol 3. New York: Plenum Press, 1985;259–329.
21. Livingstone MS, Hubel DH. Anatomy and physiology of a colour system in the primate visual cortex. *J Neurosci* 1984;4:309–356.
22. Poggio GF. Processing of stereoscopic information in monkey visual cortex. In: Edelman GM, Gall WE, Cowan WM, eds. *Dynamic aspects of neocortical function.* New York: Wiley, 1984;613–635.
23. Regan D, Cynader M. Neurons in cat visual cortex tuned to the direction of motion in depth: effect of stimulus speed. *Invest Ophthalmol Vis Sci* 1982;22:535–550.
24. Regan D, Milner BA, Heron JR. Delayed visual perception and delayed visual evoked potentials in the spinal form of multiple sclerosis and in retrobulbar neuritis. *Brain* 1976; 99:43–66.
25. Davis FA, Schauf CL. The pathophysiology of multiple sclerosis: a theoretical model. In: Klawans HK, ed. *Models of human neurological disease.* Amsterdam: Excerpta Medica, 1974.
26. Regan D, Murray TJ, Silver R. Effect of body temperature on visual evoked potential delay and visual perception in multiple sclerosis. *J Neurol Neurosurg Psychiatry* 1977;40: 1083–1091.
27. Kolb H, Nelson R. Neural architecture of the cat retina. *Prog Retinal Res* 1973;3:397–413.
28. Parsons OA, Miller PN. Flicker fusion thresholds in multiple sclerosis. *Arch Neurol Psychiatr* 1957;77:134–139.
29. Titcombe AF, Willison RG. Flicker fusion in multiple sclerosis. *J Neurol Neurosurg Psychiatry* 1961;24:260–265.
30. Galvin RJ, Regan D, Heron JR. Impaired temporal resolution of vision after acute retrobulbar neuritis. *Brain* 1976;99:255–268.
31. Galvin RJ, Regan D, Heron JR. A possible means of monitoring the progress of demyelination in multiple sclerosis: effect of body temperature on visual perception of double light flashes. *J Neurol Neurosurg Psychiatry* 1976;39:861–865.
32. Galvin RJ, Heron JR, Regan D. Subclinical optic neuropathy in multiple sclerosis. *Arch Neurol* 1976;34:666–670.
33. Brussel EM, White CW, Bross M. Multi-flash campimetry in multiple sclerosis. *Curr Eye Res* 1981;1:671–677.
34. McDonald I. Pathophysiology in multiple sclerosis. *Brain* 1974;97:179–196.
35. Regan D. New visual tests in multiple sclerosis. In: Thompson HS, ed. *Topics in neuroophthalmology.* Baltimore: Williams and Wilkins, 1980;219–242.
36. Regan D, Maxner C. Orientation-dependent loss of pattern sensitivity and flicker sensitivity in multiple sclerosis. *Clin Vision Sci* 1986;1:1–23.
37. Regan D, Silver R, Murray TJ. Visual acuity and contrast sensitivity in multiple sclerosis—hidden loss: an auxiliary diagnostic test. *Brain* 1977;100:563–579.
38. Zimmern RL, Campbell FW, Wilkinson MS. Subtle disturbances of vision after optic neuritis elicited by studying contrast sensitivity. *J Neurol Neurosurg Psychiatry* 1979;42:407–412.
39. Bodis-Wollner I, Hendley CD, Mylin LH, Thornton J. Visual evoked potentials and the visuogram in multiple sclerosis. *Ann Neurol* 1978;5:40–47.

40. Kupersmith MJ, Nelson JL, Seiple WH, Carr RE, Weiss PA. The 20/20 eye in multiple sclerosis. *Neurology* 1983;33:1015–1020.
41. Regan D, Whitlock J, Murray TJ, Beverley KI. Orientation-specific losses of contrast sensitivity in multiple sclerosis. *Invest Ophthalmol* 1980;19:324–328.
42. Camisa J, Mylin LH, Bodis-Wollner I. Meridional visual evoked potential latency changes in multiple sclerosis. *Ann Neurol* 1981;10:532–539.
43. Apkarian P, Tijssen R, Spekreijse H, Regan D. Origin of notches in the CSF: optic or neural? *Invest Ophthalmol Vis Sci* 1987;28:607–612.
44. Derrington AM, Lennie P. Spatial and temporal contrast sensitivities of neurones in lateral geniculate nucleus of macaque. *J Physiol (Lond)* 1984;357:219–240.
45. Regan D. *Human brain electrophysiology.* New York: Elsevier, 1989.
46. Regan D. Low contrast letter charts and sinewave grating tests in ophthalmological and neurological disorders. *Clin Vision Sci* 1987.

The Visual System in Alzheimer's Disease

Alfredo A. Sadun and Carl J. Bassi

Departments of Ophthalmology and Neurosurgery, University of Southern California School of Medicine, Doheny Eye Institute, Los Angeles, California 90033

Alzheimer's disease (AD) is a disorder of unknown origin afflicting more than 2 million persons in the United States. It affects more than 7% of the population over the age of 65. Institutional costs for persons with dementia probably exceed $25 billion a year. AD creates great emotional, physical, and financial tolls not only to the AD patient but to the caretakers as well (1).

The clinical diagnosis of AD can be difficult and is based on nonspecific criteria. Definitive diagnosis requires histopathological findings of neuritic plaques in neurofibrillary tangles. The diagnosis of "possible" and "probable" AD can be made by clinical diagnoses, prior to definitive histopathology. The criteria for diagnosis of possible or probable AD include the insidious onset of progressive memory loss with other cognitive impairments (2).

Visual impairments have been described in AD, usually in the form of spatial agnosia, and have been traditionally attributed to disease in the cerebral cortex (3). Other investigators have reported impairments in visual masking (4), contrast sensitivity (5), and in the flash visual evoked potential (VEP) (6–9). There has been accumulating evidence that AD involves the primary visual pathway (10–12) with associated impairments of vision (13).

This review is divided into three parts: the first describes evidence for parallel processing in humans, the second describes evidence for retinal ganglion degeneration in AD, and the third describes the clinical assessment of vision in AD patients.

PARALLEL PROCESSING

A number of lines of anatomical, physiological, and behavioral evidence demonstrate the existence of parallel visual pathways subserving different functions in cats and primates (14–17). In the cat, Enroth-Cugell and Robson (18) described two types of ganglion cells: X and Y cells. There is also a third type of ganglion cell, W cells, which do not fit into the X or Y categories. X cells are characterized by relatively small receptive fields, slower axon conduction velocity, and linear spatial summation; Y cells are characterized by larger receptive fields, faster axon conduction, and nonlinear subunit input (16).

These physiologically classified X and Y cells have beta and alpha cells as morphological counterparts. Beta cells are characterized by smaller dendritic fields and axons that project to layers A and A1 of the lateral geniculate nucleus (LGN). Alpha cells have larger dendritic fields that project to layers A, A1, and C of the LGN and superior colliculus (SC).

Similar evidence for parallel visual pathways exists in primates. Morphologically different classes of ganglion cells A and B (19) project to two different divisions of the LGN: the magnocellular and parvocellular layers. This segregation remains in the cortex; the magnocellular layer projects to 4C alpha, which eventually projects to middle temporal cortical area MT (20,21). The parvocellular projects to 4C beta to layers 2 and 3 of area 17, to the "pale stripe" region of area 18, and finally to areas V3 and V4. Like the cat, there are physiological differences between the different systems. The parvo system is characterized by color opponency, low contrast sensitivity, and high spatial resolution. The magno system is characterized by absence of color vision, high contrast sensitivity, low spatial resolution, fast temporal resolution, and sensitivity to stereoscopic depth (17).

Evidence for parallel visual pathways also exists in humans. Rodieck et al. (22) described different ganglion-cell subtypes in Golgi-stained material. Evidence for several retinofugal projections also exists in humans.

A variety of anatomical and electrophysiological techniques have been used to demonstrate retinofugal pathways in animals. However, current techniques for tracing axon pathways (such as tracer injections), immunohistological techniques, and the traditional method of utilizing silver impregnation to follow degenerating fibers (produced by an experimental lesion) cannot be used in humans. Even if one succeeds in obtaining human autopsy tissue in cases with previously documented damage to the visual system, the interval between the occurrence of the neurological lesion and tissue availability is variable and almost always prolonged. In addition, human autopsy material is usually poorly fixed. For these and other reasons, human neuropathology provides little information about human neuroanatomy. Therefore, until recently, our understanding of the human visual pathways was largely based on inferences from animal studies. Unfortunately, this indirect means of assessing the human visual system is inadequate if one takes into account the interspecies variations documented in the experimental animal literature.

We demonstrated that a modified version of an old staining technique can be successfully applied to the human brain. This technique utilizes the chemical paraphenylene diamine (PPD), which was first applied by Schultze in 1917 (23) to intensify the contrast in frozen sections of osmicated animal neural tissue. Later investigators (24,25) recognized the great advantage of the high resolution that can be obtained by staining with PPD on semithin plastic embedded sections. In 1975, we used the PPD staining method to demonstrate degenerating axon terminals in cat CNS (26). The same terminals could then be identified by resectioning the material for ultrastructural examination. In 1982 we demonstrated that this technique could be successfully applied to human autopsy specimens, even after long survival and fixation intervals (27).

The PPD method for identifying degenerated axons and axon terminals in human brain tissue has four major advantages.

1. Since the PPD method involves examination of 1-μm semithin plastic embedded sections with a very high contrast stain, the resolution is extremely high. In addition to providing sensitivity sufficient for the identification of axon terminals, the method permits the identification and measurement of the smallest myelinated axons. Thus, a histogram of the nerve fiber spectra of intact axons can be produced.

2. In addition to being extremely sensitive, the method is highly specific and reliable. Unlike silver-staining methods, which can be unpredictable, the PPD method is not contingent on stringent control of parameters of fixation, timing, or redox potentials. Most impressive, the method is not limited to a particular stage of degeneration. Silver-impregnation methods for identifying degenerating axoplasm (e.g., Nauta modifications, Fink-Heimer modifications [28–30]) take advantage of the dynamic process by which neurofibrils of an axon degenerate. The granular appearance of silver-stained degenerating axons is fugacious; the technique must be applied within a short range of time, typically 3 to 5 days after the lesion. This time constraint does not apply to the PPD method.

3. Since the PPD method is reliable, even in poorly fixed tissue, and it does not have the time constraint of being effective only during the transient neurofibrillar stage of degeneration, it is ideally suited for use in human autopsy material. We found that PPD-stained lipid remnants of axonal degeneration are found even after long survival periods in both simians and humans. We demonstrated that the PPD method can identify degenerated axons and axon terminals in the optic tracts and LGN of monkeys of 1 year after ocular enucleation (27).

4. The PPD method is very similar to the Reynold's method of preparing tissue for electron microscopic examination. Therefore, tissue prepared for PPD light microscopic examination can be resectioned for ultrastructural examination. Similarly, adjacent sections can be cut for PPD light microscopy and ultrastructural examination. This permits electron microscopic confirmation of degeneration seen by the PPD method (31,32). Moreover, such ultrastructural examination demonstrates that the products of axon degeneration remain in the primate visual system much longer than previously supposed.

By means of the PPD method we demonstrated, in humans, direct retinofugal projections to the LGN and pretectum (32). The projections to the LGN were found predominantly in the lamina corresponding to the lesioned retinofugal pathway (layers 2, 3, and 5: ipsilateral eye; layers 1, 4, and 6: contralateral eye). We also noted transsynaptic atrophy among LGN neurons when the optic nerve damage existed more than 2 years. However, transsynaptic degeneration of either neurons in the LGN or their axons in the optic radiations was not found. Nevertheless, a small amount of degenerated axon terminals was observed in layers 4b and 4c of the visual cortex following optic nerve lesions of greater than 2 years duration.

This method also provided evidence for a direct retinofugal pathway to the human pretectum (32). The fibers were found to originate from the most medial and ventral portions of the optic tract. The retinopretectal fibers bypassed the LGN and descended toward the pretectum via the brachium of the SC.

The brachium of the SC was found to also carry retinofugal fibers that projected to the SC and to the pulvinar (33). The projection to the SC consisted of two parts: a large projection was found in the deeper layers of the SC and a small projection to a very superficial reticular layer, which was organized in dominance columns separated by approximately 200 µm. A retinofugal projection to the pulvinar was also noted, with the concentration of degenerated axons seeming to be greatest in the rostral and lateral areas. As with the SC, the degeneration appeared to be greater in the pulvinar contralateral to the uniocular lesion.

Retinofugal fibers were also found projecting into the human accessory optic system. The lateral, dorsal, and medial terminal accessory optic nuclei and the interstitial nucleus of the SC all showed degeneration following retinal or optic nerve lesions (34).

Finally, retinofugal projections to three areas of the human hypothalamus were found (35). Retinofugal fibers terminating in the hypothalamus were found to originate from areas near the optic chiasm. Retinofugal projections to both the anterior and posterior lobes of the supraoptic nuclei were noted. Slightly more anteriorly, fibers from the retina were seen to course into the suprachiasmatic nucleus of the hypothalamus. Third, a fascicle of retinofugal fibers was seen to leave the most posterior areas of the optic chiasm, travel between the two lobes of the supraoptic nucleus, and terminate in the paraventricular nucleus of the hypothalamus.

Thus, we described eight primary pathways originating from the human retina and projecting to different areas of the human brain (Fig. 1). This strongly suggests that different visual functions are being mediated at different anatomical sites.

Investigations of visual function complement the anatomical studies. Livingstone and Hubel (17) provided a review of psychophysical evidence for parallel processing in humans. They demonstrated that a number of properties important for movement perception and stereopsis were noncolor selective, had high contrast sensitivity, fast temporal sensitivity, and low spatial resolution.

Thus, there is anatomical and psychophysical evidence for parallel processing in humans. Might some diseases preferentially affect these separate channels?

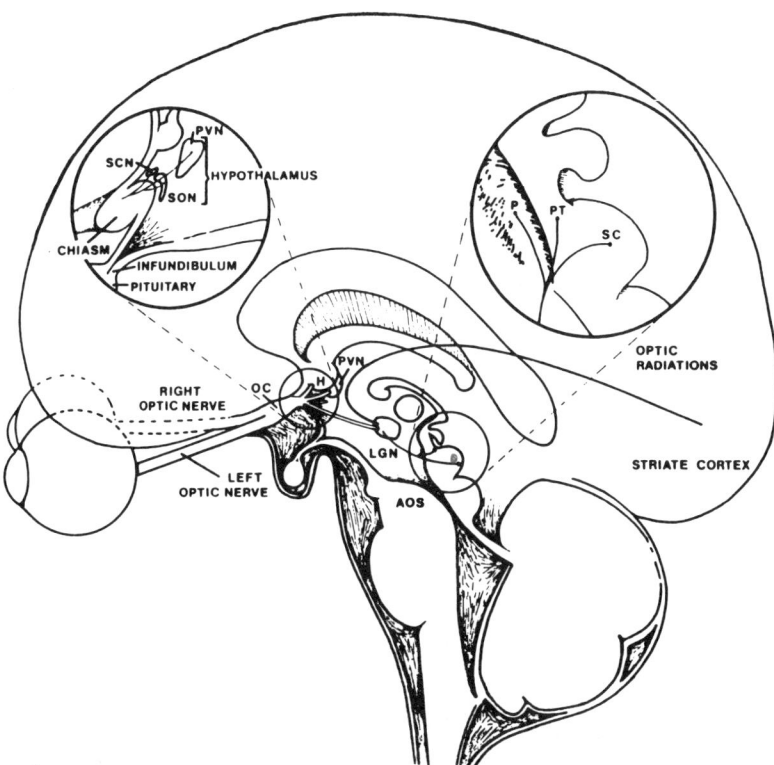

FIG. 1. Central projections of the human visual system proven by the PPD method include lateral geniculate nucleus of the thalamus (LGN), superior colliculus (SC), pretectum (PT), pulvinar (P), accessory optic nucleus (AOS), and three hypothalamic nuclei (suprachiasmatic nucleus [SCN], supraoptic nucleus [SON], and paraventricular nucleus [PVN]).

RETINAL GANGLION CELL DEGENERATION

The retinas from AD patients were compared with those obtained from age-matched controls. The retinas were evaluated through light microscopic examination of toluidine blue-stained flat-mount preparations and also of PPD-stained radial retinal sections.

Retinal whole mounts were prepared according to the method of Wong and Hughes (36). Camera lucida drawings were made of all cells in the ganglion cell layer every 0.5 mm along the horizontal and vertical meridians and along the four meridians bisecting the angles between the horizontal and vertical planes. Cells were classified into definite ganglion cells, other neurons (likely smaller ganglion cells or displaced amacrine cells), and glial cells, based on staining characteristics. Comparable areas (at 5 and 11 mm from the optic disc defining mid and far periphery) examined in the retina of a patient with AD demonstrated a lower density of retinal ganglion cells (Fig. 2). The drawings were traced on a graphics bit pad (MicroPlan II) system. Somata perimeters were calculated in more than 2,000 cells in an AD patient and an age-matched control as shown in Fig. 3. There appears to be a loss of ganglion cells with perimeters larger than 40 μm.

Examination of retinal PPD sections taken from patients with AD revealed that certain retinal ganglion cells showed degenerative changes. Particular characteristics were ganglion cell swelling with microvacuolarization. These retinal ganglion cells also stained more darkly with the PPD stain. The degenerating axon could be traced from the degenerating retinal ganglion cells to the nerve fiber layer of the retina. No degeneration was noted in the outer retinal layers.

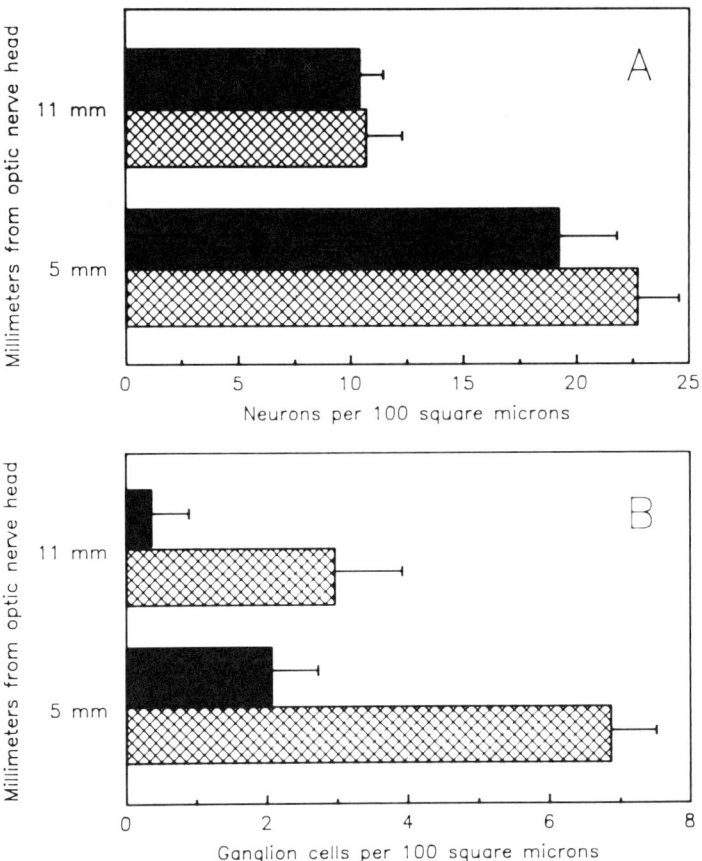

FIG. 2. Graphs comparing the mean axon diameter of neurons (**A**) and large ganglion cells (**B**) at 5 and 11 mm from the optic nerve head. ■, AD128; ▨, CON874.

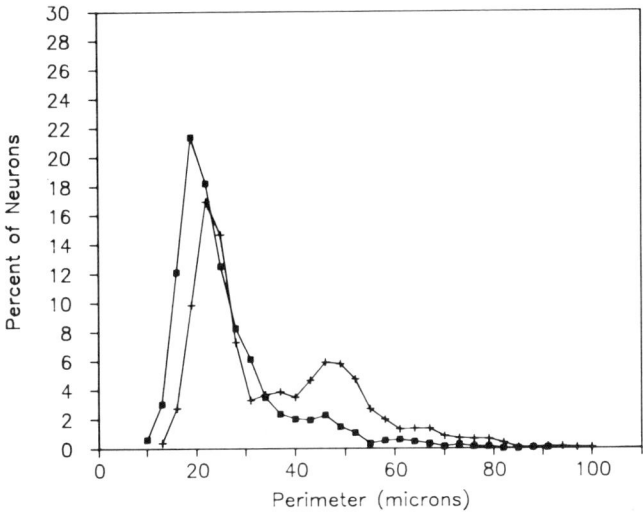

FIG. 3. Plot of percentage of neurons at different soma perimeters in the same AD and control cases as Fig. 2. Note the close match in distribution of neuron sizes observed, except in categories of neurons larger than 60 μm. ■, AD128; +, CON874.

In addition to identifying degeneration in the retinas with whole mounts and with PPD staining of AD patients, examinations were also made of the remaining intact axons in the optic nerve.

Fourteen optic nerves from 12 AD patients were compared histologically with 14 optic nerves from 12 age-matched control patients. The tissues were obtained at autopsy within 12 hr of death and fixed in buffered formaldehyde and glutaraldehyde, osmicated, dehydrated, and embedded in plastic. Each plastic block was marked by a code unknown to the histological observer. The tissue was stained and examined by the PPD method. Significant amounts of degeneration was found in 10 optic nerves. These 10 optic nerves came from 10 patients, all of whom had AD. However, four optic nerves from two patients with AD did not have significant amounts of degeneration. All 14 nerves from 12 age-matched control patients did not have significant amounts of degeneration (Table 1) (10).

The optic nerves from patients with AD demonstrated extensive degeneration as well as significant depletion of axons (a reduction, on average, of approximately 50% compared with those of the age-matched controls). These differences in the number of intact axons were reflected by decreases in axon densities in the affected optic nerves, as can be noted in Fig. 4. Note that the density of axons from the optic nerves obtained from age-matched controls averaged approximately 138 axons per 1,000 μm^2 (37). This is slightly below the 150 axons per 1,000 μm^2 noted in much younger controls. However, the

TABLE 1. *Distribution of optic nerve degeneration*

Extent of degeneration	AD	Age-matched controls
Normal	4	14
Mild	2	0
Moderate	6	0
Severe	2	0
Total	14	14

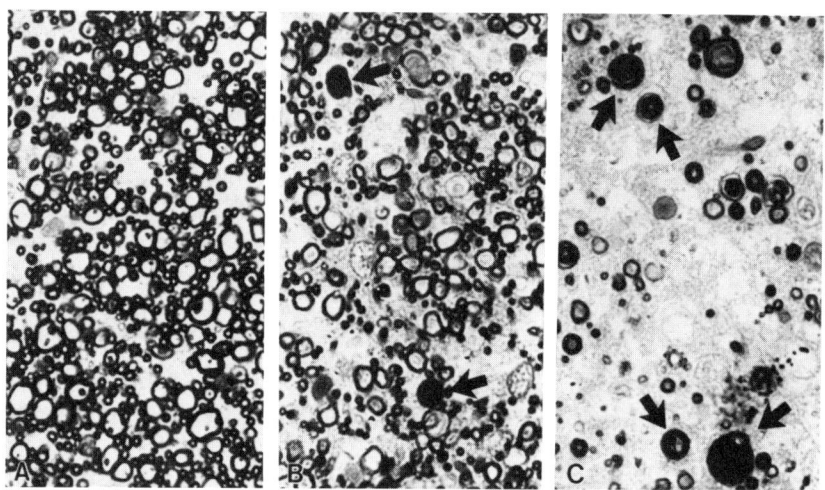

FIG. 4. Optic nerves studied by the PPD method. **A:** Normal axons from a 74-year-old control. **B:** Axons from an 89-year-old AD patient with moderate optic nerve degeneration. **C:** Axons from a 73-year-old AD patient with severe optic nerve degeneration. The degenerated profiles are seen as homogeneous dark disks that vary in size (*arrows*). Also the apparent decrease in axon density. (From ref. 10.)

lowest density of axons was found in patients in whom the presumptive diagnosis of AD was confirmed by the presence of plaques and tangles at autopsy. In this group the average axon density was only approximately 68.2 axons per 1,000 μm^2 (Fig. 5). Thus, the process of aging produced a small amount of axonal dropout whereas greater losses were observed in AD.

We also measured the cross-sectional area of the axons in the optic nerves (taken 7 mm anterior to the optic chiasm) using an enhanced video system (37). There was a significant correlation ($r = -0.74$) for nerves with a lower density of axons to have a greater mean diameter (Fig. 6). This suggests the possibility that larger axons may initially be involved with subsequent involvement of all axon sizes.

The significance of this preferential loss of retinal ganglion cell by size category is still subject to speculation. Certainly, this possibility is intriguing in

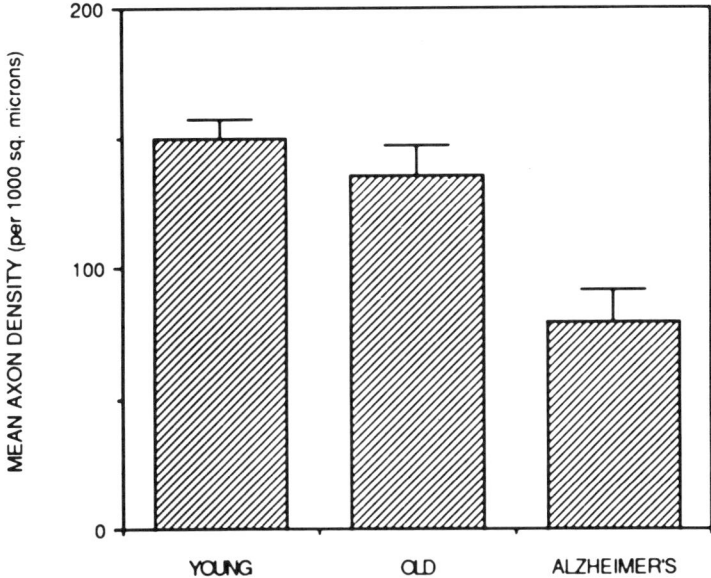

FIG. 5. Mean optic nerve axon density. A small but nonsignificant loss of optic nerve axon density is observed with age. There is a significant decrease in axon density in the AD patients.

light of the fact that animal studies and, more recently, studies on the human retina suggest that there exists a variety of different retinal ganglion cell types (22). There have been several recent investigations suggesting that at least two subgroups of retinal ganglion cells can be described that have differential projections. Thus, it is possible that in AD there is a predilection for degeneration of the larger M cells before a loss of the smaller P cells.

Such a preferential impairment of the M-cell system may have considerable clinical impact. The M-cell system derives from large retinal ganglion cells that project to the magnocellular LGN that in turn projects to certain cortical areas that eventually project to MT. There are several studies that suggest that the M-cell system subserves functions such as low contrast sensitivity and orientation. There is evidence that the P-cell system, consisting of projections to parvocellular LGN, may be more intimately related to the resolution of central vision and good visual acuity. Thus, if there was a selective involvement of one type of cell over another in early AD, one might expect to find a selective involvement of certain visual functions on clinical assessments of AD patients.

VISUAL ASSESSMENT OF AD PATIENTS

Fourteen patients with AD were given a battery of ophthalmological, neuro-ophthalmological, and psychophysical testing. These patients were clas-

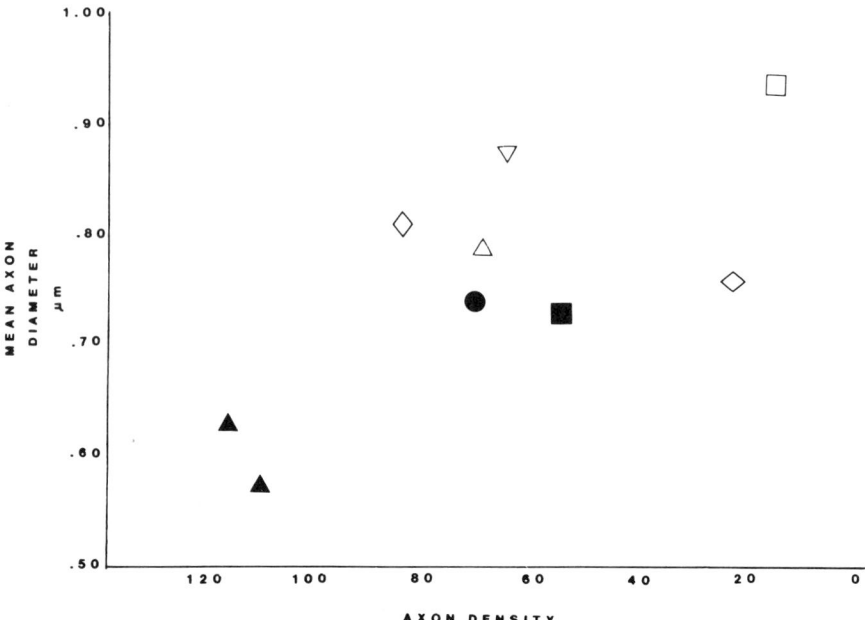

FIG. 6. Relationship between mean axon diameter and axon density (axons/1,000 μm^2) in nine AD optic nerves. There is a significant correlation ($r = -0.74$) between mean axon diameter and axon density. A decrease in axon density is associated with an increase in mean axon diameter.

sified as having AD by established protocols of neurological, neuropsychological, and laboratory tests. In general, certain patterns were noted in the clinical visual assessments of these patients. Patients who had relatively mild cognitive impairment would often complain of the inability to read. For example, a patient might mention that he used to read the newspaper but no longer can; he still finds the paper interesting, but has to have his wife read it to him. The AD patient also may note that although he can make his way past furniture by walking slowly, he has difficulties moving quickly. He may bump into furniture not seen. The AD patient, and more often his or her relatives, sometimes describes "spatial" or "perceptual" problems. By this, the family usually means that the AD patient misreaches for objects on a table, thus knocking over instead of grasping glasses, etc.

Despite these complaints, mildly impaired patients invariably had normal Snellen visual acuity. Additionally, they usually had a normal general ophthalmological examination. In particular, their fundus appeared to be normal, and there was no evidence of optic disk pallor.

Nonetheless, even patients with mild AD did display several abnormal features. The first common deficit seen in the eye movement examination was long latencies in saccadic eye movements. The second was an abnormal flash visual evoked response. Third, the pattern VEP latencies were sometimes delayed (130 msec) compared wih the age-matched controls (approximately 110 msec).

The symptoms and signs in moderate AD were often more severe. These patients had similar complaints as those with mild AD. However, their saccadic eye movements were even more delayed. Additionally, they showed dysmetria in both horizontal and vertical attempts at saccades. However, they were able to maintain fixation fairly well. In moderate AD, color vision was often impaired. Defects in contrast sensitivity functions were noted, particularly at the midspatial frequencies. Flash VEPs were often abnormal. The patients still had normal visual acuities by Snellen chart measurement and normal-appearing optic disks.

The visual symptoms and signs in severe AD were quite marked. These patients often showed very limited verbal capacities. They either said nothing or would simply say that they "can't see." Visual acuities were very hard to establish by Snellen chart measurement, and we often had to repeat them by pediatric means such as the "E game," Allen cards, picking up small white balls, or pattern VEPs. Usually we would evaluate visual acuity by at least two of these means, and typically the visual acuity would be in the 20/100 to 20/400 range. These patients also demonstrated varying degrees of dyschromatopsia. Additionally, the contrast sensitivity functions were depresssed across all spatial frequencies. These patients sometimes showed mild amounts of optic disc atrophy.

In summary, we tested 14 patients with AD; a summary of our findings appears in Table 2. Only one patient showed no visual deficits. Most mildly impaired patients showed abnormal eye movements and VEPS when reporting "spatial" problems. Most had good visual acuity. More severely impaired AD patients often showed impaired eye movements, VEPs with poor visual acuity and color vision. Contrast sensitivity, measured in three patients using Vis Tech plates, showed abnormalities. Many flash VEPs (five patients) showed a negative waveform flash characteristic of a very young infant's VEP. Electroretinograms measured in one patient were normal but with an abnormal flash VEP (Fig. 7) consistent with the anatomical findings of central pathway involvement with relative sparing of the outer retina.

Several features of these clinical evaluations were remarkable. First of all, in patients with mild or moderate AD, in whom there was histologically retinal ganglion cell dropout, no optic nerve atrophy was noted. Although initially surprising, this is understandable. Ophthalmologists who deal with optic nerve diseases, particularly glaucoma, are familiar with the fact that one can often lose more than half of the axons without clear-cut evidence of optic disc atrophy or large impairments in visual acuity (38).

Our findings are especially intriguing in light of the findings of selective psychophysical functioning of parallel pathways in monkeys (39) and humans (17). Our preliminary anatomical results suggest that larger ganglion cells

TABLE 2. Visual System Symptoms, Signs, and Laboratory Values in AD

Patient	Alzheimer classification	Subjective complaints	Acuities	Eye movements	Flash (F) VER pattern (P) VER	Other
1	Mild	Difficulty reading	OD 20/40 OS 20/30 −3	Slight delay initiating saccades	FVER: OU/loss of amplitude; delayed peak PVER: borderline delay	Mild dyschromatopsia; anosmia
2	Mild	Difficulty reading; space problems	OD 20/200 OS 20/20	Long delay in saccades; mild dysmetria	FVER: OU/abnormal asymmetric waveforms PVER: nonrecordable	Childhood amblyopia OD
3	Moderate	Difficulty reading; space problems	OD 20/20 OS 20/30 −2	Severe dysmetria	FVER: OU/low amplitude; simplification of waveform PVER: nonrecordable	Moderate/severe dyschromatopsia; mild optic atrophy; slight anosmia
4	Severe	Inability to read	OD 20/400 OS 20/400	Difficulty initiating saccades	FVER: OU/normal PVER: normal	Mild optic atrophy
5	Severe	"Blind"	OD 20/400 OS 20/100	Poor cooperation	FVER: OU/asymmetric delayed PVER: OD/nonrecordable OS/delayed	OU: Mild dyschromatopsia; disk pallor

6	Mild	None	OD 20/30 +3 OS 20/20 −1	Normal	FVER: OU/two peaks; moderate delay PVER: normal	Binasal field losses with OCTOPUS
7	Mild	"Colors appear bright"	OD 20/30 −3 OS 20/30	Normal	FVER: normal PVER: borderline delay	Inferior field losses with OCTOPUS
8	Mild	Inability to read	OU 20/40	Delay in initiating saccades	FVER: normal PVER: OD/nonrecordable OS/Borderline delay	Moderate/severe dyschromatopsia
9	Mild/moderate	Difficulty reading	OD 20/30 OS 20/25 +1	Delay in initiating saccades	FVER: normal PVER: normal	Moderate dyschromatopsia
10	Mild/moderate	Formed visual hallucinations	OD 20/40 OS 20/25	Normal	FVER: OU/slight delay PVER: borderline delay	Severe dyschromatopsia; anosmia OU: mild/moderate disk atrophy
11	Moderate	"Objects have shadows"; "Can't recognize objects"	OD 20/40 +1 OS 20/100 +1	Normal	FVER: delayed PVER: OD/delayed OS/nonrecordable	Peripheral constriction of visual fields OU: mild optic disk pallor
12	Severe	Difficulty reading; spatial problems	OD 20/100 OS 20/40	Difficulty initiating saccades	FVER: OD/normal OS/low amplitude PVER: OU/delayed	Large square wave jerks with fixation

From ref. 13.

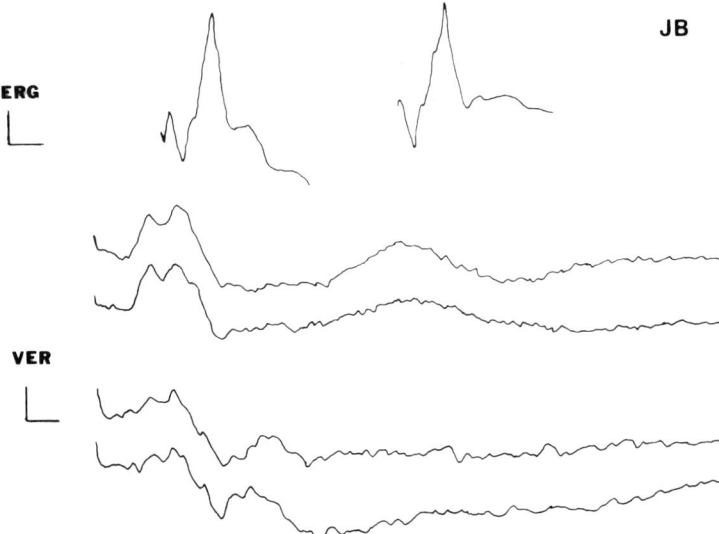

FIG. 7. Top shows flash photopic electroretinograms (ERG) from an AD patient from OS on left and OD on right. These are normal ERGs. Calibration bar is 10 μV and 5 msec. **Bottom** of figure is flash VEPs from same patient. Top two tracings are repeat tracings from OS and bottom two are repeat tracings from OD. These are low amplitude flash VEPs. Calibration bar is 2 μV and 20 msec.

with larger axon diameters may initially be involved in AD. A great deal of evidence suggests that the parvocellular projection (or P cells) are involved in high spatial frequency and color discrimination. The magnocellular projections (or M cells) are important in movement, depth, and low contrast vision. This may explain our finding that ganglion cell loss may be found without loss of visual acuity.

Further studies are needed to establish the relationship between ganglion cell loss and visual functioning in AD. Quantification of more age-matched controls in both the anatomical and psychophysical studies are required to be certain that our observations are not due to normal variation. Quantification of retinas and optic nerves from the same patients would provide converging evidence for specific ganglion cell loss. Finally, more extensive psychophysical test batteries are required to delineate the M- and P-cell pathways; specifically, tests of stereopsis and movement detection might prove useful.

CONCLUSIONS

The results of both anatomical and psychophysical tests must be interpreted cautiously. Nonetheless, several important conclusions can be drawn. Both the anatomical and clinical evidence presented is subject to several limitations. The number of anatomical examinations performed is insufficient to statistically assess the difference in the size spectra of retinal ganglion cells and their intact axons in AD. The clinical assessment of patients with AD is complicated by the problem that deterioration of the cognitive functions interferes with the ability to assess visual abilities. AD does appear, at least in many cases, to produce a primary optic neuropathy. There is good histopathological evidence for this.

Patients with AD can be clinically demonstrated to have visual impairments. However, when the disease is mild, the visual acuity remains near normal, and when the disease is severe, AD patients are difficult to evaluate due to problems with compliance, cooperation, and concentration. Thus, it is not surprising that patients with AD were not known to have lesions to their primary visual pathways.

Most intriguing is the possibility that there is a predilection in early AD for the largest retinal ganglion cells that are associated with the largest caliber axon fibers. Selective involvement of the M-cell system might explain the deficits in contrast sensitivity, spatial orientation, and eye movement control with only minimal effects on visual acuity.

It is possible to establish a pattern of impaired visual functions with AD by means of a systematic battery of visual function tests. Indeed, such visual studies may potentially aid in distinguishing AD from other common dementing illnesses of long duration. Additionally, identification of an optic neuropathy in AD may reveal the defined population of retinal ganglion cells and optic nerve fibers that are particularly susceptible to the disease. Research into this area may permit a better understanding of the biology of AD as well as of the synaptic organization of the human visual system.

ACKNOWLEDGMENTS

This work was supported by grants EY05894, P-50-AG05142, EY07087, a grant from the state of California, and MH39145 from the Alzheimer's Consortium of Southern California. We also thank Janet Blanks, Ph.D., Mark Borchert, M.D., Edward DeVita, M.D., David Hinton, M.D., Betty Johnson, M.S., and Carol Miller, M.D., for help in various stages of this project. The retinal whole mount data were done in collaboration with Janet Blanks, Ph.D.

REFERENCES

1. Katzman R. Medical progress: Alzheimer's disease. *N Engl J Med* 1986;314:964–973.
2. McKhann G, Drachman D, Folstein M, Katzman R, Price D, Stadlan EM. Clinical diagnosis of Alzheimer's disease: report of the NINCDS-ADRDA Work Group under the auspices of Department of Health and Human Services Task Force on Alzheimer's Disease. *Neurology* 1984;34:939–944.

3. Cogan DG. Visual disturbances with focal progressive dementing disease. *Am J Ophthalmol* 1985;100:68–72.
4. Schlotterer G, Moscovitch M, Crapper-McLachlan D. Visual processing deficits as assessed by spatial frequency contrast sensitivity and backward masking in normal ageing and Alzheimer's disease. *Brain* 1984;107:309.
5. Nissen MJ, Corkin S, Buonanno FS, Growden JH, Wray SH, Baur J. Spatial vision in Alzheimer's disease. General findings and a case report. *Arch Neurol* 1985;42:667.
6. Visser SL, van Tilburg W, Hooijer C, Jonker C, deRijke W. Visual evoked potentials (VEPs) in senile dementia (Alzheimer type) and in non-organic behavioural disorders in the elderly: comparison with EEG parameters. *Electroencephalogr Clin Neurophysiol* 1985;60:115.
7. Harding GFA, Doggett CE, Orwin A, Smith EJ. Visual evoked potentials in presenile dementia. *Doc Ophthalmol Proc Ser* 1981;27:193.
8. Bajalan AAA, Wright CE, van der Vliet VJ. Changes in the human visual evoked potentials caused by the anticholinergic agent hyoscine hydrobromide: comparison of the results in Alzheimer's disease. *J Neurol Neurosurg Psychiatry* 1986;49:175.
9. Wright CE, Harding GFA, Orwin A. The flash and pattern VEP as a diagnostic indicator of dementia. *Doc Ophthalmol* 1986;62:89.
10. Hinton DR, Sadun AA, Blanks JC, Miller CA. Optic nerve degeneration in Alzheimer's disease. *N Engl J Med* 1986;351:485–487.
11. Bassi CJ, Blanks JC, Sadun AA, Johnson BM. The retinal ganglion cell layer in Alzheimer's disease: a whole mount study. *Invest Ophthalmol Vis Sci* 1987;28(suppl):109.
12. Bassi CJ, Blanks JC, Hinton DR, Sadun AA, Miller CA. Retinal ganglion cell degeneration in Alzheimer's disease. *Neurosci Abstr* 1987;13:1328.
13. Sadun AA, Borchert M, DeVita E, Hinton DR, Bassi CJ. Assessment of visual impairment in patients with Alzheimer's disease. *Am J Ophthalmol* 1987;104:113–120.
14. Lennie P. Parallel visual pathways: a review: *Vision Res* 1980;20:561–594.
15. Stone J. *Parallel processing in the visual system.* New York: Plenum Press, 1983.
16. Shapley R, Perry VH. Cat and monkey retinal ganglion cells and their visual functional roles. *Trends Neurosci* 1986;9:229–235.
17. Livingstone MS, Hubel DH. Psychophysical evidence for separate channels for the perception of form, color movement, and depth. *J Neurosci* 1987;7:3416–3468.
18. Enroth-Cugell C, Robson JG. The contrast sensitivity of retinal ganglion cells of the cat. *J Physiol (Lond)* 1966;378:379–384.
19. Leventhal AG, Rodieck RW, Dreher B. Retinal ganglion cells classes in the Old World monkey: morphology and central projections. *Science* 1981;213:1139–1142.
20. Zeki SM. Representation of central visual fields in prestriate cortex of monkeys. *Brain Res* 1969;14:271–291.
21. Lund JS, Boothe RG. Intralaminar connections and pyramidal neuron organization in the visual cortex, area 17, of the Macaque monkey. *J Comp Neurol* 1975;159:305–334.
22. Rodieck RW, Binmoeller KF, Dineen J. Parasol and midget ganglion cells of the human retina. *J Comp Neurol* 1985;233:115–132.
23. Schultze WH. Uber das paraphenylenediamin in der histolgischen Farbetchnik (katalytische Farbung) und uber eine neve Schnellfarbmethode der Nervenmarkscheinen am Gefrierschnitt. *Zentrabl Allg Pathol Pathol Anat* 1917;28:257–260.
24. Holander H, Vaaland JL. A reliable staining method for semi-thin sections in experimental neuroanatomy. *Brain Res* 1968;10:120–126.
25. Estable-Puig JF, Bauer WC, Blumberg JM. Paraphenylenediamine staining of osmium-fixed plastic embedded tissue for light and phase microscopy. *J Neuropathol Exp Neurol* 1965;24:531–535.
26. Sadun AA. Differential distribution of cortical terminations in the cat red nucleus. *Brain Res* 1975;99:145–151.
27. Sadun AA, Smith LEH, Kenyon KR. Paraphenylenediamine: a new method for tracing human visual pathways. *J Neuropathol Exp Neurol* 1983;42:200–206.
28. Nauta WJH, Gygax PA. Silver impregnation of degenerating axon terminals in the central nervous system: (1) technic, (2) chemical notes. *Stain Technol* 1951;26:5–11.
29. Nauta WJH, Ryan LF. Selective silver impregnation of degenerating axon terminals in the central nervous system. *Stain Technol* 1952;27:175–179.

30. Fink RP, Heimer L. Two methods for selective impregnation of degenerating axons and their synaptic endings in the central nervous system. *Brain Res* 1967;4:369–374.
31. Sadun AA, Schaechter JD. Tracing axons in the human brain: a method utilizing TEM techniques. *J Electromicrosc Tech* 1985;2:175–186.
32. Johnson BM, Sadun AA. Ultrastructural and PPD studies of primate visual system: degenerative remnants persist for longer than expected. *J Electron Microsc Tech* (*in press*).
33. Sadun AA. Neuroanatomy of the human visual system: Part I. Retinal projections to the LGN and pretectum as demonstrated with a new method. *Neuro-ophthalmology* 1986;6:353–361.
34. Sadun AA, Johnson BM, Smith LEH. Neuroanatomy of the human visual system. Part II. Retinal projections to the superior colliculus and pulvinar. *Neuro-ophthalmology* 1986;6:363–370.
35. Sadun AA, Johnson BM, Schaechter JD. Neuroanatomy of the human visual system. Part III. Retinal projections to the hypothalamus. *Neuro-ophthalmology* 1986;6:371–379.
36. Wong ROL, Hughes A. The morphology, number, and distribution of a large population of confirmed displaced amacrine cells in the adult cat retina. *J Comp Neurol* 1987;255:159–177.
37. Johnson BM, Miao M, Sadun AA. Age-related decline of human optic nerve axon populations. *Age* 1987;10:5–9.
38. Quigley HA, Addicks EM, Green WR. Optic nerve damage in human glaucoma, ischemic neuropathy, papilledema, and toxic neuropathy. *Arch Ophthalmol* 1982;100:135–146.
39. Merigan WH, Eskin TA. Spatio-temporal vision of macaques with severe loss of P beta retinal ganglion cells. *Vision Res* 1986;26:1751–1761.

Subject Index

A

α cell
  characteristics, 332
  nicotinic acetylcholine
    immunoreactivity, 29
  size gradation, 22
N-Acetyl-aspartate-glutamate, as lateral geniculate neurotransmitter, 47–48,65
Acetylcholine
  amacrine cell release, 3,4
  as lateral geniculate neurotransmitter, 44,50–53
  in thalamic reticular nucleus, 63–64
  receptor, 98,101
    muscarinic, 91,92,93–94,95,99, 100,102–103,104
    nicotinic, 29,91,92,93–94,104
  optic nerve content, 44
Acetyl cholinesterase, as lateral geniculate neurotransmitter, 50,65,67
Acuity testing, of infants, 109–110,112
A_1-Adenosine, cortical receptor, 95,96
Adenosine 3′:5′-cyclic phosphate,
  dopamine interaction, 4,7–13
  electrical junction coupling effects, 11–13
  light responsiveness effects, 9–13
β-Adrenergic receptor
  cortical, 95,98,104–105
  of lateral geniculate nucleus pars dorsalis, 58–59
Afternystagmus, optokinetic, optic tract nucleus in
  clinical implications, 250–251
  electrical stimulation-induced, 237–242
    gravity effects, 240,241
    lesion effects, 242–247
    stimulation sites, 240,242
  theoretical basis, 236,237
Age factors
  in face/facial expression recognition, 177,178, 190
  in optic nerve degeneration, 337–338
Agnosia, spatial, 331
Alexia, 268
Alzheimer's disease
  definition, 331
  visual system, 331–347
    age factors, 337–338
    amblyopia, 342
    anosmia, 342,343
    contrast sensitivity, 331,341
    dyschromatopsia, 341,342,343
    dysmetria, 342
    optic atrophy, 342
    optic nerve degeneration, 337–338,339
    retinal ganglion cell degeneration, 335–339
    saccadic eye movement, 340, 341,342,343
    spatial agnosia, 331
    visual acuity, 340,341,345
    visual assessment, 339–344
    visual evoked potentials, 331,340–341
    visual masking impairments, 331
Amacrine cell, 19
  bipolar cell input, 312
  ganglion cell input, 26
  neurotransmitters, 27–28
    acetylcholine, 3,4
    γ-aminobutyric acid, 3
    dopamine, 312
  types, 2,3
Amblyopia
  in Alzheimer's disease, 342
  determinants, 86–91
    critical period, 88–90
    extravisual factors, 90–91
    locus of effects, 86–88
α-Amino-3-hydroxy-5-methyl-4-isoxazolepropionic acid, 47
2-Amino-4-phosphonobutyrate, on/off channel effects, 35–41
D-2-Amino-4-phosphonobutyrate, 46
D-2-Amino-5-phosphonovalerate, 46
Amino acids, acetylated, 47

349

γ-Aminobutyric acid
  amacrine cell release, 3
  cortical receptor, 91–92,95,
    98,101,102,104
  I-cell content, 67–71
  optic tract nucleus neuron content,
    235
  retinal ganglion cell content, 22–
    23
  thalamic reticular nucleus
    immunoreactivity, 61–63,64
Anosmia, in Alzheimer's disease,
    342,343
Antibody recognition, 28–30
Aphasia, face/facial recognition
  impairment in, 170
Art, depth perception in, 128,130,
    131,132,136
Aspartate, as lateral geniculate
  neurotransmitter, 44,45,46
Atrophy, optic, in Alzheimer's disease,
    342
Axotomy, retinal ganglion cell
  response, 30

B
Baclofen, cortical receptor, 95
β cell
  characteristics, 332
  nicotinic acetylcholine
    immunoreactivity, 29
  size gradation, 29
Benton line orientation test, 313
Bipolar cell, 19
  depolarizing, 1,2,3
  ganglion cell input, 26,29–30
  hyperpolarizing, 1,2,3,35
  neurotransmitters, 26–27
    glutamate, 4,29–30
  photoreceptor input, 1
  receptive field center, 3
Bird, retinal ganglion cell, 20,21
  substance-P content, 23–24,26,27
Blood flow
  cerebral, positron emission tomogra-
    phy measurement, 257–270
    anatomical localization, 259–260
    elementary stimulus variables,
      263–265
    historical background, 257–258
    low-level response detection, 261–
      262
    metabolic measurements versus,
      258–259
    response localization, 260–261
    retinoptic organization, 265,266
    spatial resolution, 260–261
    statistical analysis, 262–263
    strategy, 258–263
    visually presented word response,
      267–268
    visual system observations, 263–
      268
    voluntary saccade response, 265–
      267
  of frontal eye field, 266–267
Bombesin, retinal ganglion cell
  content, 19,23,30,31
Brain. *See also* specific areas of brain
  blood flow measurement, 257–270
    anatomical localization, 259–260
    elementary stimulus variables,
      263–265
    historical background, 257–258
    low-level response detection, 261–
      262
    metabolic measurements versus,
      258–259
    response localization, 260–261
    retinoptic organization, 265,266
    spatial resolution, 260–261
    statistical analysis, 282–283
    strategy, 258–263
    visually presented word response,
      267–268
    visual system observations, 263–
      268
    voluntary saccade response, 265–
      267
  face/facial expression/gesture recogni-
    tion mechanisms, 165–193
    age factors, 177,178,190
    in brain-lesioned subjects,
      168,169,170–172,173–
      174,175,190
    evoked potentials, 179–188,191
    left/right symmetry, 166
    limbic system and, 179,188
    neuropsychological tests, 168–170
    paraprosopia, 168
    prosopagnosia, 165,168,188
    in schizophrenia, 168,169,170,174–
      179,190
    sex factors, 168,177

visual information processing, 120–121
Brain-lesioned subjects, face/facial expression recognition, 168,190
  blace/white photograph test, 169,173
  movie test, 171–172,173–174,175
  slide test, 170–171
Brain stem, lateral geniculate transmission systems, 50–59
  cholinergic, 50–53,63–64,72
  noradrenergic, 56–59,64,72
  serotoninergic, 53–56,60,72

C

Calcium channel receptor, 95,104–105
Cat
  cortical plasticity mechanisms, 85–108
    amblyopia determinants, 86–91
    cellular mechanisms, 91–103
    critical period, 88–90,104,105–106
    neurotransmitter function effects, 88
    receptor development, 93–102
    receptor localization, 91–93
    receptor redistribution, 102–103
    second messengers, 95–97,105
    selective deprivation effects, 85–86
  dopamine-dependent visual dysfunction, 313
  lateral geniculate nucleus pars dorsalis
    N-acetyl-aspartate-glutamate content, 48
    γ-aminobutyric acid content, 67,68–69
    diencephalic innervation, 59–60,61,63
    I-cells, 67,68–69
    noradrenergic innervation, 57–58
    serotoninergic neurotransmitter, 53,55,56
    thalamic reticular nucleus innervation, 60–61
  optic nerve, glutamate content, 44
  optokinetic nystagmus/afternystagmus, 237
  pattern electroretinogram, 289–290,291–292
  retinal ganglion cells
    α cell, 29
    on-off cell, 21–22
    W cell, 331
    X cell, 3,22,331
    Y cell, 3,22,331
Catecholamine-synthesizing enzyme, 23
Cerebral cortex. See Cortex
Changing-size channels, foveal, 317
Channeling. See also Parallel processing
  changing-size channels, 317
  color channels, 317
  in multiple sclerosis, 317–329
    on/off channels, 319–320
    orientation channels, 320–324,326
    spatial channels, 320–326
    temporal channels, 320
  on/off channels, 35–41
    2-amino-4-phosphobutyrate effects, 35–41
    contrast sensitivity, 36,41
    function, 36,41
    light stimuli response, 35–37,39–41
    in multiple sclerosis, 319–320
    saccadic eye movements, 36,40
  orientation channels, 317,320–324,326
  spatial frequency channels, 317
  stereomotion channels, 317
Cholecystokinin
  amacrine cell content, 28
  cortical receptor, 95,104–105
  retinal ganglion cell content, 19,23
Choline acetyl transferase, as lateral geniculate neurotransmitter, 44,51
Cholinergic system, of lateral geniculate nucleus pars dorsalis, 50–53,63–64,72
Colineraity, 135
Color
  equiluminant
    depth perspective and, 127,128,134
    figure-ground discrimination and, 133–134
    shape discrimination and, 136
    spatial relationship and, 135
  as linking feature, 135
Color blindness, 127–128
Color channels, foveal, 317
Color contrast, 127–132
Color perception, 120,121,122,126.
  See also Spectral sensitivity
  geniculocortical visual system in, 126
  of infants, 112–114

Cone
  blue, 122
  in color blindness, 127
  green, 122
  red, 122
  in visual function development, 113,114
Contrast sensitivity in Alzheimer's disease, 331,341
  of infants, 111–112
  in monocular diplopia, 322–324
  in multiple sclerosis, 321–324
  on/off channels and, 36,41
  in Parkinson's disease, 297–304,310–311
    pattern electroretinogram, 307–310,311,312
    spatiotemporal, 299–304,310–311
Cortex. See also specific areas of cortex
  neuromagnetic localization studies, 271–287
    contrast threshold, 277–278
    extravisual area activity, 281–285
    neuromagnetic methods, 272–274
    parallel processing channels, 280–281,282
    reaction time/latency relationship, 279–280
    retinotopic sequence, 274–277
    threshold relationships, 278–279
  ocular dominance plasticity mechanisms, 85–108
    amblyopia determinants, 86-91
    cellular mechanisms, 91–103
    critical period, 88–90,104,105–106
    neuromodulator function modification effects, 88
    neurotransmitter development, 93–102
    neurotransmitter function effects, 88
    neurotransmitter localization, 91–93
    receptor development, 93–102
    receptor redistribution, 102–103
    second messengers, 95–97,105
    selective deprivation effects, 85–86
  retinotopic organization, 265,266
  during saccadic eye movements, 265–267
  visual motion processing function, 211–231
    deficit recovery, 223–224
    directional selectivity, 211–213,213–215
    extraretinal input, 216,217
    localization, 211–213
    medial superior temporal area and, 213–216,217
    middle temporal area and, 126,213–224,281–282
    optokinetic deficits, 226–229
    pursuit cells, 213–216
    pursuit initiation, 216–223
    retinal deficits, 221,222,223,225–226,228,229
    saccadic eye movements, 218,219–221,222
    superior temporal sulcus area and, 213,218,220
    word presentation task response, 267–268
Corticotrophic-related factor, 28
Critical flicker fusion. See Flicker frequency discrimination
Cusanus, Nicolaus, 165

D

da Vinci, Leonardo, 128
Delay field test, 319–320
Depth perception, 120,121
  color contrast in, 127–132
  geniculocortical pathways in
    magnocellular pathway, 127–129,132
    parvocellular pathway, 127,132
  luminance contrast in, 127–128,129–130,132
  motion processing and, 128,129,131–132
  perspective in, 130–131
  shading in, 132
  stereopsis in, 128–129
Dewar, James, 272
Diencephalon
  achromatic/chromatic systems, 212
  lateral geniculate nucleus pars dorsalis innervation, 59–64
Dihydroxyphenylacetic acid, 308
Dipeptide, acidic, 47
Diplopia, monocular, contrast sensitivity in, 322–324
Dog, lateral geniculate nucleus pars dorsalis, 56

SUBJECT INDEX

Dominance, ocular, plasticity
  mechanisms, 85–108
  amblyopia determinants, 86–91
  cellular mechanisms, 91–103
  critical period, 88–90,104,105–106
  neuromodulator function
    modification, 88
  neurotransmitter function, 88
  receptor development, 93–102
  receptor localization, 91–93
  receptor redistribution, 102–103
  second messengers, 95–97,105
  selective deprivation effects, 85–86
Dopamine
  horizontal cell effects, 4–16
    adenosine 3′:5′-cyclic phosphate
      interaction, 7–13
    in darkness, 15–16
    electrical coupling, 4,7,11–13,312
    light responsiveness, 4–7,9–13
  interplexiform cell release, 4
  as lateral geniculate
    neurotransmitter, 44
  in Parkinson's disease contrast
    sensitivity effects, 302–304
    D1 receptors, 313
    D2 receptors, 312,313
    deficiency, 307–310,311–313
    signal processing effects, 309–310
  retinal ganglion cell content, 19
Dorsal tegmental nucleus
  choline acetyl transferase active
    neurons, 51
  lateral geniculate nucleus pars
    dorsalis innervation, 60
  location, 233–235
  in optokinetic nystagmus/
    afternystagmus, 240,242–243,
    244–246,247,248–250,251–252
Dyschromatopsia, in Alzheimer's
  disease, 341,342,343
Dysmetria, in Alzheimer's disease, 342

E
Elasmobranch, retinal ganglion cell, 23
Electroretinogram (ERG). *See also* Pattern electroretinogram (PERG)
  in degenerated retinal ganglion cell,
    289–290
Enkephalin
  amacrine cell content, 28
  retinal ganglion cell content, 19,23

Equiluminance
  depth perception and,
    127,128,134,135
  figure-ground discrimination and,
    133–134
  shape discrimination and, 136
  spatial relationship and, 135
Evoked potentials. *See also* Visual
  evoked potentials
  in face/facial expression/gesture
    recognition, 179–188,191
    alternating stimuli response, 181–
      183
    black/white photograph test, 183
    direct response task, 184–185
    "famous face" response task, 185–
      186
    known versus unknown stimuli,
      186–187
    recognition task, 183–184
    upside-down stimuli, 187
Excitatory postsynaptic potential
  antagonists, 46–47
Eye movement
  saccadic. *See* Saccadic eye movement
  visual grasp reflex, 208

F
Face/facial expression, brain recognition mechanisms, 165–193
  age factors, 177,178,190
  in brain-lesioned subjects, 168,190
    black/white photograph test,
      169,173
    movie test, 171–172,173–174,175
    slide test, 170–171
  evoked potentials, 179–188,191
    alternating stimuli response, 181–
      183
    black/white photograph test, 183
    direct response task, 184–184
    "famous face" response task, 185–
      186
    known versus unknown stimuli,
      186–187
    task recognition, 183–184
    upside-down stimuli, 187
  left-right symmetry, 166
  limbic system and, 179,188
  neuropsychological tests, 168–170
  paraprosopia, 168
  prosopagnosia, 165,168,188

Face/facial expression (*contd.*)
  in schizophrenia, 168,169,174–179,190
    age factors, 177,178,190
    black/white photograph test, 169
    movie test, 170,176–178
    paranoic response correlation, 179
    sex factors, 177
    slide test, 175–176
  sex factors, 168,177
Fibroblast growth factor, retinal ganglion cell response, 31
Figure-ground discrimination, 132–134
Fish
  horizontal cell, dopamine effects, 4–16,312
  interplexiform cell, 4,5
Flicker channels, foveal, 317
Flicker frequency discrimination by infants, 112,113
  in multiple sclerosis, 320
Fovea
  channels, 317
  frontal eye field neurons, 198,200,202,204,206,207
  of infants, 112,116
Frog
  optic fiber reconnective ability, 30
  retinal ganglion cell
    neuropeptides, 23–24
    on-off, 21
Frontal eye field, 195–209
  blood flow, 266–267
  frontotectal projection, 202–207,208
    antidromic excitation, 203–205
    caudate nucleus projection, 207–208
    substantia nigra projection, 207–208
  neuron types, 195–202
    antidromic, 204–205
    auditory, 200
    foveal, 198,200,202,204,206,207
    miscellaneous nonsaccadic, 200,204
    orbital position, 200
    postsaccadic, 200,204,206
    smooth pursuit, 200
    visual, 196–198,199
    visuomovement, 198,201,204,206
  presaccadic activity, 195–198,201,207–208
Frontotectal projection. *See* Frontal eye field, frontotectal projection

G

Ganglion cells, retinal, 19–33
  α cell, 22,29,332
  in Alzheimer's disease, 335–339
  amacrine cell
    bipolar cell input, 312
    ganglion cell interaction, 19,26
    neurotransmitters, 3,4,27–28,312
    types, 2,3
  antibody receptor recognition, 28–30
  axotomy response, 30
  β cell, 22,29
  bipolar cell, 19
    depolarizing, 1,2,3
    ganglion cell input, 26,29–30
    hyperpolarizing, 1,2,3,35
    neurotransmitters, 4,26–27,29–30
    photoreceptor input, 1
    receptive field center, 3
  classification, 20,21–22,31
  degenerated
    electroretinogram, 289–290
    pattern electroretinogram, 289–295
  electrophysiology, 21–22
  growth factor response, 31
  horizontal cell, 2
    γ-aminobutyric acid release, 4
    dopamine effects, 4–16
    electrical coupling, 4,7,11–13,15–16,312
    inhibitory effects, 3
  I-cell
    γ-aminobutyric acid content, 67–71
    acetylcholinergic response, 63
    cholinergic response, 52–53
    noradrenergic response, 58–59
    presynaptic response, 54,55
    serotoninergic response, 56
  interplexiform cell
    dopamine release, 4,312
    horizontal cell modulation, 3–4,14,16
    input, 3
    neuromodulation and, 3–4,14,16
    output, 3
  M cell
    in Alzheimer's disease, 339,344
    amacrine cell input, 3
    functions, 339

off-center cell
  bipolar cell input, 1
  center-surround response, 38
  dark stimuli response, 35
on-center cell
  bipolar cell input, 1
  center-surround response, 38
  light stimuli response, 35
on-off cell, 3,21–22
P-cell, 64–67
  acetylcholine response, 63
  in Alzheimer's disease, 339,344
  amacrine cell input, 3
  γ-aminobutyric acid content, 68
  cholinergic response, 52–53
  functions, 339
  noradrenergic response, 58,59
  receptors, 47
  retrograde degeneration, 49
  serotoninergic response, 56
receptor field, 21
receptor specificity, 26–30
target specificity, 20,21
transmitter/modulators, 19,22–26,31
transmitter receptors, 28–30
W cell, 22
  target neurons, 53
X cell, 22
  amacrine cell input, 3
  characteristics, 331
  inhibitory mechanisms, 69–70,72
  light spot response, 55
  spatial frequency reaction time
    and, 280–281
Y cell, 22
  amacrine cell input, 3
  characteristics, 331
  inhibitory mechanisms, 69–70,72
  light spot response, 55
  spatial frequency reaction time
    and, 281
Geniculocortical pathway, 122–123
  magnocellular subdivision, 125
    in depth perception, 127–129,132
    evolution, 137–138
    lateral geniculate projections,
      332
    in motion processing, 126,128,
      136,138
    in shape discrimination, 136
    in spatial processing, 134–135
    in stereopsis, 126,128–129

parvocellular subdivision, 125
  in depth perception, 127,132
  evolution, 137
  in shape discrimination, 126,136
  subdivisions, 123
Gesture recognition, brain mechanisms
  in brain-lesioned subjects, 171–
    174,175
  in schizophrenia, 176–179
Gibson, James, 130
Glaucoma, pattern electroretinogram
  in, 291,293
Glucagon, amacrine cell content, 28
Glucose metabolism, cerebral, 258–259
Glutamate
  bipolar cell release, 4,29–30
  cortical receptor, 95
  horizontal cell sensitivity, 9–10
  optic nerve content, 44
  retinal ganglion cell content, 19,22
  as lateral geniculate
    neurotransmitter, 44–48,49–50
  in corticogeniculate pathway, 49–50
  norepinephrine interaction, 58
Glutamate diethyl ester, 46
γ-D-Glutamylglycine, 46
Grating acuity, of infants, 110–111
Growth factors, retinal ganglion cell
  response, 31

H
Hebephrenia, 175
Homovanillic acid, 314
Horizontal cell, 2
  γ-aminobutyric acid release, 4
  dopamine effects, 4–16
    adenosine 3':5'-cyclic phosphate
      interaction, 7–13
    in darkness, 15–16
    electrical junction coupling,
      4,7,11–13,312
    light responsiveness, 4–7,9–13
  electrical coupling
    in darkness, 15–16
    dopamine effects, 4,7,11–13,312
  inhibitory effects, 3
1-Hydroxy-3-amino-2-pyrrolidone, 46
6-Hydroxydopamine, 309
Hypothalamus
  lateral geniculate nucleus pars
    dorsalis innervation, 64
  retinofugal projection, 334

I

I-cell
  acetylcholine response, 63
  γ-aminobutyric acid content, 67–71
  cholinergic response, 52–53
  noradrenergic response, 58–59
  presynaptic response, 54,55
  serotoninergic response, 56
Infant, visual function development, 109–118
  acuity testing, 109–110,112
  color vision, 112–114
  cones, 113,114
  contrast sensitivity functions, 111–112
  flicker fusion, 112,113
  grating acuity, 110–111
  measurement techniques, 109–110
  rods, 112
  stereopsis, 115,116
  theoretical considerations, 115–117
  visual evoked potentials, 110,111,112,113,115–116
Inositol lipids, second messenger system marker, 95–97,105
Interplexiform cell
  dopamine release, 4,312
  horizontal cell modulation, 3–4,14,16
  input, 3
  neuromodulation and, 3–4,14,16
  output, 3
Intraocular pressure, pattern electroretinogram effects, 291
Ischemia, retinal, 292–293

L

Lateral geniculate nucleus
  α-cell projections, 332
  in amblyopia, 86–87
  2-amino-4-phosphonobutyrate effects, 36,37–38
  β-cell projections, 332
  magnocellular projection, 123
    ganglion-cell projections, 332
    information processing, 124–127
  M-cell system projections, 339,344
  nicotinic receptor binding sites, 92,104
  paraphenlene diamine staining, 332–334,335
  parvocellular projections, 123
    center/surround antagonism, 124–125
    ganglion-cell projections, 332
    information processing, 124–127
  P-cell system projections, 339,344
  in selective deprivation, 86
Lateral geniculate nucleus pars dorsalis
  γ-aminobutyric acid content, 68
  chemically specified systems, 43–83
    acetylcholine, 44
    aspartate, 44,45,46
    brain stem source, 50–59
    choline acetyl transferase, 44,51
    cholinergic system, 44,50–53
    cortical source, 49–50
    diencephalic source, 59–64
    dopamine, 44
    glutamate, 44–48,49–50,58
    hypothalamic source, 64
    I-cells, 67–71,72
    intrinsic components, 64–71
    noradrenergic system, 44,56–59,64,72
    P-cells, 64–67,68,69,70–71
    retinal source, 43–49
    serotoninergic system, 44,53–56
    substance P, 48–49,72
    systems of unknown nature, 59
    thalamic reticular nucleus source, 59–64
  I-cell, 64–65,72
    acetycholine response, 63
    γ-aminobutyric acid content, 67–71
    cholinergic response, 52–53
    noradrenergic response, 58–59
    presynaptic dendrites, 54,55
    serotoninergic response, 56
  P-cell, 64–67
    acetylcholine response, 63
    cholinergic response, 52–53
    noradrenergic response, 58,59
    receptors, 47
    retrograde degeneration, 49
    serotoninergic response, 56
  X cell, inhibitory mechanisms, 69–70,72
  Y cell, inhibitory mechanisms, 69–70,72
L-dopa, 311
Lightness, as linking feature, 135
Light stimuli, visual processing, 119,120–121
  on/off channel response, 35–37,39–41

SUBJECT INDEX

Limbic system, in face/facial expression recognition, 179,188
Linking features, 135
Luminance contrast, depth perception and, 127–128,129–130,132
Lysergic acid diethylamide (LSD), 55

M

Macaque
  lateral geniculate nucleus pars dorsalis innervation, 57
  middle temporal cortex neurons, 281–282
Maculopathy, pattern electroretinogram in, 293
Magnocellular pathway, 123,332
  in depth perception, 127–129,132
  information processing function, 124–127
Matisse, Henri, 132
M cell
  in Alzheimer's disease, 339,344
  amacrine cell input, 3
  functions, 339
Medial superior temporal area, visual motion processing function, 213–216,217
1-Methyl-4-phenyl 1,2,3,6-tetrahydropyridine, 297,307–310,314
Middle temporal area
  in velocity field computation, 156–159,161
  visual motion processing function, 126,213–224,281–282
Monkey
  dorsal terminal nucleus
    location, 233–234
    in optokinetic nystagmus/afternystagmus, 235–251
  frontal eye field, 195–209
    antidromic neurons, 204–205
    auditory neurons, 200
    foveal neurons, 198,200, 202,204,206,207
    frontotectal projection, 202–207,208
    miscellaneous nonsaccadic neurons, 200,204
    orbital position neurons, 200
    postsaccadic neurons, 200,204,206

presaccadic activity, 195–198,201,207–208
during saccadic eye movement, 266-267
smooth pursuit neurons, 200
visual neurons, 196–198,199
visuomovement neurons, 198,201,204,206
lateral geniculate nucleus pars dorsalis
  N-acetyl-aspartate-glutamate content, 48
  γ-aminobutyric acid immunoreactivity, 61–63
  diencephalic innervation, 61–63
  I-cells, 65,66,68,70
  noradrenergic response, 57
  P-cells, 65,66
  serotoninergic response, 53–55
  thalamic reticular nucleus innervation, 60–61
M cell, amacrine cell input, 3
optic nerve
  aspartate content, 45
  glutamate content, 44,45
optic tract, N-acetyl-aspartate-glutamate content, 48
optic tract nucleus
  location, 233–234
  in optokinetic nystagmus/afternystagmus, 235–251
optokinetic nystagmus/afternystagmus
  electrical stimulation-induced, 237–242,248
  gravity effects, 240,241
  lesion effects, 242–247
  stimulation sites, 240,242
  theoretical basis, 235–237
parkinsonian syndrome, 307–310,311
  dopaminergic deficiency, 307–310,311–312
  pattern retinogram, 307–310,311
  pattern visual evoked potentials, 307–310
P cell, 65,66
  amacrine cell input, 3
pattern electroretinogram, 289–290,292
visual motion processing, 211–231
  directional selectivity, 211–212,213–215

Monkey
  visual motion processing (*contd.*)
    extraretinal input, 216,217
    localization, 211–213
    medial superior temporal area in, 213–216,217
    middle temporal area in, 156–158
    optokinetic deficits, 226–229
    pursuit cells, 213–216
    retinal input, 216,217
    retinotopic deficits, 221,222, 223,225–226,228,229
    saccadic eye movements, 218,219–221,222
    superior temporal sulcus in, 213,218,220
Motion processing. *See* Visual motion processing
Multiple sclerosis, visual deficits, 317–329
  contrast sensitivity, 321–324
  discrimination, 324–326
  on/off mechanisms, 319–320
  orientation channels, 320–324,326
  spatial channels, 320–326
  temporal channels, 320

N

Neuritis, retrobulbar optic, 293
Nerve growth factor, retinal ganglion cell response, 31
Neuromagnetic localization, of cortical neuronal activity, 271–287
  contrast threshold, 277–278
  extravisual area activity, 281–285
  neuromagnetic methods, 272–274
  parallel processing channels, 280–281,282
  reaction time/latency relationship, 279–280
  retinotopic sequence, 274–277
  threshold relationships, 278–279
Neuromodulation. *See also* Neurotransmitters
  interplexiform cell and, 3–4,14,16
Neuron. *See also* Ganglion cell, retinal
  facial recognition-specific, 167–168
Neuropeptide(s)
  amacrine cell content, 27–28
  retinal ganglion cell content, 23–26
  as retinogeniculate neurotransmitter, 48–49

Neuropeptide Y, 23,28
Neurotensin, 23,24,28
Neurotransmitters. *See also* specific neurotransmitters
  cortical receptors, 91–103
  development, 93–102
  localization, 91–93
  redistribution, 102–103
Nicotine, cortical receptor, 95
Night vision, 122,128
Noradrenergic system, of lateral geniculate nucleus pars dorsalis, 56–59,64,72
Norepinephrine, as retinogeniculate neurotransmitter, 44,56–59,64,72
Nucleus amygdalae, face-specific neuronal connections, 167–168
Nucleus cuneiformis, as geniculate acetylcholine source, 51
Nucleus limitans, location, 234
Nystagmus, optokinetic, optic tract nucleus in
  clinical implications, 250–251
  electrical stimulation-induced, 236,237–242,248
    gravity effects, 240,248–249
    lesion effects, 242–247,249
    stimulation site location, 240–242
  theoretical basis, 235–237
  vestibular nystagmus interaction, 238–240,241
  vestibulo-ocular reflex in, 235,237

O

Off-center cell
  bipolar cell input, 1
  center-surround response, 38
  dark stimuli response, 35
On-center cell
  2-amino-4-phosphonobutyrate effects, 36,37–38
  bipolar cell input, 1
  center-surround response, 38
  light stimuli response, 35
On-off cell, 21-22. *See also* On-off channels
On-off channels
  2-amino-4-phosphonobutyrate effects, 35–41
  contrast sensitivity and, 36,41
  function, 36,41
  light stimuli response, 35–37,39–41

SUBJECT INDEX 359

in multiple sclerosis, 319–320
  saccadic eye movements, 36,40
Opiate, cortical receptor, 95,98
Optic nerve
  acetylcholine content, 44
  degeneration, 337–338,339
  glutamate content, 44
Optic nerve lesion/section, pattern electroretinogram, 289–291,293–295
Optic nucleus, accessory, paraphenlene diamine staining, 334,335
Optic system, accessory, retinofugal fiber projection, 334
Optic tract nucleus
  location, 233–235
  in optokinetic nystagmus/ afternystagmus
    clinical implications, 250–251
    electrical stimulation-induced, 237–242
    electrical stimulation sites, 240,242
    gravity effects, 240,241
    lesion effects, 242–247
    theoretical basis, 236,237
Optokinetic system. *See also* Nystagmus, optokinetic
  lesion-related deficits, 226–229
Orientation channels
  foveal, 317
  in multiple sclerosis, 320–324,326
Oxygen metabolism, cerebral, 258–259

P

Parallel processing
  evidence for, 331–335
  neuromagnetic studies, 280–281,282
Paranoic response, in schizophrenia, 179
Paraphenylene diamine staining, of central visual system projections, 332–338
  accessory optic nucleus projection, 334,335
  in Alzheimer's disease, 335–339
  lateral geniculate nucleus, 333–334,335
    retinofugal pathway, 333,334
  paraventricular nucleus, 334,335
  pretectum, 333,335
  pulvinar, 334,335
  retinofugal pathway, 333,334
  superior colliculus projection, 334

suprachiasmatic nucleus, 334,335
  supraoptic nucleus, 334,335
Paraprosopia, 168
Paraventricular nucleus, paraphenylene diamine staining, 334,335
Parkinson's disease
  contrast sensitivity, 297–304,310–311
    dopamine effects, 302–304
    pattern electroretinogram, 307–310,311,312
    spatiotemporal, 299–304,310–311
  dopamine in contrast sensitivity effects, 302–304
    D1 receptors, 313
    D2 receptors, 312,313
    deficiency, 307–310,311–313
    signal processing effects, 309–310
  visual system, 297–316
    contrast sensitivity, 297–304
    dopaminergic deficiency, 307–310,311–313
    pattern visual evoked potentials, 307–310
    visual evoked potentials, 297,304–307
Parvocellular pathway, 125
  in depth perception, 127,132
  evolution, 137
  in shape discrimination, 126,136
Pattern electroretinogram (PERG), 289–296
  in degenerated retinal ganglion cells, 289–295
    clinical aspects, 293–295
    intraocular pressure effects, 291
    optic nerve section effects, 289–291
    in optic nerve trauma, 293–295
    properties, 292–293
    retinal artery block effects, 292–293
    spatial frequency tuning, 290–291,292–293
    spike activity effects, 291–292
  historical background, 289
  in Parkinson's disease, 307–310,311,312
P-cell, 64–67
  acetylcholine response, 63
  in Alzheimer's disease, 339,344
  amacrine cell input, 3
  γ-aminobutyric acid content, 68

P-cell (*contd.*)
  cholinergic response, 52–53
  functions, 339
  noradrenergic response, 58,59
  receptors, 47
  retrograde degeneration, 49
  serotoninergic response, 56
Pedunculopontine tegmental nucleus
  choline acetyl transferase active neurons, 51
  geniculate cholinergic innervation pathways, 51,52
Peptides, cortical receptor, 98
Perspective, 130–131
Photoreceptor. *See also* Cone; Rod
  function, 120
  glutamate neurotransmitter, 35
Positron emission tomography (PET)
  brain blood flow measurement, 257–270
    anatomical localization, 259–260
    elementary stimulus variables, 263–265
    historical background, 257–258
    low-level response detection, 261–262
    metabolic measurements versus, 258–259
    response localization, 260–261
    retinotopic organization, 265,266
    spatial resolution, 260–261
    statistical analysis, 262–263
    strategy, 258–263
    visually presented word response, 267–268
    visual system observations, 263–268
    voluntary saccade response, 265–267
  definition, 257
Preferential looking techniques, 109–110,111
Pretectal olivary nucleus, location, 234
Pretectum. *See also* Dorsal terminal nucleus
  paraphenlene diamine staining, 333,335
Prosopagnosia, 165,168,199
Protein kinase C, cortical localization, 95–97,105
Pulvinar, paraphenylene diamine staining, 334,335
Purkinje's cell, in nystagmus, 237

Pursuit eye movement, cortical neuron function in
  directional selectivity, 211–212,213–215
  lesion-related deficits, 218–229
  medial superior temporal area neurons, 213–216,217,224–229
  middle temporal area neurons, 213–224
  optokinetic deficits, 226–229
  pursuit cells, 213–216
  pursuit initiation, 216–223
  retinotopic deficits, 221,222,223,225–226
  saccadic eye movements, 218,219–221,222
  superior temporal sulcus neurons, 213,218

R
Rabbit
  optic nerve
    aspartate content, 45
    glutamate content, 44,45
  retinal ganglion cell
    γ-aminobutyric acid content, 22–23
    on-off, 21
    substance-P content, 24
Rat
  lateral geniculate nucleus pars dorsalis
    γ-aminobutyric acid receptors, 70
    diencephalic innervation, 59–61,63,64
    noradrenergic response, 56–57,58–59,64
    norepinephrine content, 56
    serotoninergic response, 53,55,56
    thalamic reticular nucleus innervation, 60–61
  optic nerve, glutamate content, 44,45,47
  optic tract nucleus, 235
  optokinetic nystagmus/afternystagmus, 237
Reaction time, to spatial frequencies, 279–281
  latency relationship, 279–280
Receptor antibody recognition, 28–30
  cortical, 91–103
    acetylcholine, 29,91,92,93–94,98,99,100,101,102–103,104

adenosine, 95,98
β-adrenergic, 95,98,104–105
γ-aminobutyric acid, 91–92,95,
  98,101,102,104
baclofen, 95
calcium channel, 95,104–105
cholecystokinin, 95,104–105
development, 93–102
glutamate, 95
localization, 91–93
nicotine, 95
opiates, 95,98
peptides, 98
redistribution, 102–103
Retina
  dopamine deficiency, 307–310,311–313
  dopaminergic neurons, 311–312
  inner plexiform layer
    components, 26
    definition, 19
    laminar organization, 20
    transmitter localization, 28
  neurons. *See also* Ganglion cells, retinal
    categories, 19
  outer plexiform layer, 2
Retinal artery block, pattern electroretinogram effects, 292–293
Retinofugal pathway, 332,333,334
Retinotopic organization, of cortex, 265,266
  neuromagnetic study, 274–277
Riley, Bridget, 132,133
Rod
  light sensitivity, 122
  in visual function development, 112
Rubin, Edgar, 133

S

Saccadic eye movement
  in Alzheimer's disease, 340,341, 342,343
  cortical response during, 265–267
  frontal eye field and, 195–209
    antidromic excitation hypothesis, 200–201,203–205
    blood flow, 266–267
    frontotectal projection, 202–207,208
    neuron types, 195–202
    processing chain, 198,201

lesion-related deficits, 218,219–221,222
on/off channels in, 36,40
Schizophrenia, face/facial recognition in, 168,174–179,190
  age factors, 177,178,190
  black/white photograph test, 169
  movie test, 170,176–178
  paranoic response correlation, 179
  sex factors, 177
  slide test, 175–176
Serotoninergic system, of lateral geniculate nucleus pars dorsalis, 44,53–56,60,72
Serotonin
  as retinogeniculate neurotransmitter, 44,53–56,60,72
  retinal ganglion cell content, 19
Sex factors, in face/facial expression recognition, 168,177
Shading, 132
Shadows, 132
Shape discrimination
  equiluminance and, 136
  geniculocortical pathways in, 126,136
  luminance contrast and, 136
  shading and, 132
Somatostatin
  amacrine cell content, 28
  as retinogeniculate neurotransmitter, 49
Spatial frequency channels/tuning
  foveal, 317
  in multiple sclerosis, 320–326
  pattern electroretinogram, 290–291,292–293
Spatial perception, *See also* Depth perception
  geniculocortical pathways in, 134–135
  in Parkinson's disease, 299–304,310–311
Spatial resolution capacity, development, 111–112
Spectral sensitivity, of infants, 112–114
Spike activity, pattern electroretinogram effects, 291–292
Stereomotion channels, foveal, 317
Stereopsis
  depth perception and, 128–129
  development in infants, 115,116
  at equiluminance, 128–129

Stereopsis (*contd.*)
  geniculocortical pathways in, 126,128–129
  spatial relationship information and, 135
Substance P
  amacrine cell content, 28
  retinal ganglion cell content, 19,23,24,26,30,31
  as retinogeniculate neurotransmitter, 48–49,72
Superior colliculus
  α-cell projections, 332
  frontal eye field projection to, 202–207,208
  paraphenlene diamine staining, 334
  in saccadic eye movements, 202–207,208
Suprachiasmatic nucleus projection, paraphenlene diamine staining, 334,335
Supraoptic nucleus projection, paraphenylene diamine staining, 334,335

T
Temporal channels, in multiple sclerosis, 319–320
Temporal lobe, facial recognition-specific neurons, 167–168
Texture, as linking feature, 135
Thalamic reticular nucleus, lateral geniculate nucleus pars dorsalis innervation, 59–64
Three-dimensional image
  color representation, 137
  image motion and, 139
  retinal projection, 130–131
Thyroid-releasing hormone, 28
Turtle, horizontal cell, 312
Two-dimensional image
  retinal projection, 130–131
  velocity field computation, 139–164
    aperture problem, 139–148,156
    component cells in, 157,158,159–161
    contour-based versus area-based measurements, 143–144,151–152,155
    definition, 139–142
    middle temporal area neurons in, 156–159,161
    motion patterns in, 143

neural model, 156–161
pattern cells in, 157,158–161
perceptual study, 148–156
physiological study, 156–161
pure translation, 144–145,147–148
smoothness assumption, 146–148,152–155
solution, 144–148
two-stage measurement, 149–151,155,156
velocity vectors, 142–143
Tyrosine hydroxylase, 23,24

V
Vasoactive intestinal polypeptide, 28
Velocity field computation, 139–164
  aperture problem, 139–148,156
  contour-based versus area-based measurements, 143–144,151–152,155
  definition, 139–142
  motion patterns, 143
  pure translation assumption, 144–145,147–148
  smoothness assumption, 146–148,152–155
  solution, 144–148
  two-stage measurement, 149–151,155,156
  velocity vectors, 142–143
  neural model, 156–161
  perceptual study, 148–156
  physiological study, 156–161
    component cells in, 157,158,159–161
    middle temporal area neurons in, 156–159,161
    pattern cells in, 157,158–161
Visual evoked potentials
  in Alzheimer's disease, 331,340–341
  of infants, 110,111,112,113,115–116
  pattern, 289. *See also* Pattern electroretinogram (PERG)
  in Parkinson's disease, 307–310
Visual function, development, 109–118
  color vision, 112–114
  cones, 113,114
  contrast sensitivity, 111–112
  flicker fusion, 112
  grating acuity, 110–111
  measurement techniques, 109–110
  rods, 112

stereopsis, 115,116
theoretical considerations, 115–117
visual evoked potentials, 110,111,112,113,115–116
Visual grasp reflex, 208
Visual masking impairment, in Alzheimer's disease, 331
Visual motion processing, 121
  depth perception and, 128,129,131–132
  by extravisual area, 281–285
  function, 139
  geniculocortical pathways in, 126,128,136,138
  for oculomotor control, 211–231
    directional selectivity, 211–212,213,215,221,223,225–226,228–229
    extraretinal input, 216,217
    lesion-related deficits, 218–229
    localization, 211–213
    medial superior temporal neurons in, 213–216,217,224–229
    middle temporal area neurons in, 213–224
    optokinetic deficits, 226–229
    pursuit cells, 213–216
    retinal input, 216,217
    retinotopic deficits, 221,222, 223,225–226,228,229
    saccadic eye movements, 218,219–221,222
    superior temporal sulcus in, 213,218,220
  spatial relationship information in, 135
  velocity field computation, 139–164
    aperture problem, 139–148,156
    component cells in, 157,158,159–161
    contour-based versus area-based measurements, 143–144,151–152,155
    middle temporal area neurons in, 156–159,161
    motion patterns in, 143
    neural model, 156–161
    pattern cells in, 157,158–161
    perceptual study, 148–156
    physiological study, 156–161
    pure translation assumption, 144–145,147–148

smoothness assumption, 146–148,152–155
two-stage measurement, 149–151,155,156
velocity vectors, 142–143
Visual pathway, sequential functional stages, 317–318
Visual system
  in Alzheimer's disease
    amblyopia, 342
    anosmia, 342,343
    dysmetria, 342
    optic atrophy, 342
    saccadic eye movement, 340,341,342,343
    visual evoked potentials, 340–341
  in multiple sclerosis, 317–329
    contrast sensitivity, 321–324
    discrimination, 324–326
    on-off mechanisms, 319–320
    orientation channels, 320–324,326
    spatial channels, 320–326
    temporal channels, 320
  in Parkinson's disease, 297–316
    contrast sensitivity, 297–304,310–311
    dopaminergic deficiency, 307–310,311–313
    pattern visual evoked potentials, 307–310
    visual evoked potentials, 297,304–307
  physiological subdivisions, 318
  positron emission studies, 257–270
    anatomical localization, 259–260
    elementary stimulus variables, 263–265
    historical background, 257–258
    low-level response detection, 261–262
    metabolic measurements versus, 258–259
    response localization, 260–261
    retinotopic organization, 265,266
    spatial resolution, 260–261
    statistical analysis, 262–263
    strategy, 258–263
    visually presented response, 267–268
    voluntary saccade response, 265–267
  segregated subpathways, 120–122
    consequences, 136

Visual system
  segregated subpathways (*contd.*)
    functional differences, 123–127
    for spatial organization, 134–135

W
W cell, 22
  target neurons, 53
Word presentation task, cortical
    response, 267–268

X
X cell, 22
X cell (*contd.*)
  amacrine cell input, 3
  characteristics, 331
  inhibitory mechanisms, 69–70, 72
  light spot response, 55
  spatial frequency reaction time and, 280–281

Y
Y cell, 22
  amacrine cell input, 3
  characteristics, 331
  inhibitory mechanisms, 69–70, 72
  light spot response, 55
  spatial frequency reaction time and, 281